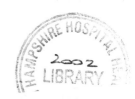

D1374662

WITHDRAWN
rked below

PLEASE ENTER ON LOAN SLIP

Author STEEL, G

Title BASIC CLINICAL
RADIO BIOLOGY

RHM0506_NS

Basic Clinical
Radiobiology

Basic Clinical Radiobiology

3rd Edition

Edited by

G Gordon Steel DSc
Emeritus Professor of Radiobiology Applied to Radiotherapy,
Department of Radiotherapy Research, The Institute of Cancer Research

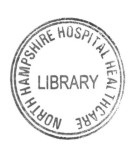

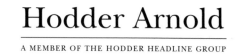

Hodder Arnold

A MEMBER OF THE HODDER HEADLINE GROUP

First published in Great Britain in 2002 by
Hodder Arnold, an imprint of Hodder Education
A member of the Hodder Headline Group,
338 Euston Road, London NW1 3BH

http://www.hoddereducation.com

Distributed in the United States of America by
Oxford University Press Inc.,
198 Madison Avenue, New York, NY10016
Oxford is a registered trademark of Oxford University Press

Whilst the advice and information in this book are believed to be true and
accurate at the date of going to press, neither the authors nor the publisher
can accept any legal responsibility or liability for any errors or omissions
that may be made. In particular (but without limiting the generality of the
preceding disclaimer) every effort has been made to check drug dosages;
however, it is still possible that errors have been missed. Furthermore,
dosage schedules are constantly being revised and new side-effects
recognized. For these reasons the reader is strongly urged to consult the
drug companies' printed instructions before administering any of the drugs
recommended in this book.

British Library Cataloguing in Publication Data
A catalogue record for this book is available from the British Library

Library of Congress Cataloging-in-Publication Data
A catalog record for this book is available from the Library of Congress

ISBN-10: 0 340 80783 0
ISBN-13: 978 0 340 80783 5

3 4 5 6 7 8 9 10

Commissioning Editor: Joanna Koster
Production Editor: James Rabson
Production Controller: Martin Kerans
Cover Design: Terry Griffiths

Typeset in 10/12 Minion by Charon Tec Pvt. Ltd, Chennai, India
Printed and bound in Great Britain by CPI Bath

What do you think about this book? Or any other Hodder Arnold title?
Please send your comments to www.hoddereducation.com

Contents

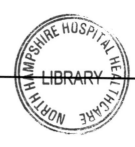

Contributors

H Bartelink
Department of Radiotherapy
Netherlands Cancer Institute
Amsterdam
The Netherlands

M Baumann
Department of Radiotherapy
Medical Faculty Carl Gustav Carus
Technical University Dresden
Dresden
Germany

AC Begg
Experimental Radiotherapy Department
Netherlands Cancer Institute
Amsterdam
The Netherlands

SM Bentzen
Gray Cancer Institute
Mount Vernon Hospital
Northwood
Middlesex, UK

MR Horsman
Department of Experimental Clinical Oncology
Aarhus University Hospital
Aarhus
Denmark

MC Joiner
Karmanos Cancer Institute
Wayne State University
Detroit
Michigan, USA

TJ McMillan
Division of Biological Sciences
Institute of Environmental and
Natural Sciences
University of Lancaster
Lancaster, UK

J Overgaard
Department of Experimental Clinical Oncology
Aarhus University Hospital
Aarhus
Denmark

MI Saunders
Department of Radiation Oncology
Mount Vernon NHS Trust
Northwood
Middlesex, UK

GG Steel
Radiotherapy Research Unit
Institute of Cancer Research
Sutton
Surrey, UK

FA Stewart
Experimental Radiotherapy Department
Netherlands Cancer Institute
Amsterdam
The Netherlands

AJ van der Kogel
Department of Radiation Oncology
University Medical Centre
Nijmegen
The Netherlands

CML West
Paterson Institute for Cancer Research
Christie Hospital NHS Trust
Manchester, UK

Preface

This is the third edition of a book first published in 1993. It is designed as a teaching book for radiation therapists, and for radiation physicists and radiobiologists who act in a support capacity.

Developments in cancer therapy are increasingly arising out of studies in basic science and it is best for their implementation to be in the hands of clinicians who are familiar with the relevant scientific areas. This book deals with the biological aspects of radiotherapy. It seeks to present in a concise and interesting way the main ideas and significant scientific developments that underlie current attempts to improve the radiotherapeutic management of cancer.

This edition has been carefully and extensively revised. New chapters have been added on three clinical topics: volume effects in radiation therapy, radiotherapy-related morbidity, and modification of the tumour microenvironment. Text relating to the mechanisms of normal-tissue injury has been brought up to date and the key chapters on the linear-quadratic approach to fractionation have been carefully revised, simplifying the recommendations on methods of calculating isoeffective schedules.

In carrying out this revision, we have once again faced the question of how much 'modern biology' to include. The last 10–15 years has seen an explosion of research interest in molecular biology, cell-cycle control, apoptosis, gene discovery, and potential gene therapy. These are widely perceived to be exciting areas of therapeutic cancer research. Although this edition contains new information related to these areas, we have decided that the emphasis of the book must remain on the basic principles of the radiation response of tumours and normal tissues. These are the principles that underlie day-to-day decision-making in oncology units. They are critically important, for it is well recognized that long-term tumour control and the incidence of serious complications both depend steeply on radiation dose, and on other factors that affect the intensity of a radiation therapy schedule.

The book is directed at an international audience. It has arisen out of teaching courses organized by the European Society for Therapeutic Radiation Oncology (ESTRO) and the material will also be of use to readers in North America and the rest of the world.

For the benefit of readers who have a visual memory, and particularly for those whose first language is not English, this book is designed with a high ratio of charts to text. There is also a substantial glossary of scientific terms. At the end of each chapter is a list of prominent published material, mainly books and reviews, which are recommended for further reading. Citations in the text sometimes refer to these works.

G Gordon Steel

1

Introduction: the significance of radiobiology for radiotherapy

G GORDON STEEL

1.1 THE ROLE OF RADIOTHERAPY IN THE MANAGEMENT OF CANCER

Radiotherapy is one of the two most effective treatments for cancer. Surgery, which of course has the longer history, is in many tumour types the primary form of treatment and it leads to good therapeutic results in a range of early non-metastatic tumours. Radiotherapy has replaced surgery for the long-term control of many tumours of the head and neck, cervix, bladder, prostate and skin, in which it often achieves a reasonable probability of tumour control with good cosmetic results. In addition to these examples of the curative role of radiation therapy, many patients gain valuable palliation by radiation. Chemotherapy is the third most important treatment modality at the present time. Following the early use of nitrogen mustard during the 1920s, it has emerged to the point where upwards of 30 drugs are available for the management of cancer, although no more than 10–15 are in common use. Many patients receive chemotherapy at some point in their management and useful symptom relief and disease arrest are often obtained.

The following is a brief outline of the role of radiotherapy in six disease sites:

- *Bladder*: the success of surgery or radiotherapy varies widely with stage of the disease; both approaches give 5-year survival rates in excess of 50%.
- *Breast*: early breast cancers, not known to have metastasized, are usually treated by surgery and this has a tumour control rate in the region of 50–70%. Radiotherapy given to the chest wall and regional lymph nodes increases control by up to 20%. Hormonal therapy and chemotherapy also have significant impact on patient survival. In patients who have evidence of metastatic spread at the time of diagnosis, the outlook is poor.
- *Cervix*: disease that has developed beyond the *in situ* stage is often treated by a combination of intracavitary and external-beam radiotherapy. The control rate varies widely with the stage of the disease, from around 70% in stage I to perhaps 7% in stage IV.
- *Lung*: most lung tumours are inoperable and in them the 5-year survival rate for radiotherapy

combined with chemotherapy is in the region of 5%.

- *Lymphoma*: In Hodgkin's disease, radiotherapy alone achieves a control rate of around 50% and when combined with chemotherapy this may rise to 80%.
- *Prostate*: where there is evidence of local invasion, surgery and radiotherapy have a similar level of effectiveness, with 10-year control rates in the region of 50%. Chemotherapy makes a limited contribution to tumour control.

Very substantial numbers of patients with common cancers achieve long-term tumour control largely by the use of radiation therapy. Informed debate on the funding of national cancer programmes requires data on the relative roles of the main treatment modalities. Broad estimates by DeVita *et al.* (1979) and Souhami and Tobias (1986) suggested that local treatment, which includes surgery and/or radiotherapy, could be expected to be successful in approximately 40% of these cases; in perhaps 15% of all cancers, radiotherapy would be the principal form of treatment. By contrast, many patients do receive chemotherapy but their contribution to the overall cure rate of cancer may be only around 2%, with some prolongation of life in perhaps another 10%. This is because the diseases in which chemotherapy does well are rare. If these figures are correct, it may be that around seven times as many patients currently are cured by radiotherapy as by chemotherapy. This is not to undervalue the important benefits of chemotherapy in a number of chemosensitive diseases, but to stress the greater role of radiotherapy as a curative agent (Tubiana, 1992).

Considerable efforts are being devoted at the present time to the improvement of radiotherapy and chemotherapy. Wide publicity is given to the newer areas of drug development such as lymphokines, growth factors, anti-oncogenes and gene therapy. But if we were to imagine aiming to increase the cure rate of cancer by, say, 2%, it would seem on a realistic estimation that this would more likely be achieved by increasing the results of radiotherapy from, say, 15% to 17% than by doubling the results achieved by chemotherapy.

There are three main ways in which such an improvement in radiotherapy might be obtained:

1. by raising the standards of radiation dose prescription and delivery to those currently in use in the best radiotherapy centres;

2. by improving radiation dose distributions beyond those that are conventionally achieved, either using techniques of conformal radiotherapy with photons, or ultimately by the use of proton beams;
3. by exploiting radiobiological initiatives.

The proportion of radiotherapists world-wide who work in academic centres is probably less than 5%. They are the clinicians who may have access to large new treatment machines, for instance for proton therapy, or to new radiosensitizers or to new agents for targeted therapy. Chapters of this book allude to these exciting developments which may well have an impact on treatment success in the future. But it should not be thought that the improvement of radiation therapy lies exclusively with clinical research in the specialist academic centres. It has widely been recognized that by far the most effective way of improving cure rates on a national or international scale is by quality assurance in the prescription and delivery of radiation treatment. Chapters 12–14 of this book deal with the principles on which fractionation schedules should be optimized, including how to respond to unavoidable gaps in treatment. For many radiotherapists this will be the most important part of this book, for in even the smallest department it is possible, without access to greatly increased funding, to move closer to optimum fractionation practices.

1.2 THE ROLE OF RADIATION BIOLOGY

Experimental and theoretical studies in radiation biology contribute to the development of radiotherapy at three different levels, moving in turn from the most general to the more specific:

- *Ideas*: providing a conceptual basis for radiotherapy, identifying mechanisms and processes that underlie the response of tumours and normal tissues to irradiation and which help to explain observed phenomena. Examples are knowledge about hypoxia, reoxygenation, tumour cell repopulation or mechanisms of repair of DNA damage.
- *Treatment strategy*: development of specific new approaches in radiotherapy. Examples are hypoxic cell sensitizers, high-LET radiotherapy, accelerated radiotherapy, hyperfractionation.
- *Protocols*: advice on the choice of schedules for clinical radiotherapy, for instance conversion formulae for changes in fractionation or dose rate,

or advice on whether to use chemotherapy concurrently or sequentially with radiation. We may also include under this heading methods for predicting the best treatment for the individual patient (individualized radiotherapy).

There is no doubt that radiobiology has been very fruitful in the generation of new ideas and in the identification of potentially exploitable mechanisms. A variety of new treatment strategies have been produced, but unfortunately few of these have so far led to demonstrable clinical gains. With regard to the third of the levels listed above, the newer conversion formulae based on the linear-quadratic equation seem to be successful. But beyond this, the ability of laboratory science to guide the radiotherapist in the choice of specific protocols is limited by the inadequacy of the theoretical and experimental models: it will always be necessary to rely on clinical trials for the final choice of a protocol.

1.3 THE TIME-SCALE OF EFFECTS IN RADIATION BIOLOGY

Irradiation of any biological system generates a succession of processes that differ enormously in time-scale. This is illustrated in Figure 1.1 where these processes are divided into three phases (Boag, 1975).

The physical phase consists of interactions between charged particles and the atoms of which the tissue is composed. A high-speed electron takes about 10^{-18} seconds to traverse the DNA molecule and about 10^{-14} seconds to pass across a mammalian cell.

As it does so, it interacts mainly with orbital electrons, ejecting some of them from atoms (ionization) and raising others to higher energy levels within an atom or molecule (excitation). If sufficiently energetic, these secondary electrons may excite or ionize other atoms near which they pass, giving rise to a cascade of ionization events. For 1 Gy of absorbed radiation dose, there are in excess of 10^5 ionizations within the volume of every cell of diameter 10 μm.

The chemical phase describes the period in which these damaged atoms and molecules react with other cellular components in rapid chemical reactions. Ionization and excitation lead to the breakage of chemical bonds and the formation of broken molecules, known as 'free radicals'. These are highly reactive and they engage in a succession of reactions that lead eventually to the restoration of electronic charge equilibrium. Free-radical reactions are complete within approximately 1 ms of radiation exposure. An important characteristic of the chemical phase is the competition between scavenging reactions, for instance with sulphydryl compounds that inactivate the free radicals, and fixation reactions that lead to stable chemical changes in biologically important molecules.

The biological phase includes all subsequent processes. These begin with enzymatic reactions that act on the residual chemical damage. The vast majority of lesions, for instance in DNA, are successfully repaired. Some rare lesions fail to repair and it is these that lead eventually to cell death. Cells take time to die; indeed, after small doses of radiation they may undergo a number of mitotic divisions before dying. It is the killing of stem cells and the subsequent loss of the cells that they would have given rise to that

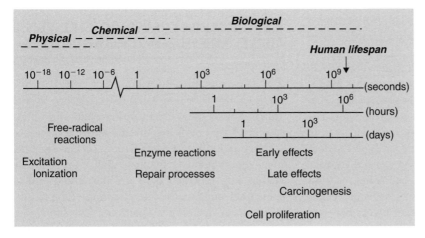

Figure 1.1 *Time-scale of the effects of radiation exposure on biological systems.*

causes the early manifestations of normal-tissue damage during the first weeks and months after radiation exposure. Examples are breakdown of the skin or mucosa, denudation of the intestine and haemopoietic damage (see Section 4.4). A secondary effect of cell killing is compensatory cell proliferation, which occurs both in normal tissues and in tumours. At later times after the irradiation of normal tissues the so-called 'late reactions' appear. These include fibrosis and telangiectasia of the skin, spinal-cord damage and blood-vessel damage. An even later manifestation of radiation damage is the appearance of second tumours (i.e. radiation carcinogenesis). The time-scale of the observable effects of ionizing radiation may thus extend up to many years after exposure.

1.4 RESPONSE OF NORMAL AND MALIGNANT TISSUES TO RADIATION EXPOSURE

Much of the text of this book focuses on effects of radiation exposure that become apparent to the clinician or the patient during the weeks, months and years after radiotherapy. These effects are seen both in tumour tissues and in the normal tissues that surround a tumour and which are unavoidably exposed to radiation. The primary tasks of radiation biology as applied to radiotherapy are to explain observed phenomena, and to suggest improvements to existing therapies (as set out in Section 1.2).

The response of a tumour is seen by *regression*, often followed by *regrowth* (or recurrence), but perhaps with failure to regrow during the normal lifespan of the patient (which we term *cure* or *local control*). These italicized terms describe the tumour responses that we seek to understand. The relationship between regression and regrowth is illustrated graphically in Figure 2.6. The cellular basis of tumour response, including tumour control, is dealt with in Section 6.6.

The responses of normal tissues to therapeutic radiation exposure range from those that cause mild discomfort to others that are life threatening. The speed at which a response develops varies widely from one tissue to another and often depends on the dose of radiation that the tissue receives. Generally speaking, the haemopoietic and epithelial tissues manifest radiation damage within weeks of radiation exposure, whereas damage to connective tissues becomes

important at later times. A major development in the radiobiology of normal tissues during the 1980s was the realization that early and late normal-tissue responses are differently modified by a change in dose fractionation and this has given rise to the current interest in hyperfractionation (Section 14.3).

The first task of a radiobiologist is to measure a tissue response accurately and reliably. The term *assay* is used to describe such a system of measurement. Assays for tumour response are described in Section 17.3. For normal tissues, the following three general types of assay are available:

- *Scoring of gross tissue effects*. It is possible to grade the severity of damage to a tissue using an arbitrary scale as is done in Figure 4.1 or Figure 11.2. In superficial tissues this approach has been remarkably successful in allowing isoeffect relationships to be determined.
- *Assays of tissue function*. For certain tissues, functional assays are available that allow radiation effects to be documented. Examples are the use of breathing rate as a measure of lung function in mice (see Figure 4.5), EDTA clearance as a measure of kidney damage (see Figure 12.4), or blood counts as an indicator of bone marrow function.
- *Clonogenic assays*. In some tumours and some normal tissues it has been possible to develop methods by which the colony of cells that derives from a single irradiated cell can be observed. In tumours this is particularly important because of the fact that regrowth of a tumour after subcurative treatment is caused by the proliferation of a small number of tumour cells that retain colony-forming ability. This important area of radiation biology is introduced in Chapter 6.

1.5 RESPONSE CURVES, DOSE–RESPONSE CURVES AND ISOEFFECT RELATIONSHIPS

The damage that is observed in an irradiated tissue increases, reaches a peak, and then may decline (Figure 1.2A). How should we quantify the magnitude of this response? We could use the measured response at some chosen time after irradiation, such as the time of maximum response, but the timing of the peak may change with radiation dose and this would lead to some uncertainty in the interpretation of the results. A common device is to calculate the *cumulative*

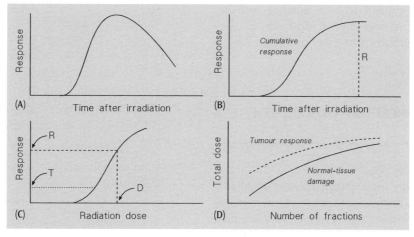

Figure 1.2 *Four types of chart leading to the construction of an isoeffect plot. (A) Time-course of development of radiation damage in a normal tissue. (B) The cumulative response. (C) A dose–response relationship, constructed by measuring the response (R) for various radiation doses (D). (D) Isoeffect plot for a fixed level of normal-tissue damage (also a similar plot for tumour response).*

response by integrating this curve from left to right (Figure 1.2B). Some normal-tissue responses give a cumulative curve that rises to a plateau, and the height of the plateau is a good measure of the total effect of that dose of radiation on the tissue. Other normal-tissue responses, in particular the late responses seen in connective and vascular tissues, are progressive and the cumulative response curve will continue to rise (Figures 11.3 and 11.4). The quantification of clinical late reactions is dealt with in Section 11.4.

The next stage in a study of the radiation response of a tissue will be to vary the radiation dose and thus to investigate the *dose–response relationship* (Figure 1.2C). Many examples of such curves are given in this book, for instance Figures 5.4, 10.6 and 11.6. Cell survival curves (see Section 6.3) are further examples of dose–response curves that are widely used in radiobiology. The position of the curve on the dose scale indicates the sensitivity of the tissue to radiation; its steepness also gives a direct indication of the change in response that will accompany an increase or decrease in radiation dose. These aspects of dose–response curves are dealt with in detail in Chapter10.

The foregoing paragraphs have for simplicity referred to 'dose' as though we are concerned only with single radiation exposures. It is a well-established fact that multiple radiation doses given over a period of a few weeks give a better curative response than

can be achieved with a single dose. Diagrams similar to Figures 1.2A, 1.2B and 1.2C can also be constructed for fractionated radiation treatment, although the results are easiest to interpret when the fractions are given over a time that is short compared with the timescale of development of the response. If we change the schedule of dose fractionation, for instance by giving a different number of fractions, changing the fraction size or radiation dose rate, we can then investigate the therapeutic effect in terms of an *isoeffect plot* (Figure 1.2D). Experimentally this is done by performing multiple studies at different doses for each chosen schedule and calculating a dose–response curve. We then select some particular level of effect (T in Figure 1.2C) and read off the total radiation dose that gives this effect. For effects on normal tissues the isoeffect will often be some upper limit of *tolerance* of the tissue, perhaps expressed as a probability of tissue failure (Sections 5.1 and 10.1). The isoeffect plot shows how the total radiation dose for the chosen level of effect varies with dose schedule. Examples are Figures 12.3 and 14.3, and recommendations for tolerance calculations are set out in Chapters 12 and 13. The dashed line in Figure 1.2D illustrates how therapeutic conclusions may be drawn from isoeffect curves. If the curve for tumour response is flatter than for normal-tissue tolerance, then there is a therapeutic advantage in using large fraction numbers: a tolerance dose given using small fraction numbers will be far short of the tumour-effective dose, whereas for large fraction numbers it may be closer to an effective dose.

1.6 THE CONCEPT OF THERAPEUTIC INDEX

Discussion of the possible benefit of a change in treatment strategy must always consider simultaneously the effects on tumour response and on normal-tissue damage. A wide range of factors enter into this assessment. In the clinic, in addition to quantifiable aspects of tumour response and toxicity, there may be a range of poorly quantifiable factors such as new forms of toxicity or risks to the patient, or practicability and convenience to hospital staff, also cost implications. These must be balanced in the clinical setting. The function of radiation biology is to address the *quantifiable biological aspects* of a change in treatment.

In the laboratory this can be done by considering dose–response curves. As radiation dose is increased, there will be a tendency for tumour response to increase, and the same is also true of normal-tissue damage. If, for instance, we measure tumour response by determining the proportion of tumours that are controlled, then we expect a sigmoid relationship to dose (for fractionated radiation treatment we could consider the total dose or any other measure of treatment intensity). This is illustrated in the upper part of Figure 1.3. If we quantify normal-tissue damage in some way for the same treatment schedule, there will also be a rising curve of toxicity (lower panel). The shape of this curve is unlikely to be the same as that for tumour response and we probably will not wish to determine more than the initial part of this curve since a high frequency of severe damage is unacceptable. By analogy with what must be done in the clinic, we can then fix a notional upper limit of tolerance (see Section 5.1). This fixes, for that treatment schedule, the upper limit of radiation dose that can be tolerated, for which the tumour response is indicated by the point in Figure 1.3 labelled A.

Consider now the effect of adding treatment with a cytotoxic drug. We expect that this will increase the tumour response for any radiation dose and this will be seen as a movement to the left of the curve for

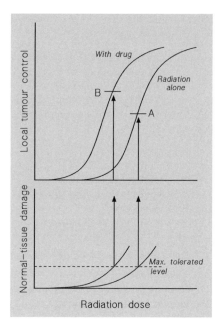

Figure 1.3 *The procedure by which an improvement in* therapeutic index *might be identified, as a result of adding chemotherapy to radiotherapy. See also Figure 20.1.*

tumour control (Figure 1.3). There will probably also be an increase in damage to normal tissues, which again will consist of a leftward movement of the toxicity curve. The relative displacement of the curves for the tumour and normal tissues will usually be different and this fact makes the amount of benefit from the chemotherapy very difficult to assess. How do we know whether there has been a real therapeutic gain? For studies on laboratory animals, there is a straightforward way of asking whether the combined treatment is better than radiation alone: for the same tolerance level of normal-tissue damage (the broken line), the maximum radiation dose (with drug) will be lower and the corresponding level of tumour control is indicated by point B in the figure. If B is higher than A, then the combination is better than radiation alone for it gives a greater level of tumour control for the same level of morbidity.

This example indicates the radiobiological concept of *therapeutic index*: it is the tumour response for a fixed level of normal-tissue damage (see Section 10.6). The term *therapeutic window* describes the (possible) difference between the tumour control dose and the tolerance dose. The concept can in principle be applied to any therapeutic situation or to any appropriate measures of tumour response or toxicity. Its application in the clinic is, however, not a straightforward matter, as indicated in Section 20.1. Therapeutic index carries the notion of 'cost–benefit' analysis. It is impossible to reliably discuss the potential benefit of a new treatment without reference to its effect on therapeutic index.

1.7 THE IMPORTANCE OF RADIATION BIOLOGY FOR THE FUTURE DEVELOPMENT OF RADIOTHERAPY

Many developments in radiotherapy have resulted from new technologies or have been made empirically by clinicians; there are few examples of developments that have begun in the radiobiological laboratory and been carried through to the point where patient survival has significantly improved. The role of oxygen is one positive example that has led to benefits (see Chapter 16), also the clinical gains obtained with accelerated fractionation and hyperfractionation (see Chapter 14).

Compared with chemotherapeutic drugs, radiation is now a well understood cytotoxic agent. Its access to tumour cells is just a matter of dosimetry, independent of the transport mechanisms that largely determine the effectiveness of chemical agents. The sequence of processes listed in Section 1.2 above are well described for radiation; some of them are equally relevant to the response of tissues to cytotoxic drug treatment, and thus research into radiation biology has brought benefits to other areas of therapeutic cancer research.

The future is likely to require greater and greater dependence on basic science. The simple empirical things have mostly been fully exploited and increasing knowledge about the cellular and molecular nature

KEY POINTS

1. Radiotherapy is an important curative and palliative modality in the treatment of cancer. Significant gains are still to be made by the optimization of biological and physical factors.
2. Therapeutic index is 'the name of the game' in curative cancer therapy.
3. The effects of radiation on mammalian tissues should be viewed as a succession of processes extending from microseconds to months and years after exposure. In choosing one end-point of effect, it is important not to overlook the rest of this process.

of radiation effects will undoubtedly lead to developments for which the radiotherapist will require a grounding in fundamental mechanisms. That is the purpose of this book.

BIBLIOGRAPHY

Boag JW (1975). The time-scale in radiation biology. 12th Failla memorial lecture. In: *Radiation Research* (eds Nygaard OF, Adler HI, Sinclair WK). Academic Press, San Diego.

DeVita VT, Goldin A, Oliverio VT *et al.* (1979). The drug development and clinical trials programs of the Division of Cancer Treatment, National Cancer Institute. *Cancer Clin Trials* **2**: 195–216.

Souhami R, Tobias J (1986). *Cancer and its Management.* Blackwell, Oxford.

Tubiana M (1992). The role of local treatment in the cure of cancer. *Eur J Cancer* **28A**: 2061–9.

Cell proliferation and growth rate of tumours

AC BEGG AND G GORDON STEEL

2.1 INTRODUCTION

The speed of development of the disease process in patients with cancer depends to a large extent on the growth rate of primary and metastatic tumours. In patients in whom treatment is unsuccessful, the speed of recurrence and thus the survival of the patient also depend on tumour growth rate. Growth rate is, however, not the only determinant of the time-course of cancer and its effect on the patient since the location, invasiveness and biochemical properties of the lesions also play a part.

Many studies have been done on what determines tumour growth rate, i.e. why one tumour grows faster than another. The three major factors are the rate at which the tumour cells go through the cell cycle, the fraction of tumour cells that are cycling, and the rate of loss of cells, or cell debris, from the tumour volume. These characteristics are determined largely by the underlying genetic profile of the tumour cells, determined in turn by the tissue of origin and the changes caused by the malignant transformation. This chapter covers methods of measuring tumour volume growth, the underlying cell proliferation kinetics, and their implications.

2.2 MEASUREMENT OF TUMOUR SIZE

The precision and frequency with which tumour size can accurately be measured varies widely from one anatomical site to another. At the time of surgery a single measurement can often be made but this gives no information on growth rate. The size of superficial lesions can be measured with engineer's callipers, within the constraints of skin thickness and depth of the lesion. Chest radiographs, CT and NMR scanning and other imaging techniques also allow repeated measurements of tumours in some sites. The greatest amount of published data on tumour growth has been on primary and metastatic tumours in the lung. However, even in this site where the difference of tissue density between tumour and surrounding tissues is considerable, the size of lesion that can be discriminated is limited. Spratt *et al.* (1963, 1999) tested the accuracy of radiologists by placing plastic balls of different sizes over various parts of the chest of patients before taking x-rays and summarized the results of their studies as follows:

> The radiologists could locate the opacities of lucite balls 10–12 mm in diameter regularly regardless of their location. They could locate the radiopacities of balls 6 mm in diameter only when they were located in intercostal spaces contrasted against aerated lung. They could distinguish the radiopacities of 3 mm diameter balls from normal pulmonary shadows in these same areas of favourable contrast only when they were shown precisely where to look.

Careful studies of the growth and regression of lung metastases were made by Breur (1966) using a series of circles engraved on Perspex, increasing in diameter by 0.5 or 1.0 mm. Thomlinson (1982) made very precise measurements of primary breast tumours using callipers (see Figure 2.5).

Various formulae have been used to transform linear dimensions into volumes, for instance:

$$V = \pi/6 \times (\text{mean diameter})^3$$
$$V = 0.5 \times \text{length} \times (\text{width})^2 \text{ [taking } \pi = 3\text{]}$$

and provided the same formula is used consistently there is probably little to choose between them. For the measurement of tumours in laboratory animals, a calibration curve can be constructed (Steel, 1977). External dimensions of tumours of varying sizes are measured, after which they are excised and weighed. Tumour weight is then plotted against the external measurements (e.g. mean diameter) and a smooth curve through these data comprises a calibration curve that can be used to interpret any further external measurements. No assumptions about the tumour's geometric form or about skin thickness need be made and the scatter of points around the calibration curve also gives a direct indication of precision.

The size and growth rate of tumours can be measured indirectly by quantifying tumour products in blood: CEA for choriocarcinomas, immunoglobulins for plasmacytomas, AFP or HCG in testicular tumours, PSA for prostate cancer (Price *et al.*, 1990a, 1990b; Fowler *et al.*, 1994; Lee *et al.*, 1995; Schmid *et al.*, 1993).

2.3 EXPONENTIAL AND NON-EXPONENTIAL GROWTH

Exponential growth is where tumour volume increases by a constant fraction in equal intervals of time. Thus, the time for tumour volume to double (the volume doubling time, T_d) is the same for lesions of size 1–2 g or 10–20 g or 100–200 g, etc. The equation of exponential growth is:

$$V = \exp(0.693 \times \text{time}/T_d)$$

where 0.693 is $\log_e 2$. The logarithm of tumour volume increases linearly with time. It is conventional to plot tumour growth curves on a logarithmic scale of volume so that departures from exponential growth can easily be seen.

Why is the idea of exponential growth so important? This is, in fact, the simplest mode of growth. One cell will produce 2 cells on division, which in turn will produce 4 after the next cycle, then 8, 16 and 32 in the next three cycles, and so on. This is exponential growth. If cells are allowed to proliferate under constant conditions, with no cell loss or infertility, their number will increase exponentially. It is *departure* from exponential growth that we have to explain! As indicated in the sections below, there are two principal processes that cause tumours to grow with a doubling time that is longer than the cell-cycle time: cell loss and decycling (i.e. proliferating cells moving into a non-proliferating state). Non-exponential growth can thus arise by any combination of three factors: increasing cell-cycle time, decreasing growth fraction and increasing rate of cell loss (Steel, 1977). The nomogram in Figure 2.1 indicates the relation between tumour volume, cell number and the number of doublings, starting from a single cell. Cells are assumed to have a mass of 10^{-9} g. The nomogram is correct for any mode of growth; exponential is the special case where the doubling time is constant.

Figure 2.2 illustrates an important feature of exponential growth. The same exponential line is drawn on a linear scale of volume (panel A) or on a logarithmic scale (panel B). On the linear scale (which is what a clinical observer will tend to see) there appears to be a long '*silent interval*' or latent period where no growth is seen. But during this time the tumour is growing regularly and with a constant doubling time. Once the tumour becomes detectable or symptomatic (at a size of perhaps 1–50 g), its size on a linear scale appears to sweep upwards, steeper and steeper. This is only a subjective and misleading impression, for growth is in many cases regular and exponential.

Exponential growth of tumours in laboratory animals is uncommon. It is more usual to find that the doubling time increases progressively as the tumour gets bigger. The growth curves (on a logarithmic scale of volume) are convex upwards, and such tumours grow progressively more slowly as they enlarge. The volume doubling time can be judged at any point by drawing a tangent to the curve and reading off its doubling time.

Such progressively slowing growth curves have often been described by the Gompertz equation:

$$V = V_0 \cdot \exp[A/B(1 - e^{-Bt})]$$

Here V_0 is the volume at the arbitrary time zero and A and B are parameters that determine the growth rate. At very early time intervals (t small) the equation becomes exponential: $V = V_0 \exp(At)$. At long time intervals $\exp(-Bt)$ becomes small compared with 1.0 and the volume tends to a maximum value of $V_0 \exp(A/B)$. The Gompertz equation is not a unique description of such growth curves. For a fuller discussion see Steel (1977).

2.4 THE GROWTH RATE OF HUMAN TUMOURS

Some examples of carefully measured human lung tumours are shown in Figure 2.3; the lines are straight or nearly so and these represent good examples of exponential tumour growth. Some human lung tumours show a Gompertzian pattern of growth, and irregular growth (a sudden increase or decrease in growth rate) is not uncommon.

Published data on the growth rate of tumours were reviewed by Steel (1977). Within any one tumour type there is a wide range of volume doubling times. For instance, the range of values for lung metastases of adenocarcinoma is shown in Figure 2.4: some double their volume in a week, some in a year or more, and the median is around 90 days. This median value is typical of other classes of human tumour. Table 2.1 gives data on the doubling times for tumours of various types. Lymphomas, teratomas and superficial breast metastases grow faster than the average; primary lung adenocarcinomas and colon tumours grow more slowly.

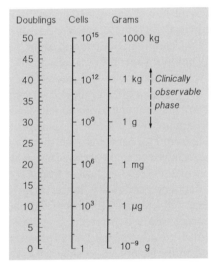

Figure 2.1 *The relationship between the weight of a tumour, the number of cells it contains (assuming 10^9 per gram) and the number of doublings from a single cell.*

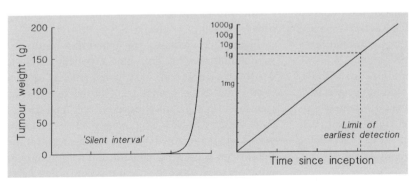

Figure 2.2 *An exponential growth curve plotted on a linear scale (left) or on a logarithmic scale (right). The clinical phase of growth is a minor part of the whole life history of the tumour.*

Table 2.1 *Volume doubling times for human tumours*

Site and type	No. tumours measured	Mean volume doubling time*	Confidence limits on mean
Metastases in lung			
Colon-rectum, adenocarcinoma	56	95	84–107
Breast, adenocarcinoma	44	74	56–98
Kidney, adenocarcinoma	14	60	37–98
Thyroid, adenocarcinoma	16	67	44–103
Uterus, adenocarcinoma	15	78	55–111
Head & neck, squamous cell carcinoma	27	57	43–75
Fibrosarcoma	28	65	46–93
Osteosarcoma	34	30	24–38
Teratoma	80	30	25–36
Lymphoma	11	27	19–39
Superficial metastases			
Breast carcinoma	66	19	16–24
Primary tumours			
Lung, adenocarcinoma	64	148	121–181
Lung, sq. cell carcinoma	85	85	75–95
Lung, undifferentiated	55	79	67–93
Colon-rectum	19	632	426–938
Breast	17	96	68–134

*Geometric mean volume doubling time in days.
From a review of early data on the growth rate of human tumours (Steel, 1977).

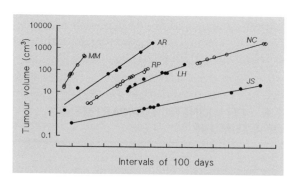

Figure 2.3 *Growth curves for primary human lung tumours. Data of Schwartz, redrawn by Steel (1977), with permission.*

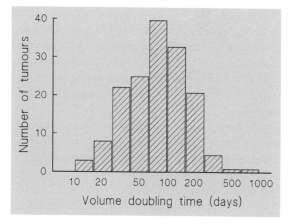

Figure 2.4 *The distribution of volume doubling times for 159 lung metastases of adenocarcinoma from various primary sites. From Steel (1977) with permission.*

2.5   THE SPEED OF TUMOUR REGRESSION

After treatment, some tumours show a rapid volume response and others respond much more slowly. It is important to distinguish between speed of shrinkage and the probability of local tumour control, for some rapidly shrinking tumours recur early. Some clinical studies have shown a correlation between shrinkage rate and local control, but this is not the case in all clinical situations. Careful studies by Thomlinson (1982) showed that among primary breast tumours there was a 50-fold range of regression halving times

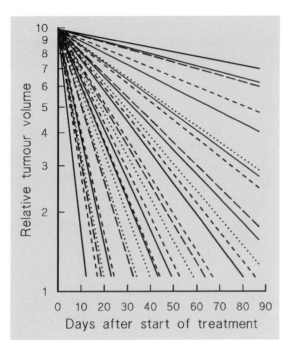

Figure 2.5 *The range of regression rates of some of the 78 primary human breast tumours studied by Thomlinson (1982).*

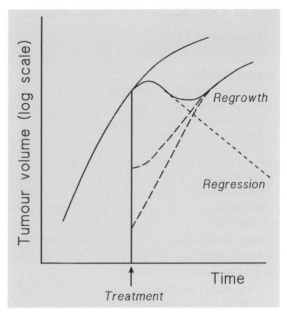

Figure 2.6 *The volume response of an uncontrolled tumour is the resultant of two processes: regression and regrowth. Repopulation during the period of regression may take place at a rate that may differ from the growth rate of the untreated tumour.*

(Figure 2.5). The rapidly shrinking tumours tended to be highly cellular, whilst those that shrank slowly had a large amount of connective tissue. He also found that in tumours that were treated by radiotherapy as well as by chemotherapy the rate of regression was independent of the treatment: it was characteristic of the biology of the tumour.

The overall volume response of a tumour to treatment is illustrated in Figure 2.6. There are two components of response, *regression* and *regrowth*, and the shape of the regrowth curve is a matter of considerable current debate (see Sections 14.4 and 22.4). The time and depth of the nadir (i.e. the minimum tumour volume) will depend upon both components. For judging the effectiveness of tumour treatment it is therefore wise to choose a measure that reflects the regrowth component rather than the speed of regression, for it is the regrowth component that depends upon the degree of tumour cell kill. *Partial remission* is an unsatisfactory criterion. *Duration of disease-free interval* is to be preferred. For measurable lesions in animals, the preferred parameter is the *tumour growth delay*: this indicates the difference between the times at which treated or untreated tumours reach a fixed multiple of the pre-treatment tumour size (e.g. twice the size at the start of treatment, see Figure 17.2A).

2.6 CELL KINETIC COMPARTMENTS OF A TUMOUR

The neoplastic cells within a tumour can be divided into four compartments based on their kinetic properties. The most important compartment is that of actively dividing cells. All cells in this compartment are going through the cell cycle and can be distinguished using cell-labelling techniques. All new tumour cells are produced from this compartment, which is therefore the major contributor to growth of the tumour volume. This compartment is called the *growth fraction* and the cells within it are sometimes called 'P' (for proliferating) cells.

In addition to actively dividing cells, there are two other compartments: resting (or G0) cells and the sterile (or differentiated) cells. The major difference between them is that G0 cells are capable of

Table 2.2 *Kinetic parameters of a typical human tumour*

Cell cycle time (~2 d) Growth fraction (~40%) Cell loss (~90%)	Potential doubling time (~5 d)	Volume doubling time (~60 d)

re-entering the cell cycle, but sterile or differentiated cells are no longer capable of division. G0 cells are often called 'Q' (for quiescent) cells. Some G0 cells may be clonogenic (and thus capable of repopulating a tumour) and are therefore dangerous and need to be killed by the applied therapy. It is often not easy to distinguish G0 cells from sterile cells on the basis of kinetic techniques, although terminally differentiated cells can sometimes be distinguished morphologically in well-differentiated tumours. Differentiated cells are no longer a danger to the patient, although their bulk contributes to the tumour volume. The other main contributor to tumour bulk is the stroma: normal-tissue cells such as blood cells and fibroblasts that in some cases can exceed the number of neoplastic cells.

In addition, there exists in most tumours a compartment consisting of dead and dying cells. Necrosis is a characteristic of tumours and is the result of an inadequate internal blood supply. The volume occupied by necrosis varies widely from one tumour to another but it can be extensive (see Figure 15.4). Apoptotic cells (see Section 8.6) are also often visible in histological sections, another sign of cell death.

Transfer of cells from one compartment to another occurs continuously. Movement of cells from the Q to the P compartment, which can occur after or during some treatments, is called *recruitment*. Transfer from P to Q must also occur, for otherwise the proportion of Q cells would decline towards zero in a growing tumour, due to the multiplication of P cells. Some cells may have an inadequate supply of nutrients such as oxygen and may fail to divide further; cells can be pushed too far away from blood vessels as a result of pressure of growth. Cells also enter the differentiated compartment by natural differentiation processes. Finally, cells can leave the volume of a primary tumour mass, either as viable cells (this can lead to metastasis) or by death followed by the lysis and removal of their constituents. These processes contribute to the general phenomenon of cell loss from tumours.

2.7   FACTORS AFFECTING TUMOUR GROWTH RATE

The volume doubling time of a tumour (T_d, Section 2.3) is determined by three main factors: the cell-cycle time (T_c), the growth fraction (GF) and the rate of cell loss. Tumours grow faster if the cycle time is short, the growth fraction is high, and cell loss is low (Table 2.2). The potential doubling time (T_{pot}) is defined as the time within which the cell population of the tumour would double if there were no cell loss (Steel, 1977). It depends on the cell-cycle time and the growth fraction. The potential doubling time can be obtained from the thymidine labelling index (LI) or S-phase fraction by the relation:

$$T_{pot} = \lambda \cdot T_s / \text{LI}$$

where T_s is the duration of the S phase. The parameter λ corrects for the non-rectangular age distribution of growing cell populations and usually lies between 0.7 and 1.0. The S-phase duration can be measured by thymidine-analogue labelling techniques (Section 2.9). The volume doubling time (T_d) is often found using callipers for superficial tumours, from radiographs, or from CT or MR scans (see above). Cell loss from a tumour can be estimated from the cell loss factor:

$$\text{Cell loss factor} = 1 - T_{pot}/T_d$$

(Steel, 1977). This factor is simply the cell loss rate as a fraction of the cell birth rate. The slow growth of many human tumours is largely the result of a high rate of cell loss. The principal mechanisms of cell loss are necrosis and differentiation: well-differentiated carcinomas (by definition) maintain some features of the hierarchical tissue structure of the tissue of origin (see Section 3.1) and cell turnover by this normal pathway probably continues in the malignant state. In many tumours it is possible to recognize individual pyknotic or apoptotic cells scattered throughout the tissue.

Evidence from studies on tumours in mice and rats suggests that the slowing of growth rate as tumours

Table 2.3 *Cell kinetic parameters of human tumours derived from* in vivo *labelling with Br-dUrd or I-dUrd and measured by flow cytometry*

Site	No. of patients	LI (%)	T_s (h)	T_{pot} (d)
Head and neck	712	9.6 (6.8–20.0)	11.9 (8.8–16.1)	4.5 (1.8–5.9)
CNS	193	2.6 (2.1–3.0)	10.1 (4.5–16.7)	34.3 (5.4–63.2)
Upper intestinal	183	10.5 (4.9–19.0)	13.5 (9.8–17.2)	5.8 (4.3–9.8)
Colorectal	345	13.1 (9.0–21.0)	15.3 (13.1–20.0)	4.0 (3.3–4.5)
Breast	159	3.7 (3.2–4.2)	10.4 (8.7–12.0)	10.4 (8.2–12.5)
Ovarian	55	6.7	14.7	12.5
Cervix	159	9.8	12.8	4.8 (4.0–5.5)
Melanoma	24	4.2	10.7	7.2
Haematological	106	13.3 (6.1–27.7)	14.6 (12.1–16.2)	9.6 (2.3–18.1)
Bladder	19	2.5	6.2	17.1
Renal cell ca	2	4.3	9.5	11.3
Prostate	5	1.4	11.7	28.0

Data derived from Haustermans *et al.* (1997); Rew and Wilson (2000).
Ranges represent variations in median or mean values between studies; ranges for individual tumours are considerably larger.

increase in size (Section 2.3) is associated with a progressive increase in the rate of cell loss, a decrease in the growth fraction, and a lengthening of the mean cell-cycle duration (Steel, 1977).

2.8 VALUES FOR KINETIC PARAMETERS IN HUMAN TUMOURS

Studies have been carried out in which [³H]thymidine ([³H]Tdr) was given to patients and multiple biopsies taken in order to measure cell-cycle parameters. Radioactive thymidine is specifically incorporated into DNA, although some of it is catabolized and lost from the tissue. Many early studies of cell proliferation were based on thymidine labelling of S-phase cells. More recently, much information on the labelling index and T_s has been obtained from *in vivo* labelling with thymidine analogues, together with flow cytometry (see below).

Cell-cycle times for human tumours from the [³H]TdR studies have ranged from 15 hours to more than 100 hours with an average of 2–3 days (Steel, 1977). These values are similar to cell population doubling times found for human tumour cells grown in culture. As described in Section 2.4, the volume doubling times for human tumours are much longer, ranging from 4 days to over a year, around a median of roughly 3 months. There are large differences between individual tumours, even within a particular

histological type. Growth fractions for the relatively few human tumours studied range between 6% and 90%, with most solid tumours having values well below 50%.

A summary of thymidine analogue/flow cytometry data is shown in Table 2.3. Values for mean LI vary widely among different tumour types, T_s is relatively constant, and T_{pot} also varies widely from less than 5 days in head and neck and cervix cancers to around 1 month in CNS and prostate cancers. It is important to note, however, that the variation within a single tumour type is considerable. Estimates of cell loss factor for a particular tumour type calculated from T_{pot} and the volume doubling time are almost always high in carcinomas, usually ranging from 70% to more than 90% (Table 2.4). This is apparent from average T_{pot} values of a few days compared with T_d values of a few months: for instance, if $T_{pot} = 5$ days and $T_d = 70$ days, the cell loss factor $= 1 - (5/70) = 0.93$, or 93%. By contrast, cell-loss factor values for sarcomas and lymphomas are relatively low.

2.9 CELL KINETIC METHODS

Percentage labelled mitoses

With this technique, cells are pulse-labelled with [³H]TdR, a radioactively labelled nucleic acid precursor that is specifically incorporated into DNA, and

Table 2.4 *Calculation of cell loss factors for human tumours based on labelling with radiolabelled thymidine or thymidine analogues and volume doubling times, in separate series*

Site	LI (%)	T_{pot} (d)	T_d (d)	Cell loss factor (%)
(A) Br/IdUrd[1]				
Head and neck	9.6	4.1	45	91
Colorectal	13.1	3.9	90	96
Melanoma	4.2	8.5	52	84
Breast[2]	3.7	9.4	82	89
Prostate[3]	1.4	28.0	1100	97
(B) [3H]Thymidine[4]				
Undifferentiated bronchus ca	19.0	2.5	90	97
Sarcoma	2.0	23.3	39	40
Childhood tumours	13.0	3.6	20	82
Lymphoma	3.0	15.6	22	29

[1] LI, T_s and T_{pot} from FCM data (Haustermans *et al.*, 1997; Rew and Wilson, 2000); calculations assume $\lambda = 0.8$ (Steel, 1977).
[2] T_d values for pulmonary metastases from Spratt *et al.* (1999).
[3] T_d from PSA doubling times; Schmid *et al.* (1993); Fowler *et al.* (1994); Lee *et al.* (1995).
[4] From Steel (1977); calculations assume $T_s = 14\,h$, $\lambda = 0.8$.

not RNA. Pulse-labelling means giving only a brief exposure to the labelled precursor: *in vivo* this occurs naturally as a result of the rapid clearance of thymidine from the circulation and *in vitro* it is achieved by wash-out. Samples are then taken at several times thereafter and labelling of mitotic figures is detected by autoradiography (i.e. coating histological slides with photographic film). The fraction of mitoses that are labelled will rise and fall as the cohort of ^{3}H-labelled cells, which were initially in S, move into, through, and out of mitosis. This pattern will be repeated one cell cycle later. From the frequency and width of the waves of labelled mitoses, the lengths of all phases of the cycle, together with their variations, can be determined (Steel, 1977). This technique was a breakthrough in quantitative cell kinetics, although the use of radiolabelled thymidine has largely been superseded by the use of non-radioactive thymidine analogues, which allow more rapid and less laborious detection.

Thymidine analogues

Replacement of the methyl group of thymidine (Figure 2.7) with halogen atoms of similar size such as iodine or bromine creates the analogues iodo- or bromo-deoxyuridine (IdUrd, BrdUrd). Enzymes

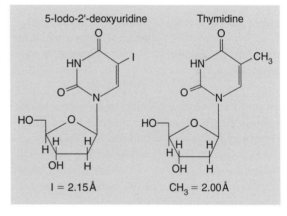

Figure 2.7 *The structure of thymidine and its analogue, IdUrd. The comparative diameters of the iodine atom and the methyl group are indicated.*

responsible for DNA synthesis cannot easily distinguish between thymidine and its analogues and these are therefore incorporated into DNA via the same pathway as thymidine. Once in DNA, they can be detected by specific antibodies, which recognize the small distortions in the DNA molecule caused by their incorporation. The development of these antibodies has led to their widespread use for cell kinetic studies. The antibodies can in turn be labelled with an enzyme (usually a peroxidase), which allows

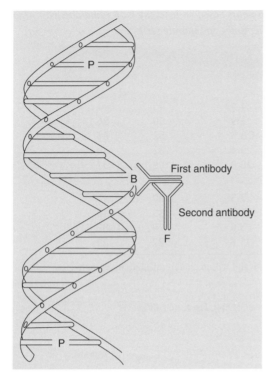

Figure 2.8 *The principle of BrdUrd staining of DNA. B, an incorporated BrdUrd molecule; P, an intercalated propidium iodide molecule; F, FITC conjugated to the second antibody.*

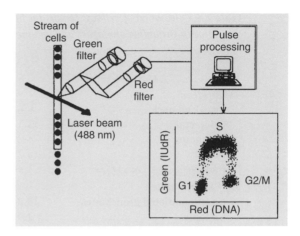

Figure 2.9 *The principle of flow cytometry.*

immunocytochemical staining, or a fluorescent label (usually the green fluorescent molecule FITC) for flow cytometry. In this way, all cells that have incorporated the analogue, and were therefore in the S phase at the time of its administration, can be detected by a brown colour on immunoperoxidase-stained sections or by green fluorescence with flow cytometry.

Flow cytometry

For cell kinetic studies using flow cytometry, IdUrd- or BrdUrd-labelled cells are stained with a mouse antibody specific for the DNA-incorporated analogue, followed by an anti-mouse antibody conjugated with FITC (Figure 2.8). Cells are counter-stained for total DNA content using propidium iodide (PI, a red fluorescent stain). In the flow cytometer, the stained cells flow through a laser beam which excites the fluorochromes, giving green fluorescent emissions from FITC and red fluorescence from the PI (Hall, 1988). These colours can be separated using

optical filters and their intensities for each cell are measured using photomultiplier tubes (Figure 2.9). The data are displayed as two-parameter cytograms, for instance green versus red fluorescence intensities. Three subpopulations, representing G1 cells (low green and low red), G2/M cells (low green and high red) and S-phase cells (high green), can readily be seen. Up to 10 000 cells per second can be analysed in this way, making this a rapid and quantitative method that also avoids the use of radioactivity.

An example of the flow cytometer output is shown in Figure 2.10. This shows green (IdUrd) versus red (DNA) fluorescence cytograms for Chinese hamster cells at different times after pulse-labelling *in vitro* with IdUrd. Movement of labelled and unlabelled cells through the cell cycle can be seen from the changing patterns. At time zero, i.e. immediately after pulse-labelling, the labelled cells should be distributed equally between the G1 and G2 positions. In Figure 2.10, movement of cells from G2/M into G1 is already visible by 2 hours, and the 'leaning' to the right of the dot pattern indicates movement through the S phase. This becomes more pronounced with increasing time. By 6 hours, all the unlabelled cells that were in G1 have moved into the S phase, and all the labelled cells have moved out of S and are now in G2 or have divided and have returned to G1. This gives an almost inverted picture compared with that at 1 hour. All phases of the cell cycle can be obtained from these pictures, in a manner similar to the analysis of labelled mitoses curves, except that the fraction of labelled cells in mid-S is measured instead of the fraction of labelled cells in mitosis.

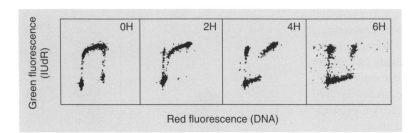

Figure 2.10 *Flow-cytometer traces from samples taken at various intervals from an* in vitro *cell population that was pulse labelled with IdUrd at time zero. Green fluorescence (IdUrd content) is plotted vertically; red fluorescence (DNA content) horizontally.*

Obtaining kinetic information from one sample

The relative movement method allows T_s, LI and T_{pot} to be estimated from one tissue sample (Begg *et al.*, 1985). This is useful for clinical application where it is often difficult to take more than one biopsy. Several hours after intravenous injection of BrdUrd or IdUrd, a tumour biopsy is taken, fixed in ethanol, and a suspension of nuclei is subsequently made, stained and analysed by flow cytometry. The average position (red fluorescence) of the labelled cells that have not yet divided, relative to the positions of G1 and G2, is measured using computer-drawn windows around the appropriate subpopulations (Figure 2.11A). The effects are quantified by the *relative movement parameter* (RM), defined to be zero for cells in G1 and 1.0 for cells in G2. Since on average the labelled cells immediately after staining will be homogeneously distributed within the S phase, it is assumed that RM at that time is 0.5. Subsequently, the cells progress towards G2 and RM increases. The recommended procedure is to measure RM in a sample taken a few hours (t) after labelling, then plot a line between RM = 0.5 at $t = 0$ and the measured RM at time t. This is extrapolated to the time required for RM to reach 1.0, which gives the estimate of T_s (Figure 2.11B). The calculation assumes that the plot of RM versus time is linear, although theoretically it is curved. There are better, more rigorous mathematical ways to calculate T_s from RM, taking into account this curvature (Terry *et al.*, 1991; White *et al.*, 2000). For accurate T_s measurements, the time interval between injection and biopsy should be longer than G2+M: 6–8 hours is recommended for most human tumours.

Endogenous proliferation markers

The use of thymidine analogues can provide dynamic, or rate, information about the cell cycle. A disadvantage

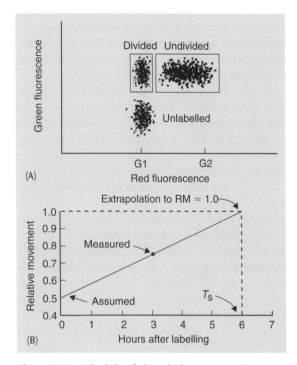

Figure 2.11 *Principle of the relative movement method. (A) The two-dimensional flow-cytometer display; (B) the principle of the method.*

for clinical studies is the need to administer a potentially toxic compound *in vivo*, although no acute or late toxicity has yet been observed from IdUrd or BrdUrd when used at low doses for cell kinetic studies. Alternative assays for proliferation that do not require drug administration have therefore been sought. There are several proteins that seem to be expressed mainly in proliferating but not quiescent cells. Examples of these are the DNA polymerases used for replication, histones H2–4, Ki67, proliferating cell nuclear antigen (PCNA), and some of the cyclins. Antibodies are available to these proteins which can therefore be used to assess proliferation by immunochemical or flow-cytometry methods.

The most commonly used marker at present is Ki67, a nuclear protein associated with proliferating cells that can be detected using the originally discovered antibody, or by MIB1, an antibody against the same protein but which works better on paraffin-embedded material. Flow cytometry can also be used for detection. The function of the molecule is presently unknown, although progress is being made since the gene has now been cloned. It may not give accurate growth fraction estimates under all circumstances, particular after cytotoxic treatments, although it is closely proliferation-related and is widely used to rank proliferative fractions of tumours and normal tissues under non-perturbed conditions.

PCNA is a protein involved in both DNA repair and DNA synthesis, being an auxiliary protein for DNA polymerase-delta. When PCNA is tightly bound in the nucleus it is associated with DNA replication. The fraction of PCNA-positive cells is therefore a measure of the S-phase fraction. PCNA is expressed in other phases of the cycle, however, where it is loosely bound. Measurement of total (tight + loose) PCNA is then in principle a measure of the growth fraction (i.e. cells in all cycle phases). Different tissue preparation techniques resulting in the removal or not of loosely bound protein will result in different PCNA indices, necessitating care in interpretation. As with Ki67, immunochemical methods or flow cytometry can be used for detection. Figure 2.12 shows flow-cytometry data for dual staining using a marker (fluorescent antibody) and total DNA content (propidium iodide). PCNA shows predominant staining in S, similar to BrdUrd, whilst Ki67 is expressed in all phases of the cycle. These lung tumour cells are also positive for cytokeratin, which could be used as a tumour marker.

Several genes are only expressed in particular phases of the cycle, allowing their use as phase markers. Histones 3 and 4 are expressed in S phase, since they are necessary for nucleosome assembly on newly synthesized DNA. The expression of histone H3 has therefore been used as a marker for the S phase and has been shown to give similar information (i.e. fraction of cells in S) as a thymidine- or BrdUrd-labelling index. In this method, gene expression is monitored by measuring mRNA levels using *in situ* hybridization (ISH), whereby an oligonucleotide or ribonucleotide probe is used which specifically hybridizes to the mRNA of histone H3. Use of a biotin- or digoxigenin-labelled probe allows detection with

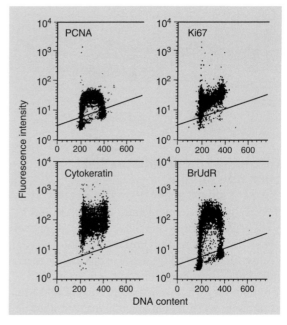

Figure 2.12 *Flow cytometry detection of proliferation markers in the human non-small cell lung cancer line MR65. Each marker was detected with a fluorescent antibody (y-axis) and plotted against total DNA content (x-axis). PCNA and BrdUrd show S-phase-specific labelling, in contrast to Ki67 which is found in all phases. Cytokeratin, a potential tumour marker, is also expressed in all phases (from Schutte et al., 1995, with permission).*

standard immunoperoxidase or immunofluorescence methods. The method can also be combined with BrdUrd labelling to give dynamic as well as static information on proliferation.

Cyclins are a class of molecule that are usually expressed in a cyclical fashion during the cell cycle, hence their name. They are instrumental in controlling the transitions between cell-cycle phases, e.g. G1 to S or G2 to M. Cyclins activate particular kinases (enzymes which phosphorylate proteins) by forming complexes with them. Cyclins D and E are G1 cyclins; cyclin A is mostly found in the S phase; cyclin B is found mostly in G2. There are several subtypes of the B and D cyclins. Antibodies are available to almost all known cyclins and these allow detection by immunochemical or flow methods. In an asynchronous population, the expression of particular cyclins can indicate the approximate position of individual cells

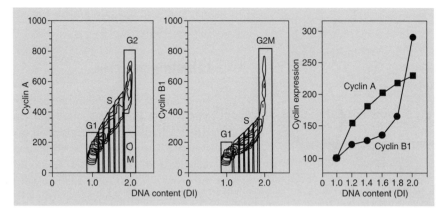

Figure 2.13 *Cyclin A and B expression in MOLT4 leukaemic cells detected using fluorescent antibodies and flow cytometry. Cyclin fluorescence in different phases of the cycle (within the vertical narrow windows drawn in the figures) was plotted in the right-hand panel, showing the S-phase specificity of cyclin A and the G2-phase specificity of cyclin B (from Gong* et al., *1995, with permission).*

in the cycle. Cyclin B, for example, has been used as a marker of G2 cells, and is also useful in distinguishing doublets of G1 cells from true G2 cells in flow cytometry. Figure 2.13 shows flow cytometry data for two cyclins in leukaemic cells, showing the G2 specificity of cyclin B and the relatively greater S-phase specificity of cyclin A. The fraction of cells containing a particular cyclin can be used as a proliferative index, e.g. to rank different tumours, assuming it is proportional to the growth fraction. The phase specificity of the cyclins, however, renders this inaccurate and a marker such as Ki67 would be preferred for this purpose. It should also be noted that cyclins control the function of cyclin-dependent kinases (CDK), but there are several other controls of this vital cellular machinery, and therefore cyclin levels do not necessarily directly reflect CDK activity.

It is important to realize that these proliferation markers on their own yield static parameters, for instance estimates of the S-phase fraction, G2 fraction or growth fraction, and do not give information on the rate of progression of the cells through the cycle. This is in contrast to the situation with labelled thymidine or thymidine analogues, which can yield both phase fractions and phase times. The most reliable, flexible and powerful methods are probably those using thymidine analogues, although the use of the markers described above can often provide useful information in clinical material, where there are considerable constraints on the number of samples, drug administration and workload.

Human tumour kinetics *in vivo* using thymidine analogue labelling

Some kinetic information can be obtained by labelling human tumour biopsy material *in vitro* with [³H]TdR or a thymidine analogue, thus obtaining the fraction of cells synthesizing DNA. Better information can be obtained by *in vivo* labelling, and this avoids some potential artefacts of the *in vitro* procedure. Human tumours can be labelled by *in vivo* injection of IdUrd or BrdUrd because these analogues produce little or no toxicity at the low doses required for pulse-labelling kinetic studies. An example of the flow-cytometer outputs following *in vivo* labelling of a human tumour with IdUrd and biopsy a few hours later is shown in Figure 2.14. Panel B shows the distribution of DNA content: the peak on the left is a diploid peak that indicates the presence of non-malignant stromal cells. The large peak is due to G1 cells and the smallest peak to G2 tumour cells. Panel A shows IdUrd uptake plotted vertically, against DNA content. The normal cells are again visible as the left-hand cluster of dots. These are not included in the analysis. Two subpopulations of labelled cells can be seen several hours after labelling, a small one at the tumour G1 position and a larger one covering most of the S phase. The kinetic parameters labelling index (LI), DNA synthesis time (T_s), and the potential doubling time can be obtained from these data. This method has been used as a predictive test for rapidly and slowly repopulating tumours (see Section 22.4).

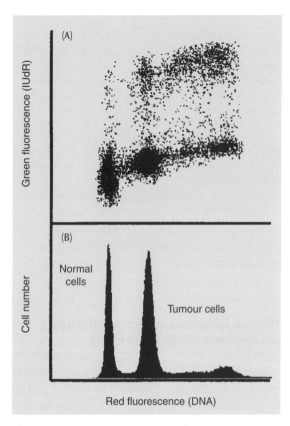

Figure 2.14 *Flow cytometry output from a human lung tumour biopsy a few hours after labelling with IdUrd. (A) The two-dimensional display of red–green fluorescence; (B) the derived distribution of DNA contents.*

The presence of non-malignant cells in a tumour biopsy can disturb the accuracy of parameter estimates for tumour cells. Attempts to overcome this have been made by using flow cytometry to measure T_s (described above) and combining it with the BrdUrd-labelling index of tumour cells counted in tissue sections using immunoperoxidase, where tumour areas can be distinguished morphologically from stromal areas (Bennett *et al.*, 1992). Alternatively, a second antibody, if available, can be used as a tumour marker, and measure the BrdUrd parameters only in cells that are positive for the tumour marker. One such marker is cytokeratin for carcinomas (Begg and Hofland, 1991; Schutte *et al.*, 1995).

No method to directly measure T_c from one biopsy has been published, although if the growth fraction were known it could be calculated from T_{pot}. A purported growth-fraction marker such as Ki67 (or MIB1) could be used for this purpose, although it may not give accurate growth fraction estimates in human tumours.

Labelling patterns

Solid tumors usually show heterogeneous labelling patters with both exogenous and endogenous cell kinetic markers such as BrdUrd or MIB1. One example is the decrease in labelling with increasing distance from a blood vessel (Tannock, 1968) because the growth fraction is highest closest to vessels and lowest for cells bordering necrosis which lack nutrients and oxygen.

In addition, some areas of human tumours show relatively high thymidine analogue labelling while others show no or low labelling in the same tumour, despite the presence of blood vessels. These regions may also be positive for an endogenous proliferation marker such as histone H3 (Gown *et al.*, 1996). The likely cause is a reduction of flow in blood vessels supplying the area, limiting access of the thymidine analogue. This is consistent with observations of acute hypoxia and transient flow changes in many tumours, including some in humans (see Chapter 15). Thymidine analogue methods may therefore underestimate proliferative potential, although in most cases the fraction of temporarily closed or 'low-flow' vessels is small.

In carcinomas, characteristic labelling patterns are often observed, including labelling in a thin layer around tumour 'islands' or gland-like structures, similar to basal-cell labelling in epithelia. Other tumours show random cell labelling, while some show intermediate patterns. These patterns can have prognostic significance for tumours treated with radiotherapy. Heterogeneous cell-labelling patterns can be due to differentiation, and the non-labelled cells lead to lower values of LI and thus contribute, correctly, to estimates of the non-growth fraction.

KEY POINTS

1. The accurate measurement of tumour size greatly helps clinical judgement on the rate of progression or response to treatment of tumours.
2. Tumour growth curves should always be plotted with size on a logarithmic scale to see

whether growth is exponential and to compare growth rates between tumours.

3. The growth rate of tumours can vary widely among tumours of the same type. Volume doubling times in the region of 3 months are common.

4. The rate of regression following treatment often varies widely among tumours of the same histopathological type. Slow regression does not necessarily mean a poor clinical response.

5. Tumour growth rate is determined by the cell cycle time, the growth fraction and the rate of cell loss. Potential doubling time indicates the cell production rate and is the predicted doubling time of the cell population with no cell loss.

6. Cell cycle times average around 2–3 days in human tumours, compared with volume doubling times of more than 2 months. Cell loss is high in many human tumours, particularly carcinomas.

7. There is a wide variation in cell kinetic parameters among human tumours even of the same histological type.

8. The movement of cells through the cell cycle can be measured using the thymidine analogues bromo- and iodo-deoxyuridine, together with flow cytometry or immuno-histochemistry.

9. Antibodies to cell-cycle regulated proteins can be used as endogenous proliferation markers. These give estimates of phase fractions or growth fractions, but not rates of progression through the cell cycle. Their advantage is that no drug needs to be administered to the patient.

10. Human tumour cell kinetics can be measured *in vitro* by labelling biopsies, or by injecting patients with low doses of thymidine analogues. Flow-cytometry analysis allows calculation of the potential doubling time from one biopsy.

BIBLIOGRAPHY

Begg AC, Hofland I (1991). Cell kinetic analysis of mixed populations using three-color fluorescence flow cytometry. *Cytometry* 12: 445–54.

Begg AC, McNally NJ, Shrieve DC, Karcher H (1985). A method to measure the duration of DNA synthesis and the potential doubling time from a single sample. *Cytometry* 6: 620–6.

Bennett MH, Wilson GD, Dische S *et al.* (1992). Tumour proliferation assessed by combined histological and flow cytometric analysis: implications for therapy in squamous cell carcinoma in the head and neck. *Br J Cancer* 65: 870–8.

Breur K (1966). Growth rate and radiosensitivity of human tumours. *Eur J Cancer* 2: 157–71.

Fowler JE, Jr, Pandey P, Braswell NT, Seaver L (1994). Prostate specific antigen progression rates after radical prostatectomy or radiation therapy for localized prostate cancer. *Surgery* 116: 302–5.

Gong J, Traganos F, Darzynkiewcz Z (1995). Discrimination of G2 and mitotic cells by flow cytometry based on different expression of cyclins A and B1. *Exp Cell Res* 220: 226–31.

Gown AM, Jiang JJ, Matles H *et al.* (1996). Validation of the S-phase specificity of histone (H3) in situ hybridization in normal and malignant cells. *J Histochem Cytochem* 44(3): 221–6.

Hall EJ (1988). *Radiobiology for the Radiologist*, 3rd edn, Chapter 11. Lippincott, Philadelphia.

Haustermans KM, Hofland I, Van Poppel H *et al.* (1997). Cell kinetic measurements in prostate cancer. *Int J Radiat Oncol Biol Phys* 37: 1067–70.

Lee WR, Hanks GE, Corn BW, Schultheiss TE (1995). Observations of pretreatment prostate-specific antigen doubling time in 107 patients referred for definitive radiotherapy. *Int J Radiat Oncol Biol Phys* 31: 21–4.

Price P, Hogan SJ, Bliss JM, Horwich A (1990a). The growth rate of metastatic non-seminomatous germ cell testicular tumours measured by marker production doubling time. II: Prognostic significance in patients treated with chemotherapy. *Eur J Cancer* 26: 453–6.

Price P, Hogan SJ, Horwich A (1990b). The growth rate of metastatic non-seminomatous germ cell testicular tumours measured by marker production doubling time. I: Theoretical basis and practical application. *Eur J Cancer* 26: 450–3.

Rew DA, Wilson GD (2000). Cell production rates in human tissues and tumours and their significance. Part II: clinical data. *Eur J Surg Oncol* 26: 405–17.

Schmid HP, McNeal JE, Stamey TA (1993). Observations on the doubling time of prostate cancer. The use of serial prostate-specific antigen in patients with untreated disease as a measure of increasing cancer volume. *Cancer* 71: 2031–40.

Schutte B, Tinnemans MMFJ, Pijpers GFP, Lenders MJH, Ramaekers FCS (1995). Three parameter flow cytometric analysis for simultaneous detection of cytokeratin, proliferation associated antigens and DNA content. *Cytometry* **21**: 177–86.

Spratt JS, Meyer JS, Spratt JA (1999). Rates of growth of human neoplasms: Part II. *J Surg Oncol* **61**: 68–83.

Spratt JS, Ter-Pogossian M, Long RTL (1963). The detection and growth of intrathoracic neoplasms. *Arch Surg* **86**: 283–8.

Tannock IF (1968). The relation between cell proliferation and the vascular system in a transplanted mouse mammary tumour. *Br J Cancer* **22**: 258–73.

Terry NHA, White RA, Meistrich ML, Calkins DP (1991). Evaluation of flow cytometric methods for determining population potential doubling times using cultured cells. *Cytometry* **12**: 234–41.

Thomlinson RH (1982). Measurement and management of carcinoma of the breast. *Clin Radiol* **33**: 481–93.

White RA, Meistrich ML, Pollack A, Terry NH (2000). Simultaneous estimation of T(G2+M), T(S), and T(pot) using single sample dynamic tumor data from bivariate DNA-thymidine analogue cytometry. *Cytometry* **41**: 1–8.

FURTHER READING

Steel GG (1977). *The Growth Kinetics of Tumours.* Oxford University Press, Oxford.

Tannock IF, Hill RP (1998). *The Basic Science of Oncology*, 3rd edn. McGraw-Hill, New York.

Proliferative and cellular organization of normal tissues

FIONA A STEWART AND ALBERT J VAN DER KOGEL

3.1 PROLIFERATIVE ORGANIZATION OF TISSUES

Cell proliferation in normal tissues is, in contrast to tumours, highly organized with cell production being homeostatically controlled. In adult tissues under non-pathological conditions the production of cells is exactly balanced by the loss of differentiated mature cells. Tissues of the body in which cell replacement is going on rapidly (e.g. intestinal epithelium, skin, haemopoietic tissues) are often called 'turnover tissues'. In the adult, these tissues can be said to have a cell loss factor (see Section 2.7) equal to 1.0. In 'post-mitotic' tissues such as neurones, the cell loss factor will be zero.

The degree of organization of cells within proliferative and functional compartments has important consequences for the response of tissues to radiation. Tissues can be divided into two main categories. First, there are tissues with a clearly recognizable separation between the proliferative compartment, comprising the stem-cell population (capable of unlimited self-renewal), the amplification population (proliferating rapidly, but for a limited number of divisions) and the post-mitotic compartment of mature functional cells (Figure 3.1A). Second, there are tissues without a recognizable separation between these compartments, in which at least some of the functional cells also have the capacity for self-renewal (Figure 3.1B).

Tissues with rapid cell turnover, such as epidermis, oral and intestinal epithelia and the haemopoietic system, are examples of a 'hierarchical' organization, with separate proliferative and functional cell compartments. In the epidermis, stem cells are located in the basal layer; in the intestine they are found in the lower half of the crypts of Lieberkühn. The stem cells in hierarchical tissues may comprise only a small fraction (less than a few per cent) of the proliferating cells, whilst the bulk of the proliferating cells make up the 'amplification compartment' and are involved in production of the cells that are needed for differentiation into mature functional cells. These differentiated cells continue to function normally after irradiation until they are lost from the tissue after their natural lifespan.

Cells that make up the amplification compartment also continue their differentiation process after irradiation. Damaged stem cells, which have lost their capacity for unlimited proliferation, may still undergo

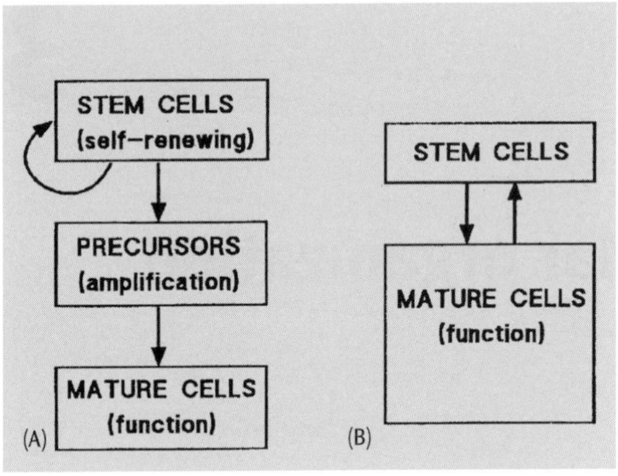

Figure 3.1 *Schematic outline of the proliferative organization of (A) hierarchical and (B) flexible normal-tissue systems.*

a limited number of (abortive) divisions before differentiating. The time at which tissue failure occurs after irradiation is therefore largely determined by the lifespan of the mature cells. Lifespan estimates for such cells range from a few days in the case of granulocytes or intestinal villus cells to more than 100 days (for example, erythrocytes).

Tissues with a slow cell turnover, such as liver, kidney, lung, and cells of the central nervous system, are examples of what Wheldon and Michalowski (1986) called a 'flexible' organization. Some degree of proliferative hierarchy may exist, but this is not as well defined as in the rapidly renewing tissues. In several slow-turnover tissues there is evidence for the existence of pluripotent, putative stem-cell populations (e.g. 0–2A glial progenitors in CNS, satellite cells in muscle) but in general there is no clear separation between stem-cell and functional compartments. Some functional, differentiated cells are also capable of proliferation but this only takes place when demand is high, due to tissue injury. After irradiation, a proportion of these functional cells will die as they attempt to go through cell division. In addition, some irradiated cells may undergo apoptosis before they reach mitosis. For example, oligodendrocytes in the adult rat CNS show a 10–20% apoptotic death rate at 1–2 days after irradiation, and early apoptotic cell death has been observed in irradiated endothelial cells of several tissue types. Moreover, some cell types, such as fibroblasts and keratinocytes, can undergo post-irradiation differentiation and retain some physiological function.

3.2 RADIATION RESPONSE IN RELATION TO PROLIFERATIVE ORGANIZATION

The most important mode of cell death following irradiation is mitotic cell death resulting from damage to the proliferative process. Lymphocytes are an exception, for they predominantly undergo interphase cell death by apoptosis. Mature (non-proliferating) functional cells of hierarchical tissues (e.g. epidermis) do not undergo necrotic cell death after irradiation. In such tissues the time between irradiation and the manifestation of tissue damage is mostly determined by the natural lifespan of the mature cells and is relatively independent of the radiation dose. The rate of recovery is, however, inversely dependent on dose. After high doses, the rapidly proliferating precursor pool is severely depleted and first needs to be replenished by the more slowly proliferating stem cells. This is clearly demonstrated in irradiated mouse epidermis, where loss of the differentiated (i.e. keratinized) layers is reflected by the development of dry and moist desquamation. The time-course for development of skin reactions (Figure 3.2A) is related to the cycle time of the proliferating basal cells (about 4.5 days) and to the number of cell layers in the mouse skin (3–4). When the cycle time of the basal cells is reduced to 2 days by plucking of the hair, the skin reactions develop faster, as is shown in Figure 3.2B. It can be seen that recovery after the higher doses was slower than after lower doses; this is because more cells have been killed and a greater number of cell divisions are required to restore the original cell number.

The relationship between cell death in the stem-cell compartment and functional injury is well established for most hierarchical tissues. In some cases (e.g. intestine), the level of cell killing required for lethal organ failure can also be estimated from a comparison of (crypt) cell survival and animal survival after a range of radiation doses. In this way it has been shown that tissue failure occurs when the surviving fraction of crypt cells is around 10^{-2} (Hornsey, 1973).

In flexible-type tissues or organs with a slow rate of renewal (e.g. kidney, lung, spinal cord), the relationship between cell death and tissue response to irradiation is not as clear as for epithelial tissues. Vascular, connective tissue and parenchymal components all contribute to the development of organ failure, which is therefore determined by many different cell types. The rate of development of radiation reactions in

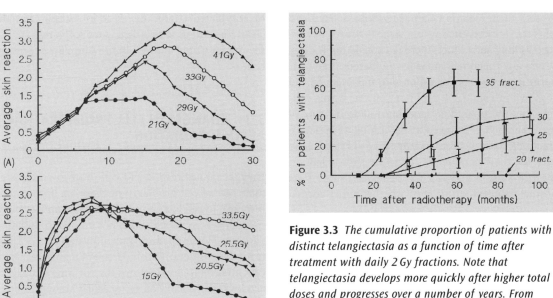

Figure 3.2 *The time-course of radiation-induced desquamation in the dorsal skin of the mouse foot: (A) normal skin; (B) plucked skin, showing a faster development of reactions due to a shorter cell cycle time. From Hegazy and Fowler (1973), with permission.*

Figure 3.3 *The cumulative proportion of patients with distinct telangiectasia as a function of time after treatment with daily 2 Gy fractions. Note that telangiectasia develops more quickly after higher total doses and progresses over a number of years. From Turesson and Notter (1986), with permission.*

these tissues depends on dose, as would be predicted in a situation in which the target cells are responsible for tissue function. In this case, the rate of functional cell loss increases with radiation dose, since the mature cells are also the proliferating cells that mainly die in mitosis. The time before expression of damage can, however, be very long, since the rate of cell loss is initially very slow. Once a certain level of cell depletion has occurred, the remaining cells are recruited into more rapid, compensatory proliferation (Section 3.3) which can result in an avalanche effect, precipitating further injury.

Late vascular effects in irradiated skin, such as telangiectasia, are examples of a flexible-type tissue response. These changes develop progressively, over a period of many years, and there is a clear, although non-linear, relationship between the rate of development of damage and total dose (Figure 3.3), in contrast to the development of acute epithelial desquamation after irradiation (Figure 3.2). One important consequence of the progressive dose-dependent development of such reactions is that the follow-up time must

be taken into account when comparing the extent of damage after different irradiation doses or schedules (see Section 11.4), since the degree of damage increases with time.

'Consequential' late effects

In addition to the generic late effects of radiation described above, consequential late effects may occur in tissues where severe breakdown of the epithelial barrier occurs during the acute phase. This may combine with infection to produce additional trauma to the target structures for late damage. Consequential late effects are predominantly seen in oral and bladder mucosae and, to a lesser extent, in skin. The consequential component of late damage follows the radiobiological principles of acute reactions, with respect to the impact of parameters such as overall treatment time and fractionation sensitivity (see Section 11.2).

The time of appearance of radiation effects in normal tissues

The latent period before the onset of radiation-induced functional damage depends on the rate of cell turnover of the tissue in question and not on its radiation sensitivity. Tissues with a high proliferative activity such as oral, intestinal and skin epithelia, express their radiation damage within a few days, whereas in radiosensitive but slow-turnover tissues, such as lung and kidney, there is a considerable delay before any functional damage is apparent. The relationship between proliferation rate and latent period is shown in Figure 3.4, proliferation rate being indicated by the thymidine labelling index. In view of the other factors involved in the timing of radiation reactions there is a remarkably smooth relationship between these parameters. Table 3.1 shows data on the relationship between the turnover times of six normal tissues of rats or mice, whether under normal

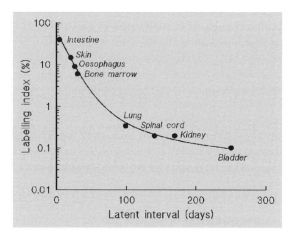

Figure 3.4 *Correlation of approximate latency times (for development of moderate to severe radiation-induced functional damage) with rate of proliferation (i.e. labelling index) in different rodent tissues. Rapidly proliferating tissues express their damage much earlier than slowly proliferating tissues. Data derived from various published sources.*

or stimulated conditions. It is interesting that the clear correlation shown in Figure 3.4 is reflected in the unstimulated and not in the stimulated turnover times.

3.3 CHANGES IN CELL PROLIFERATION AFTER IRRADIATION

Normal tissues respond to cell death by increasing their rate of cell proliferation. This is a homeostatic response to cell loss in individual cell compartments or in the entire tissue and is not unique to radiation damage. However, since radiation-induced cell loss from the proliferative compartment mainly occurs as cells attempt to divide at mitosis, the time of onset of accelerated proliferation varies widely among different tissues and is related to the turnover times of cells in the tissue (Table 3.1). For example, the cell turnover time of basal epithelial cells in unirradiated mouse skin is approximately 4 days. By 8 days after irradiation there is sufficient cell loss to trigger accelerated proliferation. At this time the cell turnover time in the basal cells is reduced to around 1 day. In addition to this increased proliferative rate, a complex reorganization of the proliferative structure takes place. This includes an increase in net stem cell production and abortive divisions of damaged cells. By contrast, accelerated proliferation in the slowly turning-over bladder urothelium does not begin until 3 months after irradiation and is not maximal until 9 months (Figure 3.5). At 9 months after irradiation the cell turnover time is reduced from over 200 days in unstimulated bladders to 9 days.

Table 3.1 *Cell turnover times and time of onset of compensatory proliferation in normal tissues*

Tissue	Cell turnover time (days)		Time of onset (days)	Authors
	Control	**Stimulated**		
Jejunum	0.6	0.4	3	Dewit *et al.* (1986)
Skin	4	1	8	Denekamp *et al.* (1976)
Lung	82	24	20/120	Coggle (1987)
Spinal cord	144	3	150	Zeman *et al.* (1964)
			20/120	Hornsey *et al.* (1981)
Kidney	144	11	120	Soranson and Denekamp (1986)
			90	Otsuka and Meistrich (1991)
Bladder	200	9	90–180	Stewart (1986)

The data in this table are approximate.

For both the epidermis and bladder there is a clear correlation between the time of onset of cell loss, functional damage and accelerated, compensatory cell proliferation. Such a relationship is not always so obvious in other organs, especially those with a flexible tissue organization. Irradiated mouse lung has two waves of accelerated proliferation in the type II pneumonocytes (see Figures 3.6 and 4.5). The early wave, at 20–40 days after irradiation, precedes the onset of functional damage but coincides with the release of surfactant from type II cells in response to increased microvascular permeability and leakage of plasma proteins onto the alveolar surface. The second wave of proliferation coincides with the onset of pneumonitis

(16–20 weeks after irradiation) and is probably a homeostatic response to cell depletion.

Two waves of accelerated proliferation are also seen in irradiated rat spinal cord (Figure 3.7). The early wave, at about 20 days, precedes functional damage but may be related to a proliferative response identified in glial progenitor cells after irradiation of the adult rat optic nerve. The late wave of proliferation beyond 120 days coincides with the onset of white-matter necrosis and paralysis after high doses to the cord. Thus, compensatory proliferative responses do occur in slowly renewing tissues but are often not so

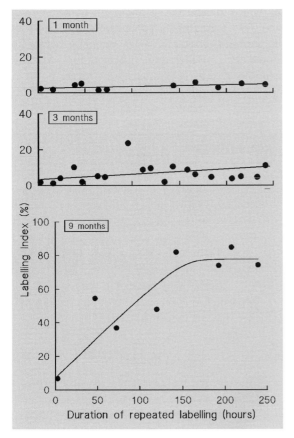

Figure 3.5 *Cell proliferation in the epithelium of the mouse bladder at 1, 3 and 9 months after irradiation with 25 Gy. The proliferation rate increased significantly from 3 months after irradiation but was not maximal until 9 months, coinciding with the histological appearance of hyperplasia and the occurrence of functional deficit. From Stewart (1986), with permission.*

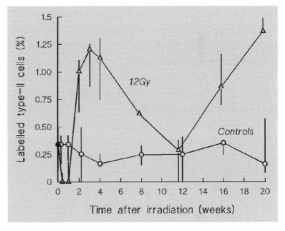

Figure 3.6 *Changes in the rate of proliferation in type-II pneumonocytes after thoracic irradiation of mice with 12 Gy, compared with unirradiated mice. From Coggle (1987) with permission.*

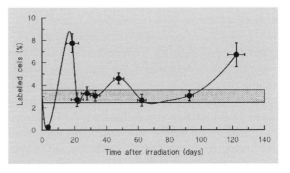

Figure 3.7 *Kinetics of glial-cell proliferation in the cervical spinal cord after a single dose of 20 Gy. In spite of the late onset of functional damage (5–6 months), an early wave of proliferation is observed. From Hornsey et al. (1981), with permission.*

clearly related to the expression of, and recovery from, functional injury as in acutely responding tissues.

3.4 MODIFIERS OF PROLIFERATION AND NORMAL-TISSUE RECOVERY

Several different growth factors are now routinely used to stimulate haematopoietic proliferation and recovery after myelosuppressive treatment with chemotherapy or after total body irradiation in preparation for bone marrow transplantation. Granulocyte colony stimulating factor (G-CSF), granulocyte/macrophage colony stimulating factor (GM-CSF) and some interleukins (IL-3, IL-6, IL-11) are effective in reducing both the depth and duration of the leucocyte or thrombocyte nadir. In some situations (e.g. acute lymphoblastic leukaemia and ovarian cancer) the use of these growth factors allows radiotherapy dose intensification. These effects can be further enhanced by other growth factors such as thrombopoietin.

Growth factors such as epidermal growth factor (EGF) and keratinocyte growth factor (KGF) have also been used to promote cell proliferation and differentiation in epidermis, oral and intestinal mucosa or lung epithelium prior to irradiation. These preclinical studies demonstrate reduced normal-tissue radiation damage, with little or no influence on tumour radiosensitivity. Such an approach may allow dose intensification in some clinical situations, e.g. radiotherapy for head and neck tumours, although clinical trials will be required to confirm the initial pre-clinical studies.

Small 'priming' doses of some chemotherapeutic drugs (e.g. cyclophosphamide or Ara-C) given before high-dose radiotherapy or chemotherapy can also protect against bone marrow or intestinal toxicity. This phenomenon is due to stimulated recruitment and repopulation of stem cells rather than to any modification of the sensitivity of the stem cells to radiation or the drugs. Substantial protection against lethal single-dose radiation toxicity has been demonstrated in animal studies but the effects are highly dependent on timing, which precludes their exploitation in fractionated clinical radiotherapy. Accelerated bone marrow recovery and reduced intestinal toxicity have, however, been demonstrated in patients given small priming doses of cyclophosphamide 1–2 weeks before high-dose chemotherapy.

Chemical stimulation of proliferation in the oral cavity has also been used as a strategy for protection against radiation-induced mucositis. Painting the oral mucosa with a weak silver nitrate solution prior to radiotherapy stimulates proliferation in the epithelium, by ablation of superficial tissue layers. This appears to reduce mucositis in accelerated split-course radiotherapy regimens, although reduced mucositis has not been demonstrated for conventional radiotherapy schedules. In contrast to the acutely responding hierarchical-type tissues, early chemical stimulation of proliferation in slow-turnover tissues (for instance cyclophosphamide treatment of the bladder or lung) tends to precipitate latent radiation damage and does not lead to a more rapid recovery from damage. It is possible that the clinical observation of a 'recall phenomenon' in which drugs like actinomycin-D, adriamycin and Taxol occasionally precipitate severe reactions in previously irradiated areas, may also be due to stimulated proliferation, perhaps in vascular endothelial cells.

KEY POINTS

1. The time of appearance and dose-dependence of radiation damage in a normal tissue depends upon its proliferative organization.
2. Rapid-renewal systems are organized in a hierarchical way with separate stem cells, a proliferating amplification compartment, and mature functional cells. The *latency* before expression of functional radiation damage is dose-independent and is related to the lifespan of the functional cells. The *rate of recovery* is dose-dependent and related to the number of surviving stem cells.
3. Slowly renewing cell systems have been termed 'flexible' because they have no clear separation between proliferative and functional compartments. The time of onset of functional damage is radiation dose-dependent.
4. Rapidly and slowly proliferating normal tissues are both capable of an accelerated rate of proliferation in response to radiation-induced cell depletion. The time of onset of accelerated proliferation ranges from a few days in rapid renewal systems to many months in slow-turnover tissues.

BIBLIOGRAPHY

Coggle JE (1987). Proliferation of type II pneumonocytes after X-irradiation on cell proliferation in mouse lung. *Int J Radiat Biol* **51**: 393–9.

Denekamp J, Stewart FA, Douglas BG (1976). Changes in the proliferation rate of mouse epidermis after irradiation: continuous labelling studies. *Cell Tissue Kinet* **9**: 19–29.

Dewit L, Oussoren Y, Bartelink H (1986). The effects of cis-diamminedichloroplatinum (II) and radiation on the proliferative kinetics of mouse duodenal crypt cells and on a partially synchronized crypt cell population. *Int J Radiat Oncol Biol Phys* **12**: 1977–85.

Hegazy MAH, Fowler JF (1973). Cell population kinetics and desquamation skin reactions in plucked and unplucked mouse skin. II. Irradiated skin. *Cell Tissue Kinet* **6**: 587–602.

Hornsey S (1973). The effectiveness of fast neutrons compared with low LET radiation on cell survival measured in mouse jejunum. *Radiat Res* **55**: 58–68.

Hornsey S, Myers R, Coultas PG, Rogers MA, White A (1981). Turnover of proliferative cells in the spinal cord after X-irradiation and its relation to time-dependent repair of radiation damage. *Br J Radiol* **54**: 1081–5.

Otsuka M, Meistrich ML (1991). Acceleration of late radiation damage of the kidney by unilateral nephrectomy. *Int J Radiat Oncol Biol Phys* **22**: 71–8.

Soranson J, Denekamp J (1986). Precipitation of latent renal radiation injury by unilateral nephrectomy. *Br J Cancer* **53**: 268–72.

Stewart FA (1986). Mechanisms of bladder damage and repair after treatment with radiation and cytostatic drugs. *Br J Cancer* **53**(Suppl VII): 280–91.

Turesson I, Notter G (1986). Dose-response and dose-latency relationship for human skin after various fractionation schedules. *Br J Cancer* **53**: 67–72.

Wheldon TE, Michalowski AS (1986). Alternative models for the proliferative structure of normal tissues and their response to irradiation. *Br J Cancer Suppl* **7**: 382–5.

Zeman W, Carsten A, Biondo S (1964). Cytochemistry of delayed radionecrosis of the murine spinal cord. In: *Response of the Nervous System to Ionizing Radiation* (eds Haley TJ, Snider RS), p. 105. Academic Press, New York.

Radiation response and tolerance of normal tissues

ALBERT J VAN DER KOGEL

4.1 THE CONCEPT OF NORMAL-TISSUE TOLERANCE

Whenever radiation therapy is given with curative intent there is the risk of serious damage to normal tissues. This risk increases with radiation dose, as does the probability of local tumour control. As described in Section 1.6, the achievable tumour control rate depends on the radiation tolerance of the unavoidably irradiated normal tissues.

Tolerance is a complex concept. In experimental studies in the clinic or on laboratory animals, it can be defined in relation to a particular end-point such as 50% moist desquamation of skin, 5% pneumonitis in lung, or 1% paralysis following spinal cord irradiation. In clinical practice, it is necessary to consider not only the measurable or life-threatening effects but also the patient's perception of morbidity. The clinical aspects of normal-tissue morbidity, the available scoring systems, and the derivation of dose–response relationships are discussed in more detail in Chapters 10 and 11.

4.2 EARLY VERSUS LATE EFFECTS

Radiation effects on normal tissues are usually divided into two categories: *early* and *late* reactions. The difference between these is important for the clinical presentation of treatment-related morbidity (see Section 11.2). The need to distinguish between these categories was stressed by the observation that early and late reactions show different patterns of response to fractionated radiotherapy, reflected in a difference in the α/β ratio. With increasing knowledge of the cellular and molecular mechanisms of radiation effects in normal tissues, the strict separation between acute or early and late effects is disappearing although it is still used on an operational basis.

The development of early effects in rapidly renewing tissues such as skin, gastrointestinal tract and the haemopoietic system is largely determined by a hierarchical cell lineage, composed of stem cells and their differentiating offspring (see Sections 3.1 and 3.2). The time of onset of early radiation reactions correlates with the lifespan of the differentiated functional cells, and the intensity of reactions reflects the balance between the rate of stem-cell killing and the rate of regeneration of surviving clonogens. For these early effects of radiation, the identity of the target cells is usually clear, in contrast to the late effects that have a long latent period. Late effects can be expected in slowly proliferating tissues, such as lung, kidney, heart, liver and central nervous system.

Late effects are, however, not necessarily restricted to these slowly renewing cell systems. For instance, in the skin, in addition to the early epidermal reactions, several later waves of injury such as fibrosis, atrophy and telangiectasia can occur (Figure 4.1). Thus, different types of injury may develop sequentially in one organ, with different underlying mechanisms and different interactions between cells. This also complicates the definition of normal-tissue tolerance, as various end-points are associated with different tolerance doses.

The distinction between early and late effects has important clinical implications. Since early reactions are usually observed during the course of a conventionally fractionated radiotherapy schedule (1.8–2 Gy per fraction, five times a week), it is possible to adjust the dose in the event of unexpectedly severe reactions, allowing a sufficient number of stem cells to survive. These surviving stem cells will repopulate and restore the integrity of the rapidly proliferating tissues. If, however, the overall treatment time is reduced, the early reactions may not reach maximal intensity before the completion of treatment. This precludes the possibility of adjusting the dose regimen to the severity of reactions. If intensive fractionation schedules reduce the number of surviving stem cells to below the level needed for effective tissue restoration, early reactions may develop into chronic injury, also called *consequential late complications* (see Section 11.2). By contrast, lengthening the overall treatment time to diminish acute toxicity may lead to increased late toxicity if total doses are increased to compensate for a reduced tumour control probability. This fine balance between acute and late toxicity in relation to dose and fractionation parameters has been well established in various treatment sites, most notably in oral mucosa.

4.3 CELLULAR AND MOLECULAR MECHANISMS OF NORMAL-TISSUE EFFECTS: FIBROSIS

The various lesions induced in normal tissues have for many years been attributed mostly to damage and depletion of specific target cells. For instance, fibrosis was related to damaged fibroblasts, demyelination to loss of oligodendrocytes, and kidney injury to renal tubular cell depletion. This 'parenchymal cell' theory was largely based on the quantitative scoring of loss

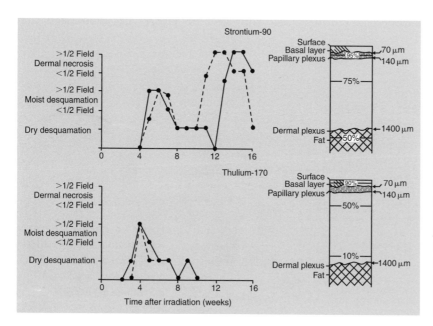

Figure 4.1 *Time-course of epithelial and dermal reactions in pig skin irradiated with single surface doses of 40 Gy ^{90}Sr or 130 Gy ^{170}Tm (solid and broken lines show results on two individual skin fields). The marked difference in radiation response is due to the greater penetration of ^{90}Sr emission into the dermis. From Hopewell (1986), with permission.*

of clonogenic cells by *in situ* assays. These assays were originally developed for acutely responding tissues (e.g. counting skin clones or regenerating intestinal crypts) but later adapted for late effects such as tubular clone formation in the kidney. The main alternative theory was that of a common vascular origin of late injury in most if not all tissues. Even this vascular mechanism was basically a target cell theory, with the slow loss of endothelial cells due to mitotic cell death as the main event leading to vascular damage, followed by secondary tissue atrophy or necrosis.

While clonogenic cell loss and lack of repopulating ability undoubtedly play major roles in the development of tissue effects, either acute or late, cascades of inflammatory and fibrogenic cytokines starting immediately after irradiation have also been identified. These events occur during the clinically silent, so-called *latent period* and they have profoundly changed the concept of late effects being irreversible and progressive events. Among the first to point out the importance of cascades of cytokines starting immediately after irradiation and ultimately leading to progressive fibrosis were Rubin and colleagues (1995). They showed that irradiation of the lung with doses in the clinical range caused an early and sustained induction of inflammatory cytokines: for example IL-1α, which is one of the triggers of radiation pneumonitis, and the various isoforms of TGF-β, including TGF-β1, which is an important fibrogenic cytokine.

In the new paradigm of normal-tissue injury, a central theme is the interaction between various cell populations mediated by cytokines and growth factors, in contrast to the target cell mechanisms which focused on the loss of a specific cell type. The cell types and pathways leading to late tissue injury show large differences between various tissues, but some common mechanisms are evolving. Radiation-induced endothelial injury is, in many organs, manifest as thrombus formation and increased vessel permeability leading to interstitial oedema. These changes may either be induced directly or by the induction of inflammatory cytokines in other cells such as macrophages or specific parenchymal cells. The mechanisms and cellular interactions are complex and are slowly being unravelled, but an important consequence of the paradigm shift is that late effects are no longer by definition regarded as progressive and irreversible but are potentially amenable to therapeutic intervention.

An example of the paradigm change is *radiation-induced fibrosis*, which is observed in many organs and generally has been regarded as an irreversible scar, characterized by fibroblast proliferation and massive production of extracellular matrix. In the last decade, the molecular biology of fibrosis has been widely studied and it is now well established that the transforming growth factor family (TGF-β1 to β3) are the most critical mediators of fibrosis. After irradiation, TGF-β is produced by a variety of cell types (e.g. macrophages and type-II pneumocytes in the lung) and this stimulates proliferation of fibroblasts, terminal differentiation and enhanced collagen synthesis. Possible interactions in the lung are illustrated in Figure 4.2 (Rodemann and

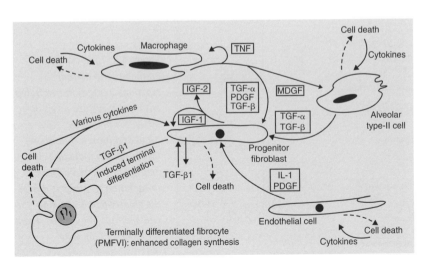

Figure 4.2 *Possible cellular interactions and events after irradiation of lung tissue. Modified from Rodemann and Bamberg (1995), with permission.*

Bamberg, 1995). The role of TGF-β in radiation fibrosis of the skin has been studied in great detail by Martin *et al.* (2000). They and others showed that the early phase of fibrosis is analogous to the wound healing process, whereby smooth-muscle-like fibroblasts (myofibroblasts) develop from fibroblasts triggered by TGF-β1. Myofibroblasts in turn are key regulatory cells in the fibrotic process, producing an abundance of inflammatory and fibrogenic growth factors, as well as the extracellular matrix proteins. In healing wounds the myofibroblasts eventually disappear by apoptosis but in radiation fibrosis these cells remain continuously activated with prolonged synthesis of various cytokines, including TGF-β and tissue-inhibitors of matrix proteinases (TIMP). In this analogy, fibrosis can be regarded as 'a wound that does not heal' (Martin *et al.*, 2000). In fibrotic lesions of human skin, sustained TGF-β expression has been observed in various cell types including myofibroblasts, endothelial cells and keratinocytes, in early as well as in late lesions. Two types of fibrotic lesions have been distinguished in irradiated human skin biopsies: early active inflammatory tissue showing many myofibroblasts actively secreting TGF-β, and late, non-inflammatory, poorly cellularized fibrotic tissue. Importantly even 'old' fibrotic lesions have shown TGF-β expression at a low level and extracellular matrix remodelling.

The recognition of long-term sustained activity of cytokine networks, of which TGF-β is a key factor but which also includes PDGF, IGF-1 and TNF-α is clinically important in that it suggests directions for therapeutic intervention. The principle of blocking TGF-β1 leading to reduced fibrosis has been demonstrated, but in view of the diverse actions of TGF-β1, it seems more advantageous to interfere with downstream events, such as the SMAD-signalling pathway or the induction of connective-tissue growth factor (CTGF). An interesting class of agents are the superoxide dismutases (SOD) which are natural scavengers of reactive oxygen species induced by radiation and various other cytotoxic agents. Over-expression of a human transgene of the mitochondrial MnSOD, as an antioxidant, in mouse lungs before and during irradiation has been shown in mice to reduce radiation pneumonitis and possibly fibrosis. Of particular interest is the recent observation that a cytosolic SOD (CuZnSOD) acts as a direct antagonist of TGF-β1 and the deposition of extracellular matrix components (Martin *et al.*, 2000).

4.4 RADIATION EFFECTS IN SPECIFIC TISSUES AND ORGANS

In this section the response and tolerance of some clinically important dose-limiting normal tissues are summarized. As a guideline to tolerance doses used in the clinic, Table 4.1 provides approximate dose levels, incidence estimates, and corresponding α/β values. The data in this table should be used with caution as they are influenced by many variables such as irradiated volume, energy of the radiation and dosimetry. The documentation and measurement of normal-tissue damage are dealt with in Chapters 10 and 11.

Skin

In the early days of radiotherapy, when orthovoltage x-rays were in common use, skin was often a dose-limiting structure as the full dose was deposited near the surface of the body. Erythema develops in the second to third week of a fractionated course of radiotherapy, followed by dry and moist desquamation due to the depletion of the basal stem-cell population; when severe, moist desquamation may lead to ulceration. With modern megavoltage equipment, the maximum dose deposition is at 0.5–4 cm below the surface and epidermal reactions are usually limited to dry desquamation and increased pigmentation. This moderate skin response is seen after conventional irradiation at a total dose of 60–66 Gy (about 40–50 Gy in the basal layer of the epidermis). Such a dose is tolerated by the skin because a substantial part of the recovery takes place by stem-cell proliferation during the 6–8 weeks of the course of radiotherapy. For skin, as well as for the oral or gastrointestinal mucosa, the total tolerated dose is less dependent on dose per fraction than is the case with most late-responding critical organs (see Section 12.6). By contrast, variation in overall treatment time can have a large but less predictable influence on the tolerance of early-responding tissues. As an approximation, skin tolerance doses decrease by about 3–4 Gy per week when treatment duration is shortened from the standard 6–8 weeks.

With high-energy x-rays, a higher dose is deposited below the surface and late damage may therefore occur in the dermis and in the absence of early reactions. These late changes are characterized by atrophy leading to contraction of the irradiated area and the clinical appearance of induration or 'radiation

Table 4.1 *Normal-tissue tolerance doses and α/β values*

Tissue	End-point	Risk (%)	Dose* (Gy)	α/β ratio (Gy)
Skin	Desquamation	50	55–60	10–12
	Fibrosis	5	60–65	2–3
	Telangiectasia	50	55–60	3–4
Oral mucosa	Confluent mucositis	50	65–70	~10
Small intestine	Late fibrosis, fistulae	5	50	3–4
Colon, rectum	Late fibrosis, fistulae	5	60	3–4
Brain, spinal cord	Necrosis	<1	50	2
		5	60	
Nerve plexus	Demyelination, fibrosis	5	65	3–4
Lung	Pneumonitis	5	20**	2–4
Heart	Pericarditis	<5	35–40	2–3
	Pericarditis	50	50–60	
	Cardiomyopathy	15–20	30–36	
	Ischaemic heart disease	<5	30	
Kidney	Glomerulosclerosis	<5	20**	2–3
Liver	Hepatitis, VOD	5	25–30**	3
Bladder	Cystitis, ulcers	<5	60–65	5–10

*Delivered as 2 Gy per fraction.
**Whole organ irradiated, partial volume tolerance usually much higher; VOD, veno-occlusive disease.
The tolerance doses and associated risks should be considered as approximations, and only for conventional daily fractionation with fraction doses of 2 Gy of high-energy photons. Irradiated volumes are generally large, and tolerance doses may increase with volume reduction, but the volume effect is widely different for different organs (see Chapter 5).

fibrosis'. Such atrophic lesions have a different aetiology from the fibrotic scars that develop after healing of a necrotic ulcer, which represent consequential late injury. However, in reality it is difficult to draw a strict distinction between the different lesions involved in the phenotype of 'late fibrosis'.

The development of telangiectasia beyond 1 year (see Figure 11.3) shows the progression of vascular injury in the late phases of radiation injury to the dermis. Telangiectasia is most clearly seen in the skin, but is also commonly observed in other irradiated tissues such as bladder and rectum; it is the result of endothelial cell loss with vessel dilation and increased blood flow in remaining vessels, combined with atrophy of the overlying dermis. The loss of smooth muscle cells surrounding larger capillaries and veins may also contribute to the development of telangiectasia.

Oral mucosa

The intensity of early mucous membrane reactions is a major factor limiting the daily and weekly dose accumulation with skin-sparing megavoltage equipment.

Early studies by GH Fletcher, using a total dose of 55 Gy in 6–6.5 weeks to the oropharynx resulted in mucosal reactions ranging from marked erythema to patchy mucositis. When the overall treatment time was reduced by 1 week for the same total dose, a few patients developed confluent mucositis but the majority experienced spotted mucositis lasting about 4 weeks. With a further reduction in overall treatment time to about 4 weeks, all patients developed confluent mucositis starting in the third week of treatment and lasting 3–6 weeks before recovery set in. One of the most commonly used radiation schedules in the curative management of head and neck cancers is administered as five fractions per week, 2 Gy per fraction, up to 68–70 Gy over 7 weeks. This regimen induces spotted-confluent mucositis in a large number of patients and clearly represents the maximal tolerable dose. Using accelerated schedules with more than 5 fractions per week, this total dose can be maintained for treatment times of at least 5 weeks but, as illustrated in Figure 4.3, further shortening needs to be accompanied by a reduction in total dose (Kaanders *et al.*, 1999).

It is now well established that the tolerance of the oral mucosa is mostly influenced by the *rate of dose*

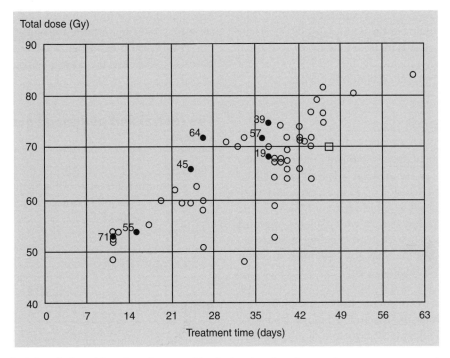

Figure 4.3 *Schedules of altered fractionation tested in the head and neck area. Open square represents conventional treatment in daily fractions of 2 Gy. Open circles represent schedules with acceptable mucosal morbidity. Closed circles represent schedules that were abandoned or modified because of excessive early mucosal toxicity. Numbers refer to references in source publication. From Kaanders* et al. *(1999), with permission.*

delivery, which for total doses >60 Gy should not exceed 12 Gy week^{-1}. The onset of regenerative proliferation in the oral mucosa occurs as early as about 1 week after the start of treatment. At a rate of dose delivery of 8–10 Gy week^{-1}, proliferation may compensate for up to 1.5–2 Gy d^{-1} (Denham *et al.*, 1996). This would suggest no dose limit for acute tolerance for standard treatment times of 6–7 weeks, but obviously late vascular and stromal tolerance will then become the limiting factor.

Salivary glands

Salivary glands are very sensitive to radiation damage and already after the first week of therapy (accumulated dose of 10–15 Gy) saliva production is significantly reduced. This effect is attributed to apoptosis of serous cells with loss of whole acini in 1–2 days. After total doses in excess of 40 Gy to both parotid glands, saliva production practically stops after about 4 weeks and does not recover after doses over 60 Gy. Volume effects are very pronounced, and sparing of partial volumes usually leads to recovery of function (see Section 5.5). These functional effects in patients have been confirmed histopathologically in rhesus monkeys, showing an almost complete loss of glandular tissue after doses in excess of 50 Gy (Price *et al.*, 1995).

The permanence of xerostomia, as the main clinical end-point of salivary dysfunction, depends not only on reduced serous fluid production, which occurs primarily in the parotid glands, but also on the mucin produced by the mucous glands. In this respect, the function of the submandibular glands may have been underestimated (Eisbruch *et al.*, 2001). The submandibular glands produce most of the mucinous components of the saliva; by their water-binding capacity they keep the mucous membranes hydrated and also provide a barrier function. Pilocarpine, which was shown to enhance saliva flow with a reduction of symptomatic xerostomia, may also stimulate mucin production, thereby further contributing to improvement in salivary gland function. Pilocarpine has also been reported to have a protective effect when given before and during irradiation. Other protective measures include the use of amifostine (WR-2721), but partial shielding of the parotid glands, especially also the minor glands in the oral cavity, by conformal techniques may provide the best means to prevent permanent xerostomia after curative doses.

Gastrointestinal tract

In the treatment of most abdominal cancers, substantial parts of the gastrointestinal (GI) tract are included in the radiation field and doses in excess of 40 Gy are often accompanied by some degree of toxicity. Acute mucositis frequently occurs, with clinical symptoms such as diarrhoea or gastritis, depending on the treatment field. When the total dose is limited to about 50–54 Gy in 2 Gy fractions, early reactions are usually not dose-limiting, and if they do occur a few days' interruption of treatment is usually sufficient to overcome acute problems. The underlying mechanism of acute mucosal injury is the depletion of mucosal precursor cells (e.g. the intestinal crypt cells) and lack of replacement of the functional villus cells. This is usually followed by rapid proliferation and regeneration. The early onset of regenerative proliferation during radiotherapy has been demonstrated in rectal biopsies taken at 2 and 6 weeks after the start of radiotherapy for prostate or bladder cancer. During the course of treatment, clinical signs of proctitis become worse but histologically a marked improvement of the rectal structures has been shown at 6 weeks (Hovdenak et al., 2000).

The loss of mucosal epithelium and its precursors leads to breakdown of the mucosal barrier and inflammation which, depending on dose, will either subside rapidly or give rise to a progressive cycle of cytokine responses with induction of necrosis, vascular sclerosis and fibrosis (Hauer-Jensen et al., 1998). An important cell type involved in these processes is the mast cell, which produces a number of inflammatory and fibrogenic cytokines. A key factor among these is TGF-β1, which plays a crucial role in the development of late fibrosis in the intestinal tract (Section 4.3). Blocking the action of TGF-β by the use of soluble receptors has shown a preserving effect on the mucosal surface as well as a reduction in collagen accumulation in the irradiated small intestine of rats.

It has long been hypothesized that pancreatic enzymes may exacerbate intestinal injury after barrier breakdown, and this has recently been confirmed experimentally by inhibition of pancreatic enzyme secretions by somatostatin analogues. Interestingly, this treatment also significantly reduced late intestinal fibrosis, underlining the consequential nature of this late effect.

The central and peripheral nervous system

The nervous system is less sensitive to radiation injury than some other late-responding tissues such as the lung or kidney. However, damage to this organ results in severe consequences such as paralysis: although tolerance doses are often quoted at the 5% complication level (TD$_5$), they generally are chosen to include a wide margin of safety.

Brain

The most important injury syndromes in the central nervous system develop a few months to several years after therapy. The often-used separation into early or late delayed injury is not very useful, as different types of lesions with overlapping time-distributions occur. Some reactions occurring within the first 6 months comprise transient demyelination ('somnolence syndrome') or the much more severe leukoencephalopathy. The more typical radiation necrosis may also occur by 6 months, but even after as long as 2–3 years. Histopathologically, changes that occur within the first year are mostly restricted to the white matter. For times beyond 6–12 months the grey matter usually also shows changes along with more pronounced vascular lesions (telangiectasia and focal haemorrhages). Radionecrosis of the brain with latent times between 1 and 2 years usually shows a mixture of histological characteristics. A schematic outline of the development of various delayed lesions in the CNS as studied in animals is given in Figure 4.4 (van der Kogel, 1991).

Spinal cord

Radiation-induced changes in the spinal cord are similar to those in the brain in terms of latent period, histology and tolerance dose. Among the relatively early syndromes, Lhermitte's sign is a frequently occurring, usually reversible, type of demyelinating injury, which develops several months after completion of

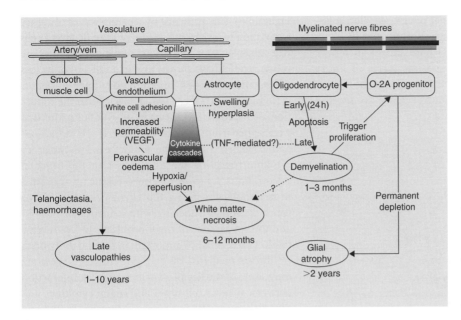

Figure 4.4 *Schematic outline of tissue components and cell types and their potential role in the pathophysiology of radiation-induced lesions in the central nervous system.*

treatment and lasts for a few months to more than a year. It may occur at doses as low as 35 Gy in 2 Gy fractions, well below tolerance for permanent radiation myelopathy when long segments of cord are irradiated, and does not predict for later development of permanent myelopathy.

As in the brain, the later types of myelopathy include two main syndromes. The first, occurring from about 6 to 18 months, is mostly limited to demyelination and necrosis of the white matter, whereas the second (with a latency of 1–4 years) is mostly a vasculopathy. The tolerance dose of the spinal cord largely depends on the size of the dose per fraction: variations in overall treatment time up to 10–12 weeks have a negligible effect in conventional schedules using one fraction per day. For longer times or intervals, substantial recovery occurs, which has important implications for retreatment (see Chapter 21).

Peripheral nerves

Radiation effects in peripheral nerves, mainly plexuses and nerve roots, are probably more common than effects in the spinal cord but are less well documented. Peripheral nerves are often quoted as being more resistant to radiation than the cord or the brain, but this view is not well supported by clinical data. As is the case for all nervous tissues, a dose of 60 Gy in 2 Gy fractions is associated with a less than 5% probability of injury, but this rises steeply with increasing radiation dose.

The brachial plexus is often included in treatments of the axillary and supraclavicular nodes in breast cancer patients. Clinically, plexopathy is characterized by mixed sensory and motor deficits, developing after a latent period ranging from 6 months to several years. The pathogenesis involves progressive vascular degeneration, fibrosis and demyelination with loss of nerve fibres.

Lung

The lung is an intermediate-to-late responding tissue, in which at least two separate radiation-induced syndromes are recognized: acute pneumonitis at 2–6 months after treatment and fibrosis, which develops slowly over a period of several months to years. The lung is among the most sensitive of late-responding organs, but because of the structural organization of the functional units, it becomes dose-limiting only when large volumes of the chest are irradiated, and when the remaining lung is not capable of providing a minimal supportive function. Thus, except in patients with severe emphysema, lung tolerance is usually only dose-limiting when both lungs are irradiated. Clinical signs or symptoms of acute radiation pneumonitis are a reduced pulmonary compliance, progressive dyspnoea, decreased gas exchange and dry cough. When there is insufficient functional reserve, cardiorespiratory failure may occur within a short time-span.

Travis and Down (1981) have shown in mouse lung the existence of two separate waves of injury and demonstrated that late fibrosis can be distinguished from early pneumonitis (Figure 4.5; see also Figure 3.6). The presence of separate waves of injury were initially attributed to loss of specific target cells (e.g. alveolar type-II cells or fibroblasts) but more recent studies have shown that in addition to the loss of specific cell types, inflammatory and fibrogenic cytokines are produced which give rise to the induction of a progressive cascade of events. In the first weeks after irradiation of the lung, IL-1α is induced and considered to be the major pro-inflammatory cytokine triggering the first phases in the onset of pneumonitis. A pro-fibrogenic cytokine up-regulated in macrophages during the latent period is TGF-α which is strongly associated with induction of TGF-β1 and the appearance of myofibroblasts. In a paracrine fashion these cells are important in driving the process of fibrosis mediated by TGF-β1. However, these are only some of the key players in a complex interaction between various cell types and many cytokines and growth factors (Rodemann and Bamberg, 1995). A schematic representation of these interactions is given in Figure 4.2. It is of potential clinical importance that a better knowledge of these inflammatory and fibrogenic pathways may lead to the development of measures to treat radiation injuries (Section 4.3).

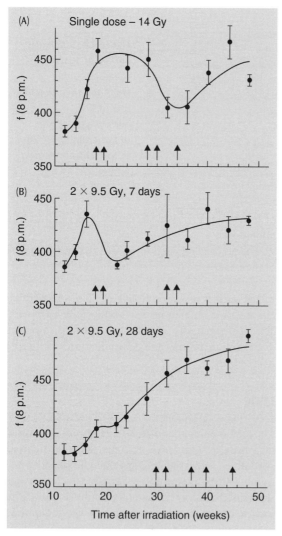

Figure 4.5 *Evidence for two phases of radiation response in the mouse lung. Using breathing rate as a measure of damage, two waves of response are seen after single doses (panel A). (B, C) Split-dose irradiation, especially with a gap of 28 days, reduced the severity of the first phase (acute pneumonitis), but had little effect on the second phase (fibrosis). Arrows indicate the death of individual mice. From Travis and Down (1981), with permission.*

Kidney

The kidney, together with the lung, is among the most sensitive late-responding critical organs. Radiation damage develops very slowly and may take years to be recognized. Radiation nephropathy usually manifests as proteinuria, hypertension and impairment in urine concentration. Anaemia is usually present, and has been attributed both to haemolysis and to a decreased production of erythropoietin. A mild form of nephritis, presenting only as a sustained proteinuria, may be observed over a period of many years. Parts of one or both kidneys can receive much higher doses without affecting excretory function. However, after partial kidney irradiation, hypertension may develop after a latent period of up to or beyond 10 years.

As observed for other typical late-responding tissues, the fractionation sensitivity of the kidney is high (i.e. the α/β ratio is low). However, in contrast to many other organs and tissues, the dose tolerated by the kidney does not increase with increasing treatment time but even declines due to a continuous progression of damage, after doses well below the threshold for induction of functional deficit (see Section 21.7).

The pathogenesis of radiation nephropathy is complex, but most current studies suggest glomerular endothelial injury as the start of a cascade leading to glomerular sclerosis and later tubulointerstitial fibrosis. Immunohistochemical studies of the pig kidney irradiated with a single dose of 10 Gy showed an early (2 weeks) activation of mesangial cells, the kidney equivalent of myofibroblasts in other tissues, but no enhanced expression of TGF-β1 (Cohen *et al.*, 2000). At 4 weeks, fibrin deposition occurred in the glomeruli, while only at 6 weeks was TGF-β1 expression seen in tubular epithelium but not in glomeruli. These and other studies showed the importance of the renin–angiotensin system in the induction of glomerular sclerosis via up-regulation of plasminogen activator inhibitor 1 (PAI-1) and enhanced fibrin deposition. Through loss of tubular epithelial cells, fibrin may then leak into the interstitium causing the onset of tubulointerstitial fibrosis.

ACE-inhibitors or angiotensin II antagonists have been shown to significantly ameliorate radiation nephropathy, possibly via a reduction in expression of PAI-1. Of importance is the observation that the maximum effectiveness of ACE inhibitors was seen when administered at 3–10 weeks after irradiation, apparently a critical period in the post-irradiation cascade of cellular events. This underlines the potential for therapeutic intervention after irradiation, when late tissue injury is already in an early stage of development.

Heart

The tolerance of the heart is intermediate between that of kidney/lung and the CNS. The most common type of radiation-induced heart injury is pericarditis with a variable degree of pericardial effusion. This complication has a relatively early onset (∼50% occurrence within the first 6 months, remainder within 2 years). It is asymptomatic and clears spontaneously in the majority of patients.

Radiation-induced cardiomyopathy is another form of complication that presents either as reduced ventricular ejection or conduction blocks and develops slowly over a period of 10–20 years. A significantly reduced cardiac function occurred in about 15–20% of patients treated for Hodgkin's disease after receiving a dose of 30–36 Gy to most of the heart (Schultz-Hector, 1991), and current estimates of doses giving a 50% complication probability are approximately 52 Gy in 2 Gy fractions. With long-term follow-up of patients treated for Hodgkin's disease or breast cancer, the enhanced risk of ischaemic heart disease after periods in excess of 10 years has increasingly been reported. The large variation in risk estimates reported in different studies suggests that volume effects are important, but also that sensitive substructures are present. In this respect, the heart auricles and the proximal parts of the coronary arteries have been suggested to be particularly sensitive to radiation damage.

Histopathologically, late damage to the myocardium is characterized predominantly by diffuse interstitial and perivascular fibrosis, and loss of cardiomyocytes. The development of fibrosis has been shown experimentally to start in the auricles as early as 1 month after irradiation, with a significantly decreased atrial volume at 4 months, whereas fibrosis of the left ventricles was only seen at 9 months and later. TGF-β1 and IL-1α were up-regulated within days following irradiation, slowly fading thereafter. Of particular importance for early detection of radiation-induced cardiac damage are enhanced plasma levels of atrial natriuretic peptide (Wondergem *et al.*, 2001).

Liver

The liver ranks in radiosensitivity immediately below kidney and lung for whole-organ irradiation. Because all these organs have their functional units organized in parallel structures, the tolerance to partial-organ irradiation can be much higher than that of the whole organ, depending on the functional reserve (see Section 5.5). Thus, liver tolerance is only dose-limiting when the whole organ is irradiated. An example is total-body irradiation preceding bone marrow transplantation. In this situation the lung is well known as a dose-limiting organ, but liver and kidney are also at risk, especially after regimens equivalent to single doses of 10 Gy or higher.

Two phases of radiation hepatopathy are recognized, with acute radiation hepatitis being the more dominant. The acute phase develops approximately 2–6 weeks after irradiation, with signs of liver enlargement and ascites. Liver function tests during this period are abnormal, especially alkaline phosphatase. Acute hepatitis usually presents as veno-occlusive disease, characterized by central vein thrombosis whereby occlusion of the centrilobular veins causes atrophy and loss of the surrounding hepatocytes. Chronic hepatopathy has a variable latency ranging from 6 months to more than 1 year post-irradiation, and shows progressive fibrotic changes in both centrilobular and periportal areas. These alterations are accompanied by blood-flow redistribution through recanalization or newly formed veins, and regenerative proliferation of hepatocytes and bile ducts.

Bladder

In contrast to most other epithelia, the mucosal lining of bladder and ureters shows very slow cell turnover (see Table 3.1). Consistent with this, radiation-induced urothelial cell loss takes a long time to develop, unless precipitated by other injury such as infection or drug-related toxicity. In clinical studies, three phases of damage have been described. An acute phase occurs 4–6 weeks after the start of fractionated irradiation and is characterized by hyperaemia and mucosal oedema. Infection may complicate this early damage which may then progress to desquamation and ulceration. A chronic phase develops from about 6 months to 2 years and presents as vascular ischaemia accompanied by progressive mucosal breakdown, ranging from superficial denudation to ulceration and even the formation of fistulae. Fibrosis of the bladder wall with a reduced urine capacity may occur up to 10 years after irradiation.

Experimentally in mice, two waves of acute injury have been observed, the first at 1–15 days after single doses of irradiation, the second at 16–30 days. Mechanistically, the first phase may be related to interference with the prostaglandin pathway, as suggested by the beneficial effect of aspirin when administered during this phase. The second acute phase is associated with changes in urothelial structural components and in its barrier function without any epithelial cell loss. These early changes correlate with the late onset of epithelial denudation, ulceration and development of fibrosis (a consequential late effect) starting at about 5–6 months. It is therefore of particular interest that restoration of barrier function by external glycosaminoglycans has been shown greatly to reduce acute effects, also late fibrosis, when heparin was instilled into the bladder during the second acute phase (Dörr et al., 2000).

KEY POINTS

1. Tolerance doses for *generic* late effects are generally more sensitive to changes in dose per fraction (low α/β ratio) when compared with early effects.
2. *Consequential* late effects are more directly correlated with acute effects, and show radiobiological characteristics similar to acute effects.
3. The latent period before late effects become apparent is not biologically silent, but a period during which cellular interactions and cytokine cascades lead to progressive tissue changes such as fibrosis.
4. Pharmacological interventions during the latent period may be effective in modifying the tolerance for late effects.

BIBLIOGRAPHY

Cohen EP, Bonsib SA, Whitehouse E, Hopewell JW, Robbins MEC (2000). Mediators and mechanisms of radiation nephropathy. *Proc Soc Exp Biol Med* **223**: 218–225.

Denham JW, Walker QJ, Lamb DS et al. (1996). Mucosal regeneration during radiotherapy. *Radiother Oncol* **41**: 10–18.

Dörr W, Krumsdorf D, Noack R (2000). Amelioration of late radiation effects in mouse urinary bladder by modulation of acute symptoms – experimental evidence for consequential late effects. *Radiother Oncol* **57**(Suppl 1): S37–8.

Eisbruch A, Kim HM, Terrell JE, Marsh LH, Dawson LA, Ship JA (2001). Xerostomia and its predictors following parotid-sparing irradiation of head-and-neck cancer. *Int J Radiat Oncol Biol Phys* **50**: 695–704.

Hauer-Jensen M, Richter KK, Wang J, Abe E, Sung C-C, Hardin JW (1998). Changes in transforming growth factor $\beta 1$ (TGF-$\beta 1$) gene expression and immunoreactivity levels during development of chronic radiation enteropathy. *Radiat Res* **150**: 673–80.

Hopewell JW (1986). Mechanisms of the action of radiation on skin and underlying tissues. *Br J Radiol Suppl* **19**: 39–51.

Hovdenak N, Fajardo LF, Hauer-Jensen M (2000). Acute radiation proctitis: a sequential clinicopathologic study during pelvic radiotherapy. *Int J Radiat Oncol Biol Phys* **48**: 1111–17.

Kaanders JHAM, van der Kogel AJ, Ang KK (1999). Altered fractionation: limited by mucosal reactions? *Radiother Oncol* **50**: 247–60.

Martin M, Lefaix J-L, Delanian S (2000). TGF-β1 and radiation fibrosis: a master switch and a specific therapeutic target? *Int J Radial Oncol Biol Phys* **47**: 277–90.

Price RE, Ang KK, Stephens LC, Peters LJ (1995). Effects of continuous hyperfractionated accelerated and conventionally fractionated radiotherapy on the parotid and submandibular salivary glands of rhesus monkeys. *Radiother Oncol* **34**: 39–46.

Rodemann HP, Bamberg M (1995). Cellular basis of radiation-induced fibrosis. *Radiother Oncol* **35**: 83–90.

Rubin P, Johnston CJ, Williams JP, McDonald S, Finkelstein JN (1995). A perpetual cascade of cytokines postirradiation leads to pulmonary fibrosis. *Int J Radial Oncol Biol Phys* **33**: 99–109.

Schultz-Hector S (1991). Heart. In: *Radiopathology of Organs and Tissues* (eds Scherer E, Streffer C, Trott KR), pp. 347–68. Springer-Verlag, Berlin.

Travis EL, Down JD (1981). Repair in mouse lung after split doses of X rays. *Radiat Res* **87**: 166–74.

van der Kogel AJ (1991). Central nervous system radiation injury in small animal models. In: *Radiation Injury to the Nervous System* (eds Gutin PH, Leibel SA, Sheline GE), pp. 91–112. Raven Press, New York.

Wondergem J, Strootman EG, Frölich M, Leer JWH, Noordijk EM (2001). Circulating atrial natriuretic peptide plasma levels as a marker for cardiac damage after radiotherapy. *Radiother Oncol* **58**: 295–301.

5

Volume effects in normal tissues

FIONA A STEWART AND ALBERT J VAN DER KOGEL

5.1 THE CONCEPT OF TOLERANCE IN RELATION TO TISSUE STRUCTURE

When considering the influence of irradiated volume on normal-tissue tolerance, it is important to discriminate between structural tissue tolerance and functional tolerance. Structural tissue tolerance depends on cellular radiation sensitivity and the ability of clonogenic cells within a defined volume to maintain the mature cell population above a critical level. Functional tolerance depends on whether the organ as a whole can continue to function, and this is determined by tissue organization as well as cellular sensitivity.

The volume of tissue irradiated can be an important determinant of clinical tolerance without having any influence on tissue sensitivity per unit volume. One example of this is skin or mucosal ulceration. If this occurs over a large area, the ulcer will lead to pain and lack of function and will heal only slowly. A small area of ulceration, by contrast, may lead only to discomfort and will heal more quickly. In this situation, the *clinical tolerance* is strongly dependent on irradiated volume although *tissue tolerance* is not. There is very little evidence for any increase in cellular radiosensitivity when the irradiated volume is increased, either in skin or in other tissues.

Clinical tolerance also depends strongly on the volume irradiated in kidney and lung; both of these organs are very sensitive to irradiation of their entire volume but small volumes can be treated to much higher doses. This is because there is considerable functional reserve capacity and only about 30% of the organ is required to maintain adequate function under normal physiological conditions. The large reserve capacity and increased tolerance to partial-volume irradiation are due to the *parallel organization* of functional nephrons and alveolar subunits. Inactivation of a small number of functional subunits (FSU) does not lead to loss of organ function. Functional damage will not occur until a critical number of FSU are inactivated by irradiation. This implies that there should also be a threshold volume of irradiation below which no functional damage will develop, even after high-dose irradiation. Above this threshold, damage is usually exhibited as a graded response, i.e. increasing severity of functional impairment with increasing dose rather than a binary, all-or-nothing response (see Section 11.2). The magnitude of the response depends on the number of FSU that are destroyed by irradiation. The risk of developing a complication depends on the dose distribution to the whole organ, rather than on the presence of small 'hot spots'.

In an attempt to categorize volume effects in tissues based on their structural organization, the *parallel organization* of organs such as kidney and lung can be contrasted with the more *serial organization* of intestine and spinal cord (Withers *et al.*, 1988). In serially organized structures, the inactivation of one subunit may cause loss of function in the whole organ. Radiation damage to such tissues is expected to show a binary response, with a threshold dose below which there is normal function and above which there is loss of function, e.g. radiation-induced myelopathy or small bowel obstruction. In this case, the probability of inactivation of any particular subunit, by a given radiation dose, will increase with increasing length of tissue irradiated. There should not be a threshold volume for the development of the end-point and the risk of complication is strongly influenced even by small hotspots of dose inhomogeneity. In reality, no organs are organized simply as a chain of functional units, and purely serially organized tissues do not exist. In addition, the simple classification of serial and parallel organization does not take into account the influence of cellular migration and regeneration from outside the irradiated area (Section 5.2). However, the modelling of volume effects on the basis of their serial or parallel organization is useful and explains the apparent paradox that radiosensitive organs, like kidney and lung, can sustain the loss of more than half their total mass without loss of function, whereas relatively radioresistant tissues such as spinal cord may be functionally inactivated by the irradiation of a small volume.

Many organs such as the brain are better described by an *intermediate type* of organizational structure which is neither serial nor parallel. Specific areas of the brain perform specific functions. The tolerance of brain tissue is therefore much more dependent on which area of brain is irradiated than the total volume irradiated. Damage to even a small area may lead to permanent loss of the particular function controlled by that area, since the undamaged parts of the brain are not able to take over these functions, but other brain functions may be unaffected.

5.2   INFLUENCE OF CELLULAR MIGRATION FROM OUTSIDE THE IRRADIATED AREA

An important factor in the influence of field size on radiation damage in small tissue volumes is the inward migration of surviving clonogenic cells. Tissues with a high cellular migratory capacity exhibit a steep increase in tolerance as the irradiated field size decreases over small distances (<2 cm) since repopulation from the surrounding, unirradiated area occurs. Above a critical field size, however, migratory repopulation is inadequate. This type of volume effect is seen in skin and in some tissues with a relatively linear or tubular structural organization, e.g. spinal cord and intestinal epithelium. Repopulation from neighbouring subunits is much less likely in tissues with a parallel type of structural organization, and this phenomenon has not been demonstrated in kidney or lung.

Irradiation experiments in pig skin have demonstrated a sharp decrease in the radiation dose required to induce moist desquamation (acute damage) or dermal thinning (late damage) with increasing field sizes up to 22.5 mm or 10 mm, respectively (Figure 5.1A).

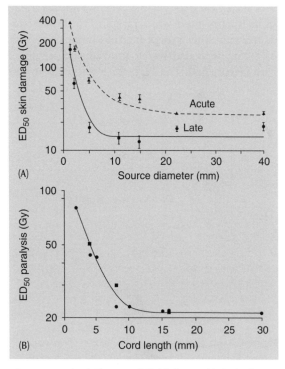

Figure 5.1 *The influence of field-size on biological response in pig skin (A) and rat spinal cord (B) after single-dose irradiation with small fields. In each case there is a steep rise in ED$_{50}$ as field-size is reduced below 10 mm, with very little change in ED$_{50}$ for larger field-sizes. From Hopewell and Trott (2000), with permission.*

For larger field sizes, there was no further increase in damage. This illustrates the fact that cellular migration from outside very small, heavily irradiated areas can protect the skin from breaking down, but that cellular migration has little effect over distances larger than about 10–12 mm. For these larger field sizes, healing after low radiation doses occurs by regeneration of surviving cells scattered randomly within the treatment volume. The extent of healing is then dependent on radiation dose, i.e. on the number of surviving cells, but not on volume.

Similar volume effects at small field sizes are seen in the rat spinal cord, with a steep rise in the ED_{50} (i.e. the radiation dose required to produce white-matter necrosis and myelopathy in 50% of treated animals) as the irradiated cord length is reduced below 10 mm (Figure 5.1B). For irradiation of cord lengths greater than 10 mm, there is little change in the ED_{50}, which again suggests that cellular migration over limited distances is responsible for the increased tolerance at very small field sizes. Further evidence for this comes from experiments in which rat spinal cords were irradiated with either a single field of 8 mm or two fields of 4 mm, separated by an unirradiated length of cord (Figure 5.2). The ED_{50} for myelopathy in rats

irradiated with 2×4 mm fields was >45 Gy, which is the same as for a single field of 4 mm, and considerably greater than the ED_{50} for a single field of 8 mm length ($ED_{50} < 26$ Gy). At these very small volumes of irradiated cord it is the *maximum field length* that determines response, rather than the total volume irradiated.

The colorectum and ureter are other examples of tissues with a tubular structure where rodent studies show a marked sparing of damage for small irradiated volumes, with a threshold length of about 10–15 mm. Repopulation by epithelial cells migrating over short distances is the likely mechanism of tissue sparing in each of these cases.

5.3 EXPERIMENTAL DATA ON VOLUME EFFECTS FOR LARGER FIELD SIZES IN ANIMAL SYSTEMS

Spinal cord

The marked volume effects described above for irradiation of very short lengths of irradiated spinal cord are less pronounced for cord lengths >2 cm, as demonstrated in pigs, monkeys and dogs.

Single radiation doses given to 2.5, 5 and 10 cm lengths of pig spinal cord showed only a small (~ 1 Gy) decrease in the ED_{50} dose for induction of white-matter necrosis with increasing field size. At low probabilities of injury, which are clinically relevant, this difference was no longer significant (van den Aardweg *et al.*, 1995). The irradiated cord length also influenced the incidence of myelopathy in monkeys given fractionated irradiation with 2.2 Gy per fraction (Schultheiss *et al.*, 1994). The incidence of myelopathy after a total dose of 70.2 Gy increased from 15% to 20% to 37.5% for field sizes of 4, 8 and 16 cm, respectively.

In an extensive study in dogs, irradiation of 4 and 20 cm lengths of spinal cord were compared using a fractionated schedule of 4 Gy per fraction (Powers *et al.*, 1998). Complete dose–response curves showed a large shift in the ED_{50} for neurological signs of injury (i.e. functional damage) from 54 Gy for the small field to 78 Gy for the large field. There was a much smaller shift in ED_{50} values for the occurrence of severe pathological lesions (Figure 5.3). This difference in volume effects for clinical morbidity compared

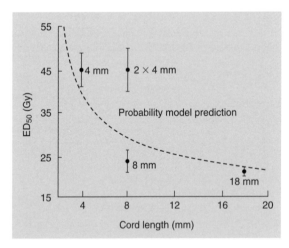

Figure 5.2 *For cord lengths below 10 mm, field-size rather than total volume determines the response of rat cervical spinal cord. The single fields (4, 8, 18 mm) were centred around C5, the two concomitant 4 mm fields were at C1/2 and C7/T1, separated by ~10 mm. Data show the ED_{50} for induction of white-matter necrosis. Statistical models predict a continuously rising curve as shown. Unpublished results, AJ van der Kogel.*

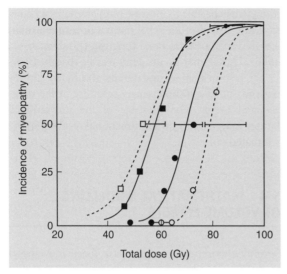

Figure 5.3 *Influence of change in field-size on spinal cord damage in dogs. Increasing the field-size from 4 cm (circles) to 20 cm (squares) had a more marked influence on the development of neurological signs of injury (dotted lines) than on the occurrence of severe pathological lesions (solid lines). Redrawn from Powers* et al. *(1998), with permission.*

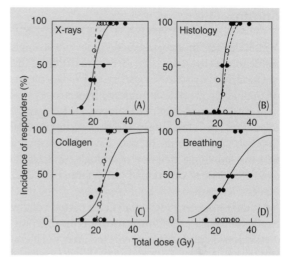

Figure 5.4 *Dose–response curves for radiation-induced lung damage in pigs after irradiation with five fractions, given to half of the right lung (○) or to the whole right lung (●). Damage was assessed from radiographic changes (A), histological evidence of fibrosis (B), elevated hydroxyproline (collagen) levels (C), or increased breathing rate (D). Only the functional end-point demonstrated a volume effect. From Herrmann* et al. *(1997), with permission.*

with histological tissue damage again emphasizes the importance of this distinction when studying volume effects.

In summary, there is a clear volume effect for severe lesions in the spinal cord which lead to irreversible signs of myelopathy; this is most pronounced at high levels of injury. At low probabilities of injury (<5%), which usually define clinical tolerance doses, a volume effect may not be detectable and should have minimal impact on the clinical practice of maintaining spinal cord dose below 45–50 Gy. However, when clinical conditions warrant the choice of higher dose levels, such as in a re-irradiation situation, the existence of a volume effect should be taken into consideration.

Lung

The influence of irradiated lung volume on structural and functional damage has been investigated in mice, rats, dogs and pigs. All studies demonstrate a pronounced volume effect for total lung function, with little or no symptomatic pneumonitis for partial irradiated volumes below 50%. These volume effects depend on the compensatory capacity of the unirradiated tissue, which enables function to be maintained despite destruction of a substantial part of one lung. By contrast, local structural lung damage, assessed by radiography, histology or collagen content, is independent of the volume irradiated (Figure 5.4). This indicates that cellular radiosensitivity is not influenced by the size of the irradiated volume, although the consequence of cell death for lung function *is* strongly dependent on volume.

A few studies have investigated regional differences in radiation sensitivity of the lung. Experiments in mice demonstrate that functional damage is more prevalent after irradiation of the base of the lung than after equivalent volume irradiation of the apex (Liao et al., 1995). This may indicate that functional subunits are not homogeneously distributed but are concentrated in basal areas. Cytokine release from partial liver irradiation, included in the basal lung field, may also contribute to these out-of-field effects. Studies in pigs have not demonstrated differences in cellular damage in apical versus basal parts of the lung.

Kidney

Volume effects in the irradiated kidney are strongly influenced by the paired, parallel organization of this organ and its large reserve capacity. Unirradiated parts of the kidney are able to undergo hypertrophy and increase their performance to compensate for damage to another part of the organ and thus maintain renal function. Experiments in pigs have demonstrated that the individual function of a single, unilaterally irradiated kidney can actually be poorer than after bilateral irradiation with equivalent doses. Total renal function is, however, much greater after partial-volume irradiation (Figure 5.5). Interestingly, if the unirradiated kidney is subsequently removed after unilateral irradiation, a previously non-functional irradiated

kidney may be able to increase both glomerular filtration rate and effective renal plasma flow to maintain a viable level of total renal function (Robbins *et al.*, 1986). These experiments demonstrate that the functional response of a unilaterally irradiated kidney depends on the compensatory response in the unirradiated organ. The presence of the unirradiated kidney may actually inhibit functional recovery in the irradiated kidney.

5.4 MATHEMATICAL MODELLING OF VOLUME EFFECTS

Several theoretical models have been developed to estimate normal-tissue complication probability (NTCP) for partial-volume irradiations and inhomogeneous dose distributions (see Section 10.9). Models using power-law functions were the earliest and were followed by models with a more biophysical basis. In the model of Lyman (1985), a power-law relationship was assumed between the tolerance dose for uniform whole- or partial-organ irradiation, where the parameter n (the exponent of the partial volume) describes the volume dependence of the tolerance dose. When $n \rightarrow 1.0$, the volume effect is large and when $n \rightarrow 0$, the volume effect is small. The Lyman model has been extended to inhomogeneous irradiation by converting the original dose-volume histogram (DVH) into an equivalent DVH for uniform irradiation, usually by the effective-volume method (Kutcher and Burman, 1989). The resulting so-called LKB model is currently one of the most commonly used models for predicting normal-tissue complication probability (NTCP).

Intermediate between the purely empirical and more biophysical models is the 'relative seriality' model of Källman *et al.* (1992). In this model, an extra parameter s is introduced as the 'degree of seriality' to describe the functional organization of a tissue. A near-zero value of s represents a parallel structure and an s value close to unity represents an organ with a serial organization. The first model that assumed that an organ is divided into physiologically discrete compartments, or functional subunits (FSU), was the 'integral response model' (Wolbarst *et al.*, 1982; Withers *et al.*, 1988). This model allows for FSU to have a non-uniform spatial distribution. A functional subunit is defined as the largest unit of cells capable

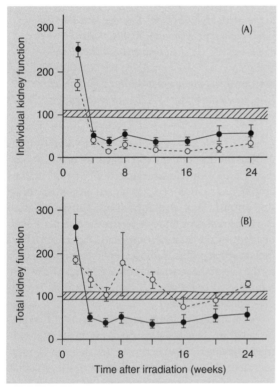

Figure 5.5 *Time-related changes in glomerular filtration rate in pigs in which one (○) or both (●) kidneys were irradiated with a single dose of 12.6 Gy. Panel A shows the change in individual kidney function, as a percentage of control values, and panel B shows the total renal function in the same pigs. Redrawn from Robbins and Hopewell (1988).*

of being regenerated from a single surviving clonogenic cell. The radiation response of each independent FSU is determined by Poisson statistics and the spatial organization of FSU determines the organ's response to partial volume irradiation.

For organs with a serial organization, every FSU is vital to the function of the organ, and irreparable damage to any one critical element will lead to a complication. Models based on serial organization predict a weak volume dependence for NTCP if the irradiated volume is larger than a few FSU and the dose–response function is steep. For organs with FSU arranged in parallel (such as acini in the lung), the integral response of the organ as a whole will depend on the fraction of FSU damaged and the functional reserve of the organ. Models based on a parallel organization predict a large volume effect, and a high dose to a small volume will fail to induce the complication. For tissues such as skin and mucosa, it was assumed that there is a mixture of structurally and functionally defined FSU. These types of tissue show a graded response to irradiation, depending on the local density of inactivated FSU.

Clinical application of dose–volume models

Rapid developments in high-precision delivery of radiation, most recently intensity-modulated radiotherapy (IMRT) and tomotherapy, have stimulated clinical trials on dose escalation, notably in lung and prostate. Data are now available for tolerance to partial-organ irradiation at doses well above the levels that were previously established. The new data obtained from prospective dose-escalation studies, combined with precise knowledge of dose distributions and dose–volume histograms, should allow the derivation of more realistic parameters and a validation of mathematical models used for describing volume effects. However, there are many limitations and uncertainties in current multi-parameter models and it seems unlikely that the biological models will quickly replace the relatively simple empirical models such as the LKB probability model.

With the rapid implementation of conformal 3D-RT, dose–volume histograms (DVH) have proved useful as a tool for the evaluation and comparison of treatment plans. However, the loss of spatial information on dose-distribution in a DVH is a serious constraint in determining the relationship between local tissue damage and overall morbidity. A high-dose region in the histogram may represent a single hotspot in the volume of interest or a number of smaller hotspots from contiguous regions or from different regions. These could have quite different implications for tissue tolerance. Dose–volume histograms also do not differentiate between functionally or anatomically different subregions or compartments within an organ, and none of the models takes account of out-of-field effects. The available models should therefore be regarded as an aid to the evaluation and comparison of clinical data using different treatment set-ups, rather than giving accurate predictions of clinical outcome.

5.5 CLINICAL DATA ON VOLUME EFFECTS AND NORMAL-TISSUE COMPLICATION PROBABILITY

Lung

Several prospective clinical studies have now described the influence of a change in irradiated lung volume on local lung damage and on NTCP. Local structural and functional lung damage can be quantified using CT-based lung-density distributions and SPECT (single-photon emission computed tomography) ventilation and perfusion distributions. By matching pre- and post-treatment SPECT scans to the 3D dose distributions in the lung, changes in perfusion and ventilation can be quantified in relation to the locally delivered radiation dose (Figure 5.6). For patients with malignant lymphoma and breast cancer, well-defined dose–response relationships were determined for local changes in lung function per SPECT voxel ($6\,mm^3$ volumes) in the irradiated areas relative to the low-dose or unirradiated regions (Figure 5.7). These and other published studies demonstrate that the magnitude of local pulmonary changes is independent of the irradiated volume but does depend on patient-related factors such as concurrent chemotherapy, smoking. Regional differences in lung radiosensitivity have not been identified in any clinical studies published to date (Theuws *et al.*, 1998a).

In an extension of these studies, the observed incidence of radiation-induced pneumonitis was related to the DVH for the irradiated lung (Kwa *et al.*, 1998). The complex 3D physical dose distribution was converted to a mean biological dose to the whole lung,

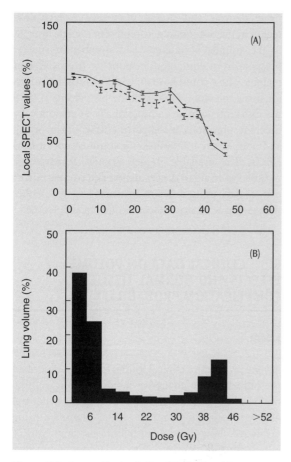

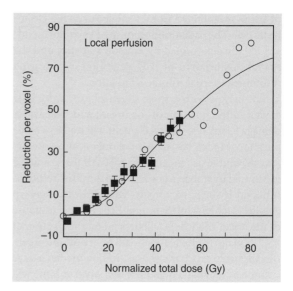

Figure 5.7 *Dose–effect relationships for the average change in local lung function (i.e. perfusion) as a function of the normalized total dose. Data are shown from functional studies carried out at Duke University (○) and The Netherlands Cancer Institute (■). From Theuws* et al. *(1998b) and including data from Marks* et al. *(1997), with permission.*

Figure 5.6 *Dose–effect relationship for local lung perfusion (solid line) and ventilation (dashed line) at 3–4 months after irradiation, as a percentage of pre-treatment value, in a patient treated for malignant lymphoma (A). The corresponding DVH of the 3D dose distribution to the lung of this patient is shown in panel B. From Boersma* et al. *(1994), with permission.*

after a normalization procedure using the linear quadratic model and α/β ratios of 2.5–3 Gy. This parameter, the 'mean normalized total lung dose', which does not use any critical-volume parameter, correlated with the incidence of pneumonitis in a large series of 540 patients treated for malignant lymphoma, lung or breast cancer in five different institutes (Figure 5.8). Other studies have shown that simple parameters such as the percentage of total lung volume irradiated to >20 Gy or >30 Gy (i.e. incorporating a critical volume parameter) can be used to predict the probability of radiation pneumonitis (Marks *et al.*, 1997;

Graham *et al.*, 1999). Further studies on patients treated with a range of different dose distributions will be required to determine which approach is best for estimation of the NTCP for pneumonitis from DVH.

Intestinal tract

Over the past 5 years the results of several large prospective trials have been published comparing conformal therapy with conventional treatments for prostate cancer. Such studies allow an evaluation of the influence of reduced-volume irradiation on intestinal damage. For example, a study from the Royal Marsden Hospital in London showed that the volume of small bowel irradiated to >90% of the prescribed dose could be reduced from 24% using conventional fields, to 18% for 3D conformal therapy and 5–8% for IMRT, depending on the number of fields used. For the rectum, the high-dose irradiated volumes could be reduced from 89% to 51% and 6–16%, respectively (Nutting *et al.*, 2000).

Several studies have now investigated the relationship between late rectal complications and DVH

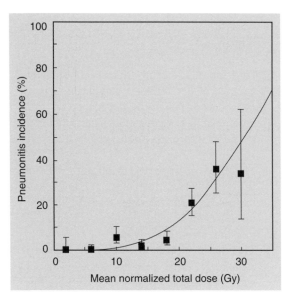

Figure 5.8 *Incidence of radiation pneumonitis as a function of mean normalized total dose to the whole lung. Pooled data are shown from a group of 264 patients with lung cancer, breast cancer or malignant lymphoma, treated in five different centres. From Kwa* et al. *(1998).*

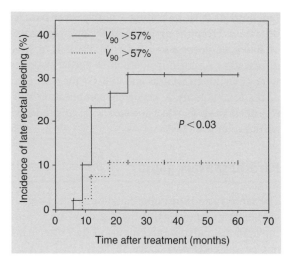

Figure 5.9 *Actuarial incidence of rectal bleeding in patients with rectal volumes irradiated to at least 90% of the isodose (~60 Gy) of greater than 57% or less than 57%. From Wachter* et al. *(2001).*

parameters for prostate cancer patients, in a similar way to the lung studies described above. The incidence of late rectal bleeding has generally been found to correlate with irradiated volume exposed to high doses, although significant volume effects have not been identified for less severe late rectal damage or for acute bowel toxicity. Some studies have demonstrated a significant dose–volume relationship for late rectal bleeding using a single cut-off value for the rectal volume irradiated to high dose (Figure 5.9). Other studies describe a more complex relationship with several cut-off levels which significantly discriminated between a high or low risk of severe rectal bleeding, or a continuous relationship between rectal bleeding and dose-volume parameters (Jackson *et al.*, 2001). Volume effects for small-bowel obstruction have been demonstrated in patients treated with extended field radiotherapy (bowel volumes $>500\,\mathrm{cm}^3$) combined with abdominal surgery. In these patients, the incidence of bowel obstruction may rise above 30%, compared with 10% or less for smaller-field irradiation. For patients treated with radiotherapy alone, no volume effect has been demonstrated for bowel

obstruction, although some studies do show a significant volume effect for diarrhoea if the total dose exceeds 45 Gy (Letschert *et al.*, 1994). In this study the actuarial incidence of diarrhoea at 5 years varied from 31% to 42% in patients treated with small bowel volumes $<77\,\mathrm{cm}^3$ and $>328\,\mathrm{cm}^3$, respectively.

Liver

The liver is usually regarded as a prime example of a parallel-type organ, with liver acini as functional subunits. Whole-liver irradiation with doses around 30 Gy (2 Gy/fraction) is generally associated with the induction of 5–10% hepatitis. Until the introduction of 3D treatment planning, clinical data on the relation between tolerance dose and partial volume irradiation were very conservatively estimated (Emami *et al.*, 1991). So far, the most extensive clinical data on liver tolerance to partial organ irradiation has been accumulated by Lawrence and colleagues at the University of Michigan for close to 200 patients (summarized by Dawson *et al.*, 2001). Step-wise dose-escalation studies in combination with 3D dose planning and dose prescription based on DVH has shown that the liver truly behaves as a parallel-type organ with a large reserve capacity. The data obtained were fitted with the LKB-NTCP probability model, resulting in a volume effect parameter (the *n* exponent in a power-law function) of 0.94, indicating a near-perfect parallel behaviour. From the derived NTCP values, estimates of tolerance doses associated with 5% risk of liver disease after uniform irradiation to partial volumes were 47 Gy for two-thirds and >90 Gy for one-third of the total volume. A negligible complication risk, regardless of dose, was associated with an irradiated partial volume of 25%.

Parotid salivary glands

The parotid glands are important dose-limiting organs in radiation treatments of the head and neck with conventional radiation techniques as they often cannot be spared. Doses above 40–50 Gy lead to permanent loss of function contributing to xerostomia and impairment of quality of life. One of the major advantages of the introduction of 3D-conformal techniques in the head and neck area is the possibility of limiting the irradiated volume to parts of the parotids, and this has resulted in a marked reduction of permanent xerostomia. A DVH-based prospective trial showed complete recovery of salivary flow at 1 year after mean doses to the parotid of ~26 Gy (Eisbruch *et al.*, 1999). The anatomical organization in acini as functional units was clearly reflected in the outcome of modelling the partial-volume data as derived from the DVH. The LKB model showed the volume-effect parameter n to be close to 1.0, which indicates a nearly parallel behaviour whereby the mean dose determines NTCP. In these studies partial-volume thresholds were ~45 Gy for 25%, ~30 Gy for 50% and ~15 Gy for 67% of the total volume.

KEY POINTS

1. *Structural* tissue tolerance depends on cellular radiation sensitivity and is independent of volume irradiated. *Functional* tolerance depends on tissue organization and functional reserve capacity.
2. Tissues with a parallel organization (e.g. lung) have a large reserve capacity and show a pronounced volume effect, with a threshold volume below which functional damage does not occur. The risk of developing a complication depends on dose distribution throughout the whole organ rather than the maximum dose to a small area.
3. Tissues with a serial organization (e.g. spinal cord) have little or no functional reserve and the risk of developing a complication is less dependent on volume irradiated than for tissues with a parallel organization. The risk of complication is strongly influenced by high-dose regions and hotspots.
4. Migration of surviving clonogenic cells into the edge of irradiation fields can lead to a steep increase in tissue tolerance for field diameters up to 20 mm in some tissues (e.g. spinal cord, intestine, skin).
5. Theoretical models have been developed to estimate NTCP for partial-volume irradiations and inhomogeneous dose distributions. Simple power-law and probability models have been expanded to incorporate parameters relating to tissue architecture and reserve capacity. These models need to be validated against clinical data emerging from conformal treatment schedules.

BIBLIOGRAPHY

Boersma LJ, Damen EM, de Boer RW *et al.* (1994). Dose-effect relations for local functional and structural changes of the lung after irradiation for malignant lymphoma. *Radiother Oncol* **32**: 201–9.

Boersma LJ, van den BM, Bruce AM, Shouman T, Gras L, te Velde A, Lebesque JV (1998). Estimation of the incidence of late bladder and rectum complications after high-dose (70–78 GY) conformal radiotherapy for prostate cancer, using dose–volume histograms. *Int J Radiat Oncol Biol Phys* **41**: 83–92.

Dawson LA, Ten Haken RK, Lawrence TS (2001). Partial irradiation of the liver. *Semin Radiat Oncol* **11**: 240–6.

Eisbruch A, Ten Haken RK, Kim HM, Marsh LH, Ship JA (1999). Dose, volume, and function relationships in parotid salivary glands following conformal and intensity-modulated irradiation of head and neck cancer. *Int J Radiat Oncol Biol Phys* **45**: 577–87.

Emami B, Lyman J, Brown A *et al.* (1991). Tolerance of normal tissue to therapeutic irradiation. *Int J Radiat Oncol Biol Phys* **21**: 109–22.

Graham MV, Purdy JA, Emami B *et al.* (1999). Clinical dose-volume histogram analysis for pneumonitis after

3D treatment for non-small cell lung cancer (NSCLC). *Int J Radiat Oncol Biol Phys* **45**: 323–9.

Herrmann T, Baumann M, Voigtmann L, Knorr A (1997). Effect of irradiated volume on lung damage in pigs. *Radiother Oncol* **44**: 35–40.

Hopewell JW, Trott KR (2000). Volume effects in radiobiology as applied to radiotherapy. *Radiother Oncol* **56**: 283–8.

Jackson A, Skwarchuk MW, Zelefsky MJ *et al.* (2001). Late rectal bleeding after conformal radiotherapy of prostate cancer. II. Volume effects and dose-volume histograms. *Int J Radiat Oncol Biol Phys* **49**: 685–98.

Källman P, Agren A, Brahme A (1992). Tumour and normal tissue responses to fractionated non-uniform dose delivery. *Int J Radiat Biol* **62**: 249–62.

Kutcher GJ, Burman C (1989). Calculation of complication probability factors for non-uniform normal tissue irradiation: the effective volume method. *Int J Radiat Oncol Biol Phys* **16**: 1623–30.

Kwa SL, Theuws JC, Wagenaar A *et al.* (1998). Evaluation of two dose-volume histogram reduction models for the prediction of radiation pneumonitis. *Radiother Oncol* **48**: 61–9.

Letschert JG, Lebesque JV, Aleman BM *et al.* (1994). The volume effect in radiation-related late small bowel complications: results of a clinical study of the EORTC Radiotherapy Cooperative Group in patients treated for rectal carcinoma. *Radiother Oncol* **32**: 116–23.

Liao ZX, Travis EL, Tucker SL (1995). Damage and morbidity from pneumonitis after irradiation of partial volumes of mouse lung. *Int J Radiat Oncol Biol Phys* **32**: 1359–70.

Lyman JT (1985). Complication probability as assessed from dose–volume histograms. *Radiat Res Suppl* **8**: S13–19.

Marks LB, Munley MT, Spencer DP *et al.* (1997). Quantification of radiation-induced regional lung injury with perfusion imaging. *Int J Radiat Oncol Biol Phys* **38**: 399–409.

Nutting CM, Convery DJ, Cosgrove VP *et al.* (2000). Reduction of small and large bowel irradiation using an optimized intensity-modulated pelvic radiotherapy technique in patients with prostate cancer. *Int J Radiat Oncol Biol Phys* **48**: 649–56.

Powers BE, Thames HD, Gillette SM, Smith C, Beck ER, Gillette EL (1998). Volume effects in the irradiated canine spinal cord: do they exist when the probability of injury is low? *Radiother Oncol* **46**: 297–306.

Robbins ME, Hopewell JW (1988). Effects of single doses of X-rays on renal function in the pig after the irradiation of both kidneys. *Radiother Oncol* **11**: 253–62.

Robbins ME, Hopewell JW, Golding SJ (1986). Functional recovery in the irradiated kidney following removal of the contralateral unirradiated kidney. *Radiother Oncol* **6**: 309–16.

Schultheiss TE, Stephens LC, Ang KK, Price RE, Peters LJ (1994). Volume effects in rhesus monkey spinal cord. *Int J Radiat Oncol Biol Phys* **29**: 67–72.

Theuws JC, Kwa SL, Wagenaar AC *et al.* (1998a). Dose-effect relations for early local pulmonary injury after irradiation for malignant lymphoma and breast cancer. *Radiother Oncol* **48**: 33–43.

Theuws JC, Kwa SL, Wagenaar AC *et al.* (1998b). Prediction of overall pulmonary function loss in relation to the 3-D dose distribution for patients with breast cancer and malignant lymphoma. *Radiother Oncol* **49**: 233–43.

van den Aardweg GJ, Hopewell JW, Whitehouse EM (1995). The radiation response of the cervical spinal cord of the pig: effects of changing the irradiated volume. *Int J Radiat Oncol Biol Phys* **31**: 51–5.

Wachter S, Gerstner N, Goldner G, Potzi R, Wambersie A, Potter R (2001). Rectal sequelae after conformal radiotherapy of prostate cancer: dose–volume histograms as predictive factors. *Radiother Oncol* **59**: 65–70.

Withers HR, Taylor JM, Maciejewski B (1988). Treatment volume and tissue tolerance. *Int J Radiat Oncol Biol Phys* **14**: 751–9.

Wolbarst AB, Chin LM, Svensson GK (1982). Optimization of radiation therapy: integral-response of a model biological system. *Int J Radiat Oncol Biol Phys* **8**: 1761–9.

FURTHER READING

Ten Haken RK (2001). Partial organ irradiation. *Semin Radiat Oncol* **11**(4).

Cell survival as a determinant of tumour response

G GORDON STEEL

6.1   CONCEPT OF CLONOGENIC CELLS

As indicated in Section 3.1, the maintenance of tissue size and therefore of tissue function in the normal renewal tissues of the body depends upon the existence of a small number of primitive 'stem cells' – cells that have the capacity to maintain their numbers whilst at the same time producing cells that can differentiate and proliferate to replace the rest of the functional cell population. Stem cells are at the base of the hierarchy of cells that make up the epithelial and haemopoietic tissues.

Carcinomas are derived from such hierarchical tissues, and our ability to recognize this in histological sections derives from the fact that these tumours often maintain many of the features of differentiation of the tissue within which they arose. Well-differentiated tumours do this to a greater extent than anaplastic tumours. It follows that not all the cells in a tumour are neoplastic stem cells: some have embarked on an irreversible process of differentiation. In addition, carcinomas contain many cells that make up the

stroma (fibroblasts, endothelial cells, macrophages, etc.). Stem cells thus may comprise only a small proportion of the cells within a tumour.

When a tumour regrows after non-curative treatment, it does so because some neoplastic stem cells were not killed. Radiobiologists have therefore recognized that the key to understanding tumour response is to ask: how many stem cells are left? (If we can eradicate the last neoplastic stem cell then the tumour cannot regrow.) It is almost impossible to recognize tumour stem cells *in situ*, and therefore assays have been developed that allow them to be detected after removal from the tumour. These assays generally detect stem cells by their ability to form a colony within some growth environment. We therefore call these 'clonogenic' or 'colony-forming' cells – cells that form colonies exceeding about 50 cells within a defined growth environment. The number 50 represents 5–6 generations of proliferation. It is chosen in order to exclude cells that have a limited growth potential as a result of having embarked on differentiation, or having been sublethally damaged by therapeutic treatment.

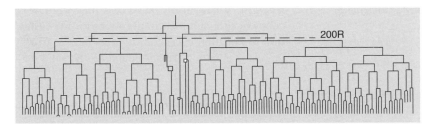

Figure 6.1 *Pedigree of a clone of mouse L-cells irradiated with a dose of 200 R (i.e. roentgens) at the four-cell stage, illustrating the concept of surviving and non-surviving clonogenic cells. From Trott (1972), with permission.*

After exposure to radiation, damaged cells do not die immediately and they may produce a modest family of descendants. This is illustrated in Figure 6.1. The growth of single mouse L-cells was observed under the microscope and one selected colony was irradiated with 200 roentgens (R) of x-rays at the four-cell stage (Trott, 1972). The roentgen is an old radiation unit, roughly equivalent to 1 cGy. Subsequent growth was carefully recorded and in the figure each vertical line indicates the lifetime of a cell from birth at mitosis to its subsequent division. The two irradiated cells on the left and the right of this figure produced continuously expanding colonies, although some daughter cells had long intermitotic times. The other two irradiated cells fared badly: they underwent a number of irregular divisions, including a tripolar mitosis. But note that at the end of the experiment cells are present from each of the original four cells: the difference is that two produced expanding colonies and the other two did not. The first two were 'surviving clonogenic cells' and the other two are usually described as 'killed' by radiation, since their regrowth is probably unimportant for clinical outcome. It would be more precise to say that two of the cells *lost their proliferative ability* as a result of irradiation. Some cells fail to undergo even one division after irradiation. Interphase cell death occurs in many cell types at very high radiation doses, and at conventional therapeutic dose levels it is characteristic of lymphoid cells, parotid acinar cells and some cells in the intestinal crypts. Although interphase cell death and apoptosis are related concepts (see Sections 8.6 and 9.8) they are not synonymous for the same process. But the conventional radiobiological view is that it is loss of reproductive integrity that is the critical response to irradiation (either in tumour or normal-tissue cells): this occurs within a few hours of irradiation through damage to the genome, and the subsequent metabolic and death processes are 'downstream' of this event.

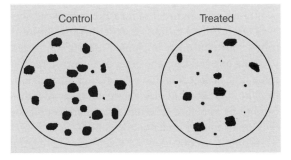

Figure 6.2 *Illustrating the principle of measuring a surviving fraction.*

6.2 CLONOGENIC ASSAYS

Clonogenic assays have formed the basis of cellular response studies in tumours, and also in some normal tissues. The basic idea is to remove cells from the tumour, place them in a defined growth environment and test for their ability to produce a sizeable colony of descendants. Many types of assay have been described; we illustrate the principle by a simple assay in tissue culture that is analogous to a microbiological assay.

A single-cell suspension of tumour cells is prepared and divided into two parts. One is irradiated, the other kept as an unirradiated control. The two suspensions are then plated out in tissue culture under identical conditions, except that since we anticipate that radiation has killed some cells we will have to plate a larger number of the irradiated cells. We here envisage plating 100 control cells and 400 irradiated cells. After a suitable period of incubation, the colonies are scored (Figure 6.2). There are 20 control colonies, and we therefore say that the plating efficiency was 20/100 = 0.2. The plating efficiency of the treated cells is lower: 8/400 = 0.02. We calculate a surviving fraction as the ratio of these plating efficiencies:

$$\text{Surviving fraction} = \frac{\text{PE}_{\text{treated}}}{\text{PE}_{\text{control}}} = \frac{0.02}{0.2} = 0.1$$

thus correcting for the efficiency with which undamaged clonogenic cells are detected and for the different numbers of cells plated. Surviving fraction is often given as a percentage (10% in this case).

The above description started with a suspension of tumour cells. In order to measure *in vivo* cell survival we take two groups of experimental tumours (often subcutaneously implanted tumours in mice), irradiate one and keep the other as a control, then at some time after irradiation we make cell suspensions from both groups and plate them out under identical conditions as before. The difference here is that the cells are irradiated under *in vivo* conditions.

Although colony assays have formed a central place in tumour radiobiology, they are not without artefacts. Bearing in mind that the numbers of cells plated will often differ between control and treated cultures, a key question is whether colony counts increase linearly with the number of cells plated. If they do not, then this will lead to errors in cell survival. The colonies in Figure 6.2 have been drawn to illustrate a feature of colony assays that was mentioned in the previous section. Irradiation not only reduces the colony numbers; it also increases the number of small colonies. Some of these small colonies may represent clones that eventually die out; others may arise from cells that have suffered non-lethal injury that reduces colony growth rate. Unless they reach the usual cut-off of 50 cells they will not be counted, although their implications for the evaluation of radiation effects on tumours may be worthy of greater attention (Seymour and Mothersill, 1989).

6.3 CELL SURVIVAL CURVES

A cell survival curve is a plot of surviving fraction against dose (of radiation, cytotoxic drug or other cell-killing agent). Figure 6.3A shows that when plotted on linear scales the survival curve for cells irradiated in tissue culture is often sigmoid: there is a shoulder followed by a curve that asymptotically approaches zero survival. To indicate the sensitivity of the cells to radiation we could just read off the dose that kills, say, 90% of the cells. This is sometimes called the ED_{90} (i.e. effect dose 90%). In doing this we need make no assumptions about the shape of the curve.

There are two reasons why survival curves are always plotted on a logarithmic scale of survival:

1. If cell killing is random, then survival will be an exponential function of dose, and this will be a straight line on a semi-log plot.
2. A logarithmic scale more easily allows us to see and compare effects at very low survivals.

Such a plot is illustrated in Figure 6.3B. The shapes of radiation survival curves and ways of describing their steepness are dealt with in Chapter 7.

Note that for the data shown in Figure 6.3, radiation doses above 5 Gy reduce the survival of clonogenic cells to below 10%. Measurement of radiosensitivity

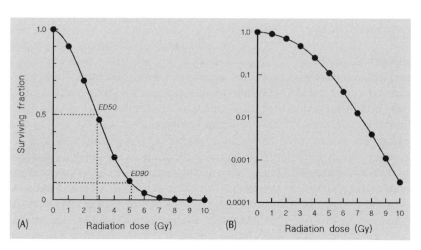

Figure 6.3 *A typical cell survival curve for cells irradiated in tissue culture, plotted (A) on a linear survival scale. (B) Shows the same data plotted on a logarithmic scale.*

in terms of the parameter D_0 (see Section 7.3) is made on the exponential part of the survival curve, which in this case is above 5 Gy. These measurements are therefore made in a dose range where the surviving fraction is very low. Such D_0 values are relevant to the problem of exterminating the last few clonogenic cells, but if the cell population contains cells of differing radiosensitivity these values may not be typical of the radiosensitivity of the bulk of the tumour cell population.

6.4 ASSAYS FOR THE SURVIVAL OF CLONOGENIC CELLS

Many techniques have been described for detecting colony formation by tumour cells and thus for measuring cell survival. They almost all require first the production of single-cell suspensions. This is not a simple matter, for tumour tissues differ widely in the ease with which they can be disaggregated. Enzymes such as trypsin, collagenase and pronase are often used, and some tissues can be disaggregated mechanically.

Such techniques can also be used for the assay of colony-forming cells in normal tissues, especially the haemopoietic tissues that can easily be sampled and made into cell suspensions. In addition, a variety of *in situ* assays for normal-tissue stem cells have been described (Potten, 1983). The following are some of the principal assays that have been used for tumour cells.

In vitro colony assays

Some tumour cells grow well attached to plastic tissue culture dishes. Others can be encouraged to do so by first laying down a feeder layer of lethally irradiated connective-tissue or tumour cells. For cells that have been established as an *in vitro* cell line, this often works well, but for studies on tumour samples taken directly from patients or animals it is commonly observed that normal-tissue fibroblasts grow better than the tumour cells and overgrow the cultures.

An alternative is to thicken the growth medium with agar or methylcellulose. This inhibits the growth of anchorage-requiring cell types, but many epithelial cells will still grow. A widely used assay of this type is that of Courtenay and Mills (1978) for human tumour cells. Agar cultures are grown in 15 ml plastic tubes overlaid with liquid medium that can regularly be replenished. The addition of rat red blood cells to the agar was found to promote the growth of a number of human tumour cell types. An important feature of the Courtenay–Mills assay was the use of a low oxygen tension (a gas phase of 90% nitrogen, 5% oxygen and 5% carbon dioxide), which enhanced the plating efficiency of human tumour cells.

Spleen colony assay

Till and McCulloch (1961) showed that when mouse bone marrow cells were injected intravenously into syngeneic recipients that had received sufficient whole-body irradiation to suppress endogenous haemopoiesis, colonies were produced in the spleen that derived from the stem cells in the graft. The colonies varied in morphology (erythroid, granulocyte or mixed) and these stem cells are therefore termed *pluripotent*. Their precise identity was not known and they are therefore often called colony-forming units (CFU). Using this assay, Till and McCulloch obtained the first survival curve for bone marrow cells and found it to be very steep. The spleen colony assay has also been used for some types of mouse lymphoma cells.

The lung colony assay

This is analogous to the spleen colony assay and is applicable to any transplanted mouse tumour that readily forms colonies in the lung following intravenous injection of a single-cell suspension. The cloning efficiency can often be increased by mixing the test cells with an excess ($\sim 10^6$ per injection) of lethally irradiated tumour cells or plastic microspheres, which perhaps act by increasing the trapping of injected tumour cells in the lung. Not all the tumour cells grow: a few colonies per thousand tumour cells injected would be regarded as satisfactory. Although colonies are formed throughout the lung, they are usually scored only on the lung surface. The method was used by Hill and Stanley (1975) on two experimental tumours and they give further experimental details.

Limiting-dilution assay

This is a non-cloning assay that was used in early radiation cell survival studies and which for some experimental tumours has the advantage of high sensitivity. The principle of the method is to prepare a suspension of tumour cells and to make a large number of subcutaneous implants into syngeneic animals, covering a range of inoculum sizes and, if possible, spanning the level of 50% tumour takes. The animals, usually mice, are then observed for a long enough period to record nearly every tumour that can grow from a single-cell implant. Take rate is plotted against inoculum size and the point of 50% takes is interpolated; this is usually called the 'TD$_{50}$' cell number. The experiment is performed simultaneously on treated cells and control cells and the surviving fraction is given by the ratio of the TD$_{50}$ values. The addition of an excess of lethally irradiated cells improves the take rate; using this manoeuvre, Steel and Adams (1975) found a TD$_{50}$ of one to three cells for the Lewis lung tumour and were thus able to measure survival down to 10^{-6}. The method only works well in the absence of an immune response against the tumour grafts, a relatively uncommon situation especially with chemically and virally induced tumours.

Short-term *in vitro* assays

The need to develop *in vitro* assays that yield a quicker result than a true clonogenic assay arises from the current interest in prediction of tumour response to treatment (see Chapter 22). A variety of assays has been proposed but their reliability has often been in doubt. Three common pitfalls are:

1. Biopsy samples of human tumours contain both tumour cells and normal connective-tissue cells; both may grow under the assay conditions and it may be difficult to distinguish colony formation by tumour cells.
2. If the method requires the production of single-cell suspensions, great care must be taken to exclude cell clumps, for these may preferentially give rise to scorable colonies.
3. Radiation-killed cells take time to die and in a short-term assay they may be confused with surviving tumour cells; if this is not done, the method may not distinguish between radiosensitive cells and cells that die rapidly after irradiation.

Many aspects of the prediction of tumour response are dealt with in the book edited by Chapman *et al.* (1989). Non-clonogenic assays for tumour cells have

been reviewed by Mitchell (1988) and they include the following.

The micronucleus test

Tumour cells are cultured in the presence of cytochalasin-B, which blocks cytokinesis, creates binucleate cells, and thus allows nuclei that have undergone one post-treatment division to be identified. Micronuclei can be scored as small extranuclear bodies. Their frequency is linearly related to radiation dose and gives a measure of radiation sensitivity (Streffer *et al.*, 1986). The reliability of the method is limited by the fact that diploid, polyploid and aneuploid cells may differ in their tolerance of genetic loss and therefore of micronucleus formation.

The adhesive tumour cell culture system

Human tumour biopsy specimens are disaggregated into a single-cell suspension and plated out in 24-well culture plates that have been coated with a commercially patented adhesive coating (Baker *et al.*, 1986). The medium is supplemented with added growth factors. Two weeks after irradiation or drug treatment, the cultures are stained with crystal violet and the absorbance is measured using an image analyser.

Growth assays

A variety of methods has been used to measure the growth of cultures derived from treated and control tumour specimens, thus to derive a measure of radiosensitivity or chemosensitivity. Incorporation of radioisotopes such as [^{3}H]thymidine has been widely used. MTT is a tetrazolium salt that can be used to stain cell cultures and thus by a colorimetric assay to estimate the extent of growth (Carmichael *et al.*, 1987; Wasserman and Twentyman, 1988). It can be used to evaluate growth in microtitre plates and with careful attention to technical factors it can yield a measure of radiosensitivity. Such methods are vulnerable to the variable growth of fibroblasts and for studies on leukaemic cells it may be preferable to stain the cells differentially and analyse the cultures microscopically (Bosanquet, 1991).

Cell sorter or DMIPS methods

All the methods so far described involve the plating of an aliquot of a cell suspension that on average will contain a known number of cells. The *actual* number of cells will vary according to Poisson statistics. For studies of the effects of low radiation doses (where the effects are small) greater precision can be achieved by knowing *exactly* how many cells have been plated. This has been done using two main methods (see Section 7.8). A fluorescence-activated cell sorter (FACS) allows counted numbers of cells to be plated into culture dishes (Durand, 1986). An alternative is to use a 'dynamic microscopic image processing scanner' (DMIPS) (Marples and Joiner, 1993), which allows the spatial coordinates of plated cells to be recorded; subsequently, the colony formation by each individual cell can be examined. Both these methods give high precision in the initial region of a cell survival curve and their use has led to the identification of the hyper-radiosensitivity (HRS) phenomenon (see Section 7.8).

6.5   COMPARISON OF ASSAYS

Intercomparison of the results of assays of cell survival provides an important check on their validity, yet it has seldom been done. The information can be valuable both at a practical and a fundamental level. At the practical level, it is logical to check a rapid short-term assay against the results of a more laborious but more reliable clonogenic assay. The more general question is whether assay of cell survival in two different growth environments does actually identify the same population of surviving tumour cells. It is usually cell survival *in situ* in the patient or in the experimental animal that we seek to determine, and to subject tumour cells to extraction procedures and to artificial growth environments might well produce artefacts. It is therefore reassuring that some careful comparisons between clonogenic assays *in vitro*, in the mouse lung, and by subcutaneous transplantation, have demonstrated good agreement for mouse tumours (Steel and Stephens, 1993).

6.6   THE RELATIONSHIP BETWEEN CELL SURVIVAL AND GROSS TUMOUR RESPONSE

The objective of studies of clonogenic cell survival is to be able to understand, or to make predictions about,

the main features of tumour response to therapy: tumour growth delay and tumour cure.

Tumour growth delay

Inadequate treatment of a tumour leads to a temporary phase of tumour regression that is subsequently followed by tumour recurrence. This pattern is illustrated in Figure 2.6. Regression is due to the death and disappearance of cells killed by radiation, also to the loss of those differentiated cells of limited lifespan that would have been produced by the killed stem cells. The rate of tumour regression differs widely from one tumour to another, as illustrated in Figure 2.5.

The regrowth component in Figure 2.6 is due to repopulation by surviving clonogenic cells. The speed of regrowth probably varies considerably from one tumour to another, and the broken lines in the figure illustrate the possibilities of a lag period before repopulation gets fully under way, or repopulation at the speed of a small untreated tumour. Fowler (1991) expressed the view that rapid repopulation may be the norm. He has postulated that irradiation will arrest the proliferation of tumour cells and that if this is the driving force behind the loss of cells to necrosis (see Section 15.2), then this loss will temporarily be interrupted. The result will be a period of tumour cell repopulation at a rate that is close to the potential doubling time (see Section 2.7) and faster than would have been the case in the absence of treatment. Fowler describes this as the 'unmasking' of rapid tumour cell proliferation.

Growth delay is defined as the difference in time for treated and untreated tumours to reach a fixed multiple of the size at the time of treatment (see Figure 17.1A). This has been widely used as a measure of tumour response in transplanted animal tumours.

What is the relationship between growth delay and cell survival following treatment? For a particular radiation dose, Figure 17.4 shows that the colony-forming ability of tumour cells is depressed immediately after irradiation but that the tumour volume response takes time to appear. In that study, a radiation dose that reduced survival to 0.01 gave only partial remission of tumour growth. This observation is significant for the converse of this comparison: a partial remission observed clinically in response to chemotherapy may be associated with two or more logs of cell kill.

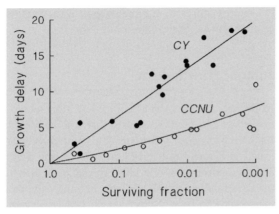

Figure 6.4 *Relationship between tumour growth delay and surviving fraction, for B16 mouse melanomas treated either with cyclophosphamide (CY) or CCNU. For a particular level of cell killing, greater growth delay was observed after CY than CCNU. From Steel and Stephens (1983), with permission.*

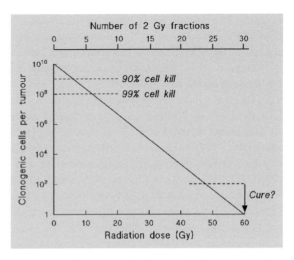

Figure 6.5 *Illustrating the idea that '99% tumour cell kill is complete failure'.*

As the dose of radiation or cytotoxic drug is increased, this leads to greater cell kill and to a longer growth delay. The results of a representative dose–response study (for chemotherapy) are shown in Figure 6.4. Transplanted B16 mouse melanomas were treated either with cyclophosphamide or the nitrosourea CCNU and both parameters were measured over a range of drug doses. Following cyclophosphamide treatment, there was an almost linear relationship between log(survival) and the time the tumours took to reach four times the treatment size. The curve for CCNU was much flatter: reducing survival to 10^{-2} gave a growth delay of roughly 4 days, as compared with around 14 days for cyclophosphamide. The explanation appeared to lie in a reduced rate of repopulation after cyclophosphamide. These results illustrate the general principle that growth delay is a function both of the level of clonogenic cell survival and of the rate of regeneration.

Local tumour control

The eradication of every clonogenic tumour cell must lead to tumour cure; this is, however, a daunting objective. Every gram of tumour may contain 10^9 cells of which perhaps 1% might be clonogenic. A human tumour at presentation could weigh some tens or hundreds of grams and the total number of clonogenic cells might therefore exceed 10^9. Cell kill by radiotherapy or chemotherapy is roughly exponential with dose. Thus, when treatment has reduced survival to 10^{-2} (which could lead to complete disappearance of all visible tumour), we would expect that four or five times this dose will be needed to reach a curative level. This is the basis of the popular saying: '99% tumour cell kill is complete failure' (Figure 6.5). A nomogram relating cell number to tumour size is given in Figure 2.1. Whether it is always necessary to eradicate the last clonogenic tumour cell in order to achieve local tumour control has been a matter of intense debate. During the 1970s there was a widespread belief that the immune responses of patients against their tumours may be strong and this gave rise to many attempts at immunotherapy. Unfortunately, it has subsequently been realized that the animal tumours used to support the optimistic claims for immunotherapy were not truly syngeneic (i.e. genetically identical) and were misleading (Alexander, 1977; Hewitt, 1979). Thus, whilst it is possible that weak tumour-directed immune responses may exist within cancer patients, sufficient perhaps to eradicate the last decade or so of surviving tumour cells, this cannot be relied upon.

6.7 REPAIR AND RECOVERY

Most of the damage induced in cells by radiation is satisfactorily repaired. Evidence for this comes from studies of strand breaks in DNA, the vast majority of

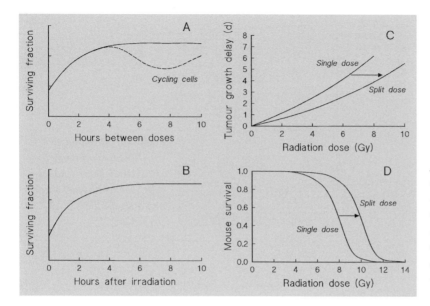

Figure 6.6 *Illustrating four ways of measuring recovery from radiation damage (see text). Panels A, C and D show three types of split-dose experiment; panel B shows the results of a 'delayed-plating experiment'. The arrows in panels C and D indicate the measurement of $(D_2 - D_1)$ values.*

which disappear during the few hours after irradiation (see Section 8.2). Further evidence for repair comes from the wide variety of recovery experiments that have been done, both on *in vitro* cell lines and on normal and tumour tissues *in vivo*. It is useful to draw a distinction between these two sources of evidence:

- *Repair*: refers to the process by which the function of macromolecules is restored. Rejoining of DNA strand breaks provides some evidence for this, although the rejoining of a break does not necessarily mean that gene function is restored. Rejoining can leave a genetic defect (i.e. a mutation) and specific tests of *repair fidelity* are needed to detect this. 'Repair' has often loosely been used for cellular or tissue recovery.
- *Recovery*: refers to an increase in cell survival or a reduction in the extent of radiation damage to a tissue when time is allowed for this to occur.

There is a number of experimental sources of evidence for recovery, including the following.

Split-dose experiments

The effect of a given dose of radiation is less if it is split into two fractions delivered a few hours apart. This effect has been termed 'recovery from sublethal damage' (SLD), or 'Elkind recovery' (Elkind and Sutton, 1960). SLD recovery can be observed using various experimental end-points: for instance using cell survival (Figure 6.6A), tumour growth delay (Figure 6.6C) or mouse lethality after irradiating a vital normal tissue (Figure 6.6D). The typical timing of split-dose recovery is shown in Figure 6.6A. Considerable recovery occurs within 15 minutes to 1 hour, and recovery often seems to be complete by roughly 4 hours. Recovery seems to be slower than this in some normal tissues such as the spinal cord (see Table 13.2). When the split-dose technique is applied to cycling cells there is usually a wave in the data caused by cell-cycle progression effects (Section 6.8).

Delayed-plating experiments

If cells are irradiated in a non-growing state and left for increasing periods of time before assaying for survival, an increase in survival is often observed (Figure 6.6B). During this delay the cells are recovering the ability to divide when called upon to do so. This has been termed 'recovery from potentially lethal damage' (PLD). The kinetics of PLD recovery and SLD recovery are similar.

Dose-rate effect

Reduction in radiation damage as dose rate is reduced to around 1 Gy h^{-1} is primarily due to cellular recovery (see Sections 18.1 and 18.2).

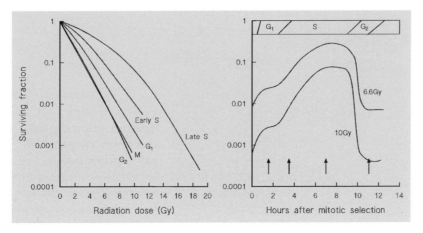

Figure 6.7 *Variation of radiosensitivity through the cell cycle of Chinese hamster cells. Adapted from Sinclair and Morton (1965), with permission.*

Fractionation

The sparing effect of fractionating radiation treatment within a relatively short overall time is primarily due to recovery. This is therefore the main reason why iso-effect curves slope upwards as the fraction number is increased (see Figures 12.1 and 12.2).

Summary

What is the relationship between these various ways of detecting recovery? The damage induced in cells by ionizing radiation is complex, as are the enzymatic processes that immediately begin to repair it. The various types of 'recovery experiment' listed above evaluate this complex repair process in different ways. For instance, the evaluation based on giving a second dose (i.e. SLD recovery) may be different from that obtained by asking irradiated non-dividing cells to divide (i.e. PLD recovery). There is only one complex entity, but a variety of ways of detecting it.

6.8 VARIATION OF CELL KILLING THROUGH THE CELL CYCLE

The radiosensitivity of cells varies considerably as they pass through the cell cycle. Although this has not been studied in a large number of cell lines, there seems to be a general tendency for cells in the S phase (in particular the latter part of the S phase) to be the most resistant and for cells in G2 and mitosis to be

the most sensitive. The reason for the resistance in S is thought to be due to homologous recombination, increased as a result of the greater availability of undamaged sister template through the S phase, per-haps also due to conformational changes in DNA facilitating repair processes. Sensitivity in G2 prob-ably results from the fact that those cells have little time to repair radiation damage before the cell is called upon to divide.

The classic results of Sinclair and Morton (1965) are illustrated in Figure 6.7. They synchronized Chinese hamster cells at five different points in the cell cycle and performed cell survival experiments. The survival curves showed that it was mainly the shoulder of the curve that changed: there was little shoulder for cells in G2 or mitosis and the shoulder was greatest for cells in S. The right-hand panel shows the profile of variation in cell killing through the cell cycle, constructed from these data.

The effect of this phenomenon is that it must create a degree of synchrony in the cells that survive irradi-ation. Immediately after a dose of x-rays, all the cells will be at precisely the same point in the cell cycle as they were before irradiation, but some will have lost their reproductive integrity and it is the number that retain this which will be greatest in the S phase.

Mitotic delay and cell-cycle progression

Important effects become apparent during the course of the cell cycle within which cells are irradiated. Mitotic delay (i.e. delay in the entry of cells into mito-sis from G2) is very commonly observed, as also is a

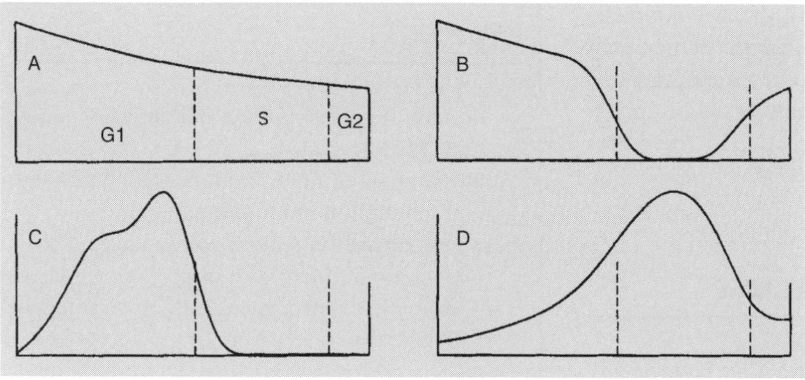

Figure 6.8 *Cell-cycle progression (i.e. reassortment) induced in an exponentially growing cell population by an S-phase-specific cytotoxic agent. From Steel (1977), with permission.*

delay from G1 into the S phase. The genetic control mechanisms involved in these processes are receiving much research attention (see Section 9.3).

The phenomena of induced cell synchrony and cell-cycle progression are illustrated in Figure 6.8 for cells treated with an S-phase-specific cytotoxic drug. Untreated cells in exponential growth have a distribution through the cell cycle shown by Figure 6.8A. Immediately after treatment the distribution of *surviving clonogenic cells* will be as shown by Figure 6.8B. S-phase killing agents also tend temporarily to block the movement of cells into the S phase, and a few hours later there may be a pile-up of survivors in the latter part of the G1 phase (Figure 6.8C). Later, these cells will begin to recover and move on in a semi-synchronous wave through the S phase (Figure 6.8D), when the effect of a second dose of the drug would be greatest. Similar effects occur after irradiation and this is the basis of *reassortment*, as described in the next section.

In the 1970s there was much interest in *synchronization therapy*. This was the attempt to exploit cell-cycle progression phenomena by treating with a second agent (usually a cytotoxic drug) at the optimum time interval after a priming treatment with drug or radiation. In the example illustrated in Figure 6.8, a second treatment with an S-phase-specific agent would be expected to be most effective at the time of panel D. Although this approach to improving tumour therapy was thoroughly researched, it proved in most cases to be disappointing. One possible reason for this is that tumours tend to be very heterogeneous from a kinetic point of view: cells move at very different speeds through the phases of the cell cycle and induced cell synchrony is therefore quickly lost (see Chapter 8 in Steel, 1977).

6.9 THE FIVE Rs OF RADIOTHERAPY

The biological factors that influence the response of normal and neoplastic tissues to fractionated radiotherapy were summarized by Withers (1975) in the 'four Rs of radiotherapy':

- *Repair*: as evidenced by cellular recovery during the few hours after exposure (Section 6.7).
- *Reassortment*: cell-cycle progression effects, otherwise known as '*redistribution*'. Cells that survive a first dose of radiation will tend to be in a resistant phase of the cell cycle and within a few hours they may progress into a more sensitive phase (Section 6.8).
- *Repopulation*: during an extended course of radiotherapy, cells that survive irradiation may proliferate and thus increase the number of cells that must be killed (see Sections 13.6 and 14.4).
- *Reoxygenation*: in a tumour, cells that survive a first dose of radiation will tend to be hypoxic but thereafter their oxygen supply may improve, leading to an increase in radiosensitivity (see Section 15.5).

Note that two of these processes (repair and repopulation) will tend to make the tissue *more resistant* to a second dose of radiation; the other two (reassortment and reoxygenation) tend to make it *more sensitive*. These four factors modify the response of a tissue to repeated doses of radiation and are responsible for the slope of an isoeffect curve (see Figure 12.1). The overall radiosensitivity of the tissue (i.e. the height of the isoeffect curve on the page) depends on a fifth 'R': *radiosensitivity*. Thus for a given fractionation course (or for single-dose irradiation) the haemopoietic system shows a greater response than the kidney, even allowing for the different timing of response. Similarly, tumours such as lymphomas are more radioresponsive than others, and this is largely due to differences in radiosensitivity (Steel *et al.*, 1989).

6.10 REMISSION AND RELAPSE

The concept of clonogenic cells provides a basic understanding of the main features of the time-course of cancer in response to treatment (Figure 6.9). At the time of presentation, the patient may well be carrying in the region of 10^{10}–10^{12} clonogenic tumour cells. During a course of treatment with radiation or cytotoxic drugs this number will be reduced. If the total body burden of tumour cells is significantly reduced, this is often described as a *partial remission*. If it falls below the limit of detection by physical and imaging techniques, then such a response is described as *complete remission*. If treatment leads to the elimination of all clonogenic cells, then the disease will be *controlled*. If not, then in the majority of cases there will be a period of remission followed by relapse. The duration of remission will depend greatly on the level of cell kill achieved by the treatment, i.e. on the depth of the nadir in the curve in Figure 6.9 (see also Figures 2.6 and 17.4).

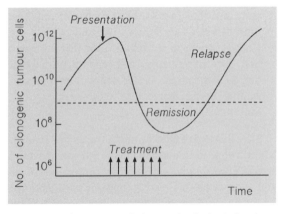

Figure 6.9 *Time-course of changes in the body burden of clonogenic cells through the four main phases of uncontrolled cancer: presentation, treatment, remission and relapse. The broken line indicates the limit of detection.*

KEY POINTS

1. Tumour recurrence after treatment depends upon the survival of clonogenic cells, which may comprise only a small proportion of the total cells within the tumour.
2. Evaluation of the survival of clonogenic cells following treatment is an important aspect of experimental cancer therapy. In experimental situations this is relatively simple to perform, but for cells removed directly from human tumours great care is necessary in the selection and performance of the assays.
3. In tumour therapy, as with tumour growth, it is important to *think logarithmically*. Partial or complete tumour remission may involve only perhaps two decades of clonogenic cell reduction, yet over nine decades of cell kill may be necessary before long-term tumour control can be assured.
4. Repair of radiation damage is an important feature of irradiated tissues. It can be assessed by a variety of experimental tests.
5. Variation of cell killing through the cell cycle is considerable and may give rise to cell-cycle progression phenomena.
6. The 5 Rs of radiotherapy.

BIBLIOGRAPHY

Alexander P (1977). Back to the drawing board – the need for more realistic model systems for immunotherapy. *Cancer* **40**: 467–70.

Baker FL, Spitzer G, Ajani JA *et al.* (1986). Drug and radiation sensitivity measurements of successful primary monolayer culturing of human tumour cells using cell-adhesive matrix and supplemented medium. *Cancer Res* **46**: 1263–74.

Bosanquet A (1991). Correlations between therapeutic response of leukaemias and *in vitro* drug-sensitivity assay. *Lancet* **337**: 711–14.

Carmichael J, DeGraff WG, Gazdar AF *et al.* (1987). Evaluation of a tetrazolium-based semiautomated colorimetric assay: assessment of radiosensitivity. *Cancer Res* **47**: 943–6.

Chapman JD, Peters LJ, Withers HR (1989). *Prediction of Tumour Response to Treatment*. Pergamon, New York.

Courtenay VD, Mills J (1978). An *in vitro* colony assay for human tumours grown in immune-suppressed mice and treated *in vivo* with cytotoxic agents. *Br J Cancer* **37**: 261–8.

Durand RE (1986). Use of a cell sorter for assays of cell clonogenicity. *Cancer Res* **46**: 2775–8.

Elkind MM, Sutton H (1960). Radiation response of mammalian cells grown in culture: I. Repair of X-ray damage in surviving Chinese hamster cells. *Radiat Res* **13**: 566–93.

Fowler JF (1991). The phantom of tumour treatment – continually rapid proliferation unmasked. *Radiother Oncol* **22**: 156–8.

Hewitt HB (1979). A critical examination of the foundations of immunotherapy for cancer. *Clin Radiol* **30**: 361–9.

Hill RP, Stanley JA (1975). The lung colony assay: extension to the Lewis lung tumour and the B16 melanoma. *Int Radiat Biol* **27**: 377–87.

Marples B, Joiner MC (1993). The response of Chinese hamster V79 cells to low radiation doses: evidence for enhanced sensitivity of the whole cell population. *Radiat Res* **133**: 41–51.

Mitchell JB (1988). Potential applicability of nonclonogenic assays to clinical oncology. *Radiat Res* **114**: 401–14.

Potten CS (ed.) (1983). *Stem Cells, their Identification and Characterisation*. Churchill Livingstone, Edinburgh.

Seymour CB, Mothersill C (1989). Lethal mutations, the survival curve shoulder and split-dose recovery. *Int J Radiat Biol* **56**: 999–1010.

Sinclair WK, Morton RA (1965). X-ray and ultraviolet sensitivity of synchronised Chinese hamster cells at various stages of the cell cycle. *Biophys J* **5**: 1–25.

Steel GG (1977). *The Growth Kinetics of Tumours*. Oxford University Press, Oxford.

Steel GG, Adams K (1975). Stem-cell survival and tumour control in the Lewis lung carcinoma. *Cancer Res* **35**: 1530–5.

Steel GG, Stephens TC (1983). Stem cells in tumours. In: *Stem Cells* (ed. Potten CS), pp. 271–94. Churchill Livingstone, Edinburgh.

Steel GG, McMillan TJ, Peacock JH (1989). The 5 Rs of radiobiology. *Int J Radiat Biol* **56**: 1045–8.

Streffer C, van Beunigen D, Gross E *et al.* (1986). Predictive assays for the therapy of rectum carcinoma. *Radiother Oncol* **5**: 303–10.

Till JE, McCulloch EA (1961). A direct measurement of the radiation sensitivity of normal mouse bone marrow. *Radiat Res* **14**: 213–22.

Trott KR (1972). Relation between division delay and damage expressed in later generations. *Curr Topics Radiat Res* **7**: 336–7.

Wasserman TH, Twentyman P (1988). Use of a colorimetric microtiter (MTT) assay in determining the radiosensitivity of cells from murine tumors. *Int J Radiat Oncol* **15**: 699–702.

Withers HR (1975). The four R's of radiotherapy. *Adv Radiat Biol* **5**: 241–7.

FURTHER READING

Elkind MM, Whitmore GF (1967). *The Radiobiology of Cultured Mammalian Cells*. Gordon and Breach, New York.

Potten CS (ed.) (1983). *Stem Cells, their Identification and Characterisation*. Churchill Livingstone, Edinburgh.

Steel GG (1977). *The Growth Kinetics of Tumours*. Oxford University Press, Oxford.

Tannock IF, Hill RP (1992). *The Basic Science of Oncology*, 2nd edn. Pergamon, New York.

7

Models of radiation cell killing

MICHAEL C JOINER

7.1 INTRODUCTION

Research in experimental radiobiology covers studies at the cellular, animal and human levels. It deals at the fundamental level with the molecular, biochemical and biophysical nature of radiation damage. Models are a necessary part of radiobiological research: they provide a framework in which to analyse and compare data and ultimately to assist in building up a consistent theory of radiation action both *in vitro* and *in vivo*. Models and mathematics are also sometimes necessary to relate experimental studies to clinical cancer treatment with the aim of improving therapy. This chapter describes some of the models that are used to analyse the relationship between cell survival and radiation dose.

7.2 A NOTE ON RADIATION RESPONSE AT THE MOLECULAR LEVEL

Radiation kills cells by producing secondary charged particles and free radicals in the nucleus, which in turn produce a variety of types of damage in DNA. Evidence that damage to DNA is the primary cause

of radiation cell killing and mutation is set out in Section 8.2. Each 1 Gy dose of low linear energy transfer (LET) radiation produces over 1000 base damages, about 1000 initial single-strand breaks and 40 initial double-strand breaks. Some lesions are more important than others and radiation lethality correlates most significantly with the number of residual, unrepaired double-strand breaks (DSB) several hours after irradiation. Table 8.2 shows that if cell kill is modified by changing LET, oxygen level, thiol concentration or temperature, then for a fixed radiation dose only the number of DSB reliably correlates with the change in cell kill. Single-strand breaks, base damage and DNA–protein cross-links do not reflect the change in cell kill for all of these modifiers. The DNA double-strand break is therefore thought to be the most important type of cellular damage. Just one residual DSB (or 'hit') in a vital section of DNA may be sufficient to produce a significant chromosome aberration and thus to sterilize the cell.

7.3 TARGET THEORY

A simple way of picturing how radiation might kill cells is the idea that there may be specific regions of

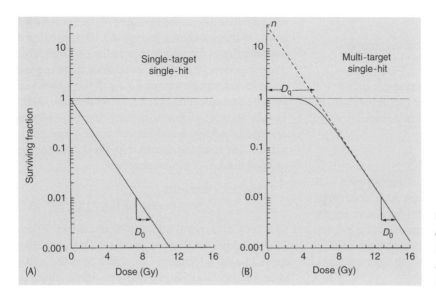

Figure 7.1 *The two most common types of target theory. (A) Single-target inactivation; (B) multi-target inactivation.*

the DNA that are important to maintain the reproductive ability of cells. These sensitive regions could be thought of as specific targets for radiation damage so that the survival of a cell after radiation exposure would be related to the number of targets inactivated. There are two versions of this idea that have commonly been used. The first version of the theory proposed that just one hit by radiation on a single sensitive target would lead to death of the cell. This is called single-target single-hit inactivation, and it leads to the form of survival curve shown in Figure 7.1A. The survival curve is exponential (i.e. a straight line in a semi-logarithmic plot of survival against dose). To derive an equation for this survival curve, Poisson statistics can be applied. The presumption is that during irradiation there is a very large number of hits on different cells taking place, but the probability (P) of the next hit occurring in a given cell is very small. Thus for each cell,

$$P(\text{survival}) = P(0 \text{ hits}) = \exp(-D/D_0)$$

where D_0 is defined as the dose that gives an average of one hit per target. A dose of D_0 Gy reduces survival from 1 to 0.37 (i.e. to e^{-1}), or from 0.1 to 0.037, etc. D/D_0 is the average number of hits per target (and in this case per cell). This is the reason why (as in Figure 7.4) a scale of cell survival is sometimes labelled $-\ln(S)$: this is a scale of the natural logarithm of surviving fraction and it is also the equivalent number of 'lethal lesions' per cell.

In this example (Figure 7.1A), $D_0 = 1.6$ Gy. Straight survival curves of this sort are usually found for the inactivation of viruses and bacteria. They may also be appropriate in describing the radiation response of some very sensitive human cells (normal and malignant) and also the radiation response at very low dose rates (see Section 18.3) and response to high LET radiations (see Section 19.3). This type of 'single-target single-hit' survival curve model is therefore actually valid outside of the 'target theory' framework. It describes the simple situation where if an individual cell receives an amount of radiation greater than D_0 then it will die, otherwise it will survive.

For mammalian cells in general, their response to radiation is usually described by 'shouldered' survival curves of the form introduced in Section 6.3. In an attempt to model this type of response, a more general version of target theory was proposed called multi-target single-hit inactivation. In this extended target idea, just one hit by radiation on each of n sensitive targets in the cell is required for death of the cell. The shape of this survival curve is shown in Figure 7.1B. Again, the argument can be developed using Poisson statistics,

$$P(0 \text{ hits on a specific target}) = \exp(-D/D_0)$$

Thus,

$$P(\text{specific target inactivated}) = 1 - \exp(-D/D_0)$$

As there are n targets in the cell,

$$P(\text{all } n \text{ targets inactivated}) = [1 - \exp(-D/D_0)]^n$$

Thus,

$$P(\text{survival}) = P(\text{not all targets inactivated})$$
$$= 1-[1-\exp(-D/D_0)]^n \quad (7.1)$$

Figure 7.1B shows that multi-target single-hit survival curves have a shoulder whose size can be indicated by the quasi-threshold dose (D_q). This is related to n and D_0 by the relation:

$$D_q = D_0 \log_e n \quad (7.2)$$

For the example in Figure 7.1B we have chosen $n = 30$ and $D_0 = 1.6\,\text{Gy}$, giving $D_q = 5.4\,\text{Gy}$. Such multi-target survival curves have proved useful for describing the radiation response of mammalian cells at high doses, 'off the shoulder'. They do not describe the survival response well at lower more clinically relevant doses.

7.4 THE PROBLEM WITH TARGETS

The derivation of simple cell survival relationships in terms of targets and hits, particularly the straight survival curve shown in Figure 7.1A, is an intellectually attractive idea and it dominated radiobiological thinking for a long time. The key difficulty with this concept is that so far the specific radiation targets have not been identified for mammalian cells, despite considerable effort to search for them. Rather, what has emerged is the key role of DNA strand breaks and their repair, with sites for such DNA damage being generally dispersed throughout the cell nucleus (see Sections 8.2

and 8.8). An obvious shortcoming of the multi-target model is that, as shown in Figure 7.1B, it predicts a response that is flat for very low radiation doses. This is not supported by experimental data: there is good evidence for significant cell killing at low doses and for cell survival curves that have a finite initial slope. To take account of this, the multi-target model was adjusted by adding an additional single-target component. The resulting equation for the survival curve is called the two-component model:

$$P(\text{survival}) = \exp(-D/D_1)$$
$$\times (1-\{1-\exp[-D(1/D_0-1/D_1)]\}^n) \quad (7.3)$$

This type of survival curve is illustrated in Figure 7.2A. In addition to the parameters n, D_0 and D_q, this curve also has a parameter D_1, which fixes the initial slope, i.e. the dose required in the low-dose region to reduce survival from 1 to 0.37. In this example, $n = 30$ and $D_0 = 1.6\,\text{Gy}$, and $D_1 = 4.6\,\text{Gy}$. This type of curve now correctly predicts finite cell killing in the low-dose region but it still has the drawback that the change in cell survival over the range 0 to D_q occurs almost linearly. This implies that no sparing of damage should occur as dose per fraction is reduced below 2 Gy, which is usually not found to be the case either experimentally or in clinical radiotherapy (see Figures 12.1 and 12.2, and Section 14.3). A way of overcoming this limitation would be to use a multi-target instead of single-target component as the initial slope. However, this would make the model far too complicated to be of much use in comparing survival responses. It would require at least four parameters, and would be

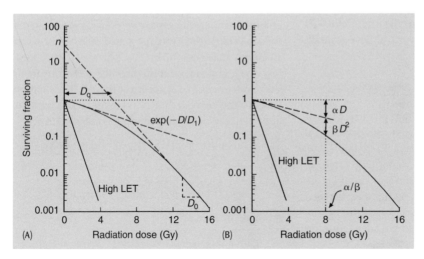

Figure 7.2 *Models with non-exponential cell killing but a finite initial slope. (A) The two-component model and (B) the linear-quadratic model.*

of little value in helping to understand the fundamental mechanisms determining radiation effect.

7.5 THE LINEAR-QUADRATIC MODEL

The continually downward bending form of a cell survival can simply be fitted by a second-order polynomial, with a zero constant term to ensure that SF = 1 at zero dose. This is exactly the formulation that is termed the linear-quadratic (LQ) model. Although we can regard this as based on pure mathematics, it has also been possible to attach radiobiological mechanisms to this model. The formula for cell survival is:

$$-\ln(S) = \alpha D + \beta D^2$$
$$P(\text{survival}) = \exp(-\alpha D - \beta D^2) \qquad (7.4)$$

and the cell survival curve is drawn in Figure 7.2B. Although the shapes of the LQ model and the complicated two-component model are superficially similar (compare Figures 7.2A and 7.2B), the simple LQ formula gives a better description of radiation response in the low-dose region (0–3 Gy): LQ survival curves are continuously bending with no straight portion either at low or high radiation doses. The shape (or 'bendiness') is determined by the ratio α/β.

Since the dimensions of the parameters are α: Gy^{-1} and β: Gy^{-2}, the dimensions of α/β are Gy: as shown in Figure 7.2B, this is the dose at which the linear contribution to damage (αD on the logarithmic scale) equals the quadratic contribution (βD^2). The response of cells to densely ionizing radiations like neutrons or α-particles is usually a steep and almost exponential survival curve (see Figure 19.2). As shown in Figure 7.2, this would be explained in the two-component model by the ratio D_1/D_0 being near to 1.0, or in the LQ model by a high α/β ratio.

The LQ model is now in widespread use in both experimental and clinical radiobiology and generally works well in describing responses to radiation *in vitro* and also *in vivo*. What could be its mechanistic justification? One simple idea is that the linear component [$\exp(-\alpha D)$] might be due to single-track events while the quadratic component [$\exp(-\beta D^2)$] might arise from two-track events. This interpretation is supported by studies of the dose-rate effect (see Section 18.3) which show that as dose rate is reduced, cell survival curves become straight and tend

to extrapolate the initial slope of the high dose-rate curve: the quadratic component of cell killing disappears, leaving only the linear component. This would be expected, for at low dose rate single-track events will occur far apart in time and the probability of interaction between them will be low. Although this interpretation of the LQ equation seems reasonable, the nature of the interactions between separate tracks is still a matter of considerable debate. Chadwick and Leenhouts (1973) postulated that separate tracks might hit opposite strands of the DNA double helix and thus form a double-strand break. We now know that this is unlikely in view of the very low probability of two tracks interacting within the dimensions of the DNA molecule (diameter ~2.5 nm) at a dose of a few Gy. Interaction between more widely spaced regions of the complex DNA structure, or between DNA in different chromosomes, may be a more plausible mechanism (see Section 8.4).

7.6 THE LETHAL, POTENTIALLY LETHAL DAMAGE (LPL) MODEL

Curtis (1986) proposed this model as a 'unified repair model' of cell killing. Ionizing radiation is considered to produce two different types of lesion: repairable (i.e. *potentially* lethal) lesions and non-repairable (i.e. lethal) lesions. The non-repairable lesions produce single-hit lethal effects and therefore give rise to a linear component of cell killing [= $\exp(-\alpha D)$]. The eventual effect of the repairable lesions depends on competing processes of repair and binary misrepair. It is this latter process that leads to a quadratic component in cell killing. As shown in Figure 7.3, the model has two sensitivity parameters (η_L determines the number of non-repairable lesions produced per unit dose, and η_{PL} the number of repairable lesions). There are also two rate constants (ϵ_{PL} determines the rate of repair of repairable lesions, and ϵ_{2PL} the rate at which they undergo interaction and thus misrepair).

This model produces almost identical cell survival curves to the LQ equation, down to a survival level of perhaps 10^{-2}. It can therefore be taken to provide one possible mechanistic interpretation of the LQ equation. It predicts that as dose rate is reduced, the probability of binary interaction of potentially lethal lesions will fall and parameter values can be found that allow the model to simulate accurately cell survival data

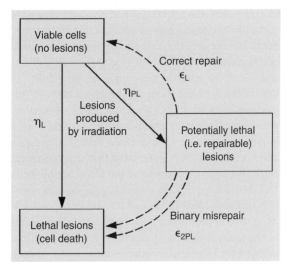

Figure 7.3 *The lethal, potentially lethal (LPL) damage model of radiation action.*

on human and animal cells irradiated at various dose rates (see Sections 18.3 and 18.5).

7.7 REPAIR SATURATION MODELS

Curtis's LPL model is an example of a lesion-interaction model that also incorporates repair processes. Figure 7.4A shows how this produces the downward-bending cell survival curve: the dashed curve indicates the component of cell killing that is due to single-track non-repairable lesions. It is the *extra* lethal lesions produced by the binary interaction of potentially lethal lesions that give the downward-bending curve.

Another class of models are the repair saturation models, which propose that the shape of the survival curve depends only on a dose-dependent rate of repair. Figures 7.4B and 7.4C demonstrate this idea. Only one type of lesion and single-hit killing are postulated, and in the absence of any repair these lesions produce the steep dashed survival curve in Figure 7.4B. The final survival curve (solid line) results from repair of some of these lesions but if the repair enzymes become saturated (Figure 7.4C), there is not enough repair enzyme to bind to all damaged sites simultaneously and so the reaction velocity of repair no longer increases with increasing damage. Therefore at higher doses (more lesions) there is proportionally less repair during the time available before damage becomes fixed; this will lead to more residual damage

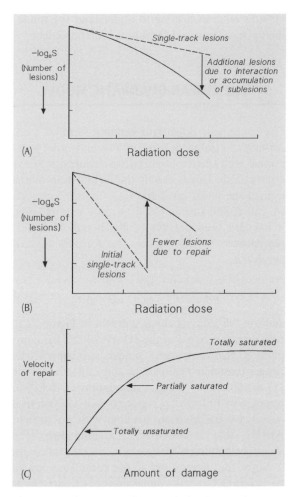

Figure 7.4 *The contrast between lesion-interaction models and repair-saturation models. (A) The LPL model; (B) the effect of repair becoming less effective at higher radiation doses; (C) the basic concept of repair saturation. Adapted from Goodhead (1985), with permission.*

and to greater cell kill. The mechanisms of fixation of non-repaired damage are not understood but they may be associated with the entry of cells carrying such damage into DNA synthesis or mitosis. It should be noted that an alternative 'saturation' hypothesis, leading to the same consequence, is that the pool of repair enzymes is used up during repair, so that at higher doses the repair system is depleted and is less able to repair all the induced damage. Table 7.1 illustrates how the basic conceptual difference between the lesion accumulation/interaction models such as Curtis's LPL and the dose-dependent repair models

Table 7.1 *Different interpretations of radiobiological phenomena by lesion-interaction and saturable-repair models*

Observation	Explanation	
	Lesion interaction	Repair saturation
Curved dose–effect relationship	Interaction of sublesions	Saturation of capacity to repair sublesions
Split-dose recovery	Repair of sublesions (sublethal damage repair)	Recovery of capacity to repair sublesions
RBE increase with LET	More non-repairable lesions at high LET	High-LET lesions are less repairable
Low dose rate is less effective	Repair of sublesions during irradiation	Repair system not saturating

Adapted from Goodhead (1985).

affects the interpretation of some radiobiological phenomena (Goodhead, 1985). Both types of model predict linear-quadratic cell survival curves in the clinically relevant dose region. They also provide good explanations of split-dose recovery (see Section 6.7), changing effectiveness with LET (see Section 19.4) and the dose-rate effect (see Section 18.2). At present, radiation scientists are uncertain whether lesion interaction or repair saturation really exist in cells but it may well be that molecular and microdosimetric studies will eventually determine which explanation (maybe both!) is correct.

7.8 LOW-DOSE HYPER-RADIOSENSITIVITY

The LQ model and its mechanistic interpretations (Curtis's LPL and repair saturation) adequately describe cellular response to radiation above about 1 Gy. It has been difficult to make accurate measurements of cell killing by radiation below this dose, but this problem has been partially overcome by methods that determine exactly the number of cells 'at risk' in a colony-forming assay (see Section 6.4). This can be achieved using a fluorescence-activated cell sorter (FACS) to *plate* an exact number of cells, or microscopic scanning to identify an exact number of cells *after* plating. Using such techniques, it can be shown that many mammalian cell lines actually exhibit the type of radiation response shown in Figure 7.5 at doses less than 1 Gy. Below about 10 cGy, the cells show hyper-radiosensitivity (HRS) which can be characterized by a slope (α_s) that is considerably steeper than the slope expected by extrapolating back the response from high-dose

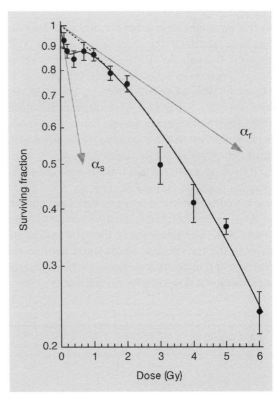

Figure 7.5 *Survival of asynchronous T98G human glioma cells irradiated with 240 kVp x-rays, measured using a cell-sorter protocol (Short et al., 1999). Each data point represents 10–12 measurements. The solid line and dashed lines show the fits of the induced-repair (IndRep) model and linear-quadratic (LQ) models respectively. At doses below 1 Gy the LQ model, using an initial slope α_r, substantially underestimates the effect of irradiation and this domain is better described by the IndRep model using a much steeper initial slope α_s.*

measurements (α_r). The transition (over about 20–80 cGy) from a sensitive to resistant response has been termed a region of increased radioresistance (IRR). This phenomenon was originally discovered in mammalian cells by Marples and Joiner (1993) using V79 hamster fibroblasts and is thought to be due to an increase in the DNA repair capability of the cells in the IRR region, although it is not yet known by what mechanism this occurs (Joiner *et al.*, 2001).

The LQ model can be modified to take account of this phenomenon and the result is called the induced repair (IndRep) model:

$$P(\text{survival}) = \exp\{-\alpha_r D[1 + (\alpha_s/\alpha_r - 1) \\ \times \exp(-D/D_c)] - \beta D^2\} \quad (7.5)$$

In this equation, D_c is around 0.2 Gy and describes the dose at which the transition from the HRS response through the IRR response starts to occur. At very high doses ($D \gg D_c$), Eqn 7.5 tends to an LQ model with active parameters α_r and β. At very low doses ($D \ll D_c$), Eqn 7.5 tends to an LQ model with active parameters α_s and β. The IndRep model thus comprises two LQ models with different α sensitivities merged into a single equation.

It has been proposed that this curious HRS phenomenon might be exploitable clinically if it is practicable to deliver radiotherapy as a very large number of dose fractions each smaller than 0.5 Gy. The aim would be to take advantage of the extra radiosensitivity in the HRS region, which could improve the response of tumours that are known to be resistant to radiotherapy at doses of 2 Gy per fraction.

KEY POINTS

1. A number of different mathematical models adequately simulate the shape of cell survival curves for mammalian cells. So far it has not been possible to strongly prefer one model to others.
2. Target theory proposes that a specific number of targets or DNA sites must be inactivated or damaged to kill the cell. This approach is only satisfactory if a component of single-hit killing is also introduced. So far it has not been possible to identify the location of these vital 'targets' within the cell nucleus.
3. Lesion-interaction models explain downward-bending cell survival curves by postulating two classes of lesion. One class is directly lethal, but the other type is only *potentially* lethal and may be repaired enzymatically or may interact with other potentially lethal lesions to form lethal lesions.
4. Repair-saturation models also provide a plausible explanation of cell survival phenomena.
5. The recently discovered hyper-radiosensitivity phenomenon at very low radiation doses illustrates that the older explanations of radiation cell killing cannot be taken as absolute.

BIBLIOGRAPHY

Chadwick KH, Leenhouts HP (1973). A molecular theory of cell survival. *Phys Med Biol* **13**: 78–87.

Curtis SB (1986). Lethal and potentially lethal lesions induced by radiation: a unified repair model. *Radiat Res* **106**: 252–70.

Goodhead DT (1985). Saturable repair models of radiation action in mammalian cells. *Radiat Res* **104**: S58–67.

Joiner MC, Marples B, Lambin P, Short SC, Turesson I (2001). Low-dose hypersensitivity: current status and possible mechanisms. *Int J Radiat Oncol Biol Phys* **49**: 379–89.

Marples B, Joiner MC (1993). The response of Chinese hamster V79 cells to low radiation doses: evidence of enhanced sensitivity of the whole cell population. *Radiat Res* **133**: 41–51.

Short S, Mayes C, Woodcock M, Johns H, Joiner MC (1999). Low dose hypersensitivity in the T98G human glioblastoma cell line. *Int J Radiat Biol* **75**: 847–55.

FURTHER READING

Alpen EL (1998). *Radiation Biophysics*, 2nd edn. Academic Press, San Diego.

Douglas BG, Fowler JF (1976). The effect of multiple small doses of X-rays on skin reactions in the mouse and a basic interpretation. *Radiat Res* **66**: 401–26.

Elkind MM, Sutton H (1960). Radiation response of mammalian cells grown in culture: I. Repair of X-ray damage in surviving Chinese hamster cells. *Radiat Res* **13**: 556–93.

Ward JF (1990). The yield of DNA double-strand breaks produced intracellularly by ionizing radiation: a review. *Int J Radiat Biol* **57**: 1141–50.

DNA damage and cell killing

TREVOR J McMILLAN AND G GORDON STEEL

8.1 INITIAL PROCESSES OF RADIATION DAMAGE

Irradiation of a biological system initiates a series of processes that can be classified in terms of the time-scale over which they act (Figure 1.1). The physical, chemical and biological phases of this process have been described in Section 1.3.

An electron with an energy of 1 MeV has a range in soft tissue of a few millimetres. In the early part of its track the particle moves very quickly and its rate of energy deposition is low; the result is a relatively straight track in which the ionizations may be separated by distances of around 0.1 mm on average. We describe this as radiation with a low linear energy transfer (low LET, see Section 19.2). As the electron slows down, it interacts more strongly with the orbital electrons in the medium. Its rate of energy loss increases, the track becomes more tortuous due to stronger collisions, and the ionization density increases. Figure 8.1A shows a computer simulation of the tracks of 1 keV electrons, representing a very small terminal part of the tracks of 1 MeV electrons. The important feature is the tendency towards clustering of the ionization events at the ends of the tracks, each cluster having the size of a few nanometres. Within

each electron track there is opportunity for interactions between the products of separate ionization events and it may be, particularly at low dose rate or following acute radiation doses up to a few Gy, that the main biological effects of radiation (i.e. cell killing and mutation) are predominantly due to damage that is produced by these 'hot spots'. Within perhaps 10^{-10} seconds of exposure to either photon or particle beams, the irradiated volume will contain atoms that have been ionized and a corresponding number of free electrons, all produced by the cascade of atomic reactions just described and with a rather non-uniform spatial distribution. The numbers of ionizations produced at therapeutic dose levels is very large – approximately 10^5 ionizations per cell per Gy – but the vast majority of these produce no cytotoxic damage. The biological effect of ionizations is influenced by three main factors: free-radical scavenging processes, the number of ionizations that are close enough to DNA to damage it, and cellular repair processes.

Free-radical processes

Since biological systems consist largely of water, the bulk of the ionizations produced by irradiation occur

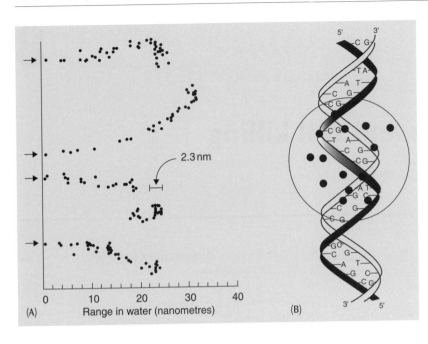

Figure 8.1 *(A) Computer-simulated tracks of 1 keV electrons. Note the scale in relation to the 2.3 nm diameter of the DNA double helix (adapted from Chapman and Gillespie, 1981). (B) Illustrating the concept of a local multiply-damaged site produced by a cluster of ionizations impinging on DNA.*

in water molecules. Negatively charged free electrons (e^-) that are produced by ionization will rapidly become associated with polar water molecules, greatly reducing their mobility. The configuration of an electron surrounded by water molecules (a 'hydrated electron', e_{aq}^-) has a degree of stability and a lifetime under physiological conditions of a few microseconds. The water molecule that has lost an electron is a highly reactive positively charged ion. It quickly breaks down to produce a hydrogen ion (H^+) and an (uncharged) OH radical. OH is a molecule that normally does not exist in water. Oxygen has valency 2, hydrogen 1, and the stable configuration is H_2O. The uncharged OH radical has an unpaired electron ('unattached valency') that makes it highly reactive. We designate it as a free radical thus: OH$^{\cdot}$. Free radicals are simply fragments of broken molecules. OH$^{\cdot}$ is different from OH$^+$, which is a positively charged ion: the OH radical has equal numbers of protons and orbital electrons but because of the unpaired electron it is chemically reactive (note that some ions may also be radicals, for example a water molecule that has lost an electron is actually H_2O^+, a radical cation). Similarly, H^+ is a bare proton, positively charged, whilst H$^{\cdot}$ is a proton plus an electron (neutral charge) but again highly reactive because the stable form of hydrogen is H_2.

Around 10^{-10} seconds after irradiation there will be three principal radiolysis products of water: e_{aq}^-, H$^{\cdot}$ and OH$^{\cdot}$. These highly reactive species will go on to take part in further reactions. An important one is:

$$OH^{\cdot} + OH^{\cdot} \rightarrow H_2O_2$$

the production of hydrogen peroxide. Oxygen, if present, plays an important part in the free-radical reactions that follow irradiation. Molecular oxygen has a high affinity for free radicals (R$^{\cdot}$):

$$R^{\cdot} + O_2 \rightarrow RO_2^{\cdot}$$

giving rise to further reactive products and acting to fix the free-radical damage. The oxygen effect in radiation cell killing has often been explained in terms of this type of process.

In biological systems, the free radicals produced in water may react with essential macromolecules. A vast range of reactions takes place, most of which are unimportant for the survival and functioning of the cell. The most important reactions are those with DNA, because of the uniqueness of the function of many parts of this molecule. Damage to DNA from free radicals produced in water is called the *indirect* effect of radiation; ionization of atoms that are part of the DNA molecule is the *direct* effect.

There has been some debate as to whether effects in water that is tightly bound to DNA are direct or indirect.

Compounds containing sulphydryl (–SH) groups have a particular affinity for free radicals. Their presence within the cell may therefore act to 'mop up' a proportion of radicals, thus decreasing radiation effects. The principal non-protein thiols in mammalian cells are:

- cysteine – a natural amino acid;
- cysteamine – decarboxylated cysteine;
- glutathione – the commonest non-protein thiol.

Administration of these compounds to animals or to cells in tissue culture immediately before irradiation reduces the extent of damage; the radiation dose required to produce a given level of damage can go up by as much as a factor of 2.0.

During the first millisecond after radiation exposure, a competition takes place between damage-fixing and scavenging reactions for radicals in key target molecules. There is considerable interest in the possibility of manipulating the levels of cellular thiols either to protect normal tissues or, by depressing thiol levels, to increase the radiosensitivity of tumour cells. Thiol depression can be achieved experimentally by blocking the synthesis of glutathione using such agents as diamide or buthionine sulphoximine (BSO).

The development and radiobiological properties of hypoxic cell radiosensitizers are dealt with in Section 16.3. The most important class of sensitizers are the electron-affinic compounds, principally the nitroimidazoles, which act like oxygen in promoting the fixation of free-radical damage. Since they are less rapidly metabolized than oxygen, they can diffuse further in tumour tissue and thus reach hypoxic cells.

8.2 RADIATION DAMAGE TO DNA

The structure of DNA

Deoxyribonucleic acid (DNA) is a large molecule that has a characteristic double-helix structure consisting of two strands, each made up of a sequence of nucleotides (Figure 8.2). A nucleotide is a subunit

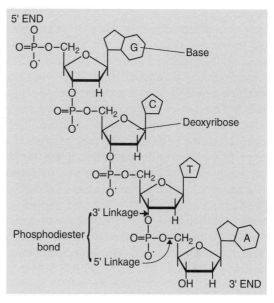

Figure 8.2 *The structure of DNA, in which the 4 bases (G, C, T, A) are linked through sugar groups to the sugar-phosphate backbone.*

in which a 'base' is linked through a sugar group to a phosphate group. The sugar is deoxyribose, which has a five-atom ring: four carbons and one oxygen. The 'backbone' of the molecule consists of alternating sugar–phosphate groups. Note that by the conventional numbering system the connection points of the phosphates to the sugar ring are labelled 5' and 3': this leads to the ends of a sequence of nucleotides also being labelled in this way and it defines the direction in which the sequence is read during transcription. There are four different bases. Two are single-ring groups (pyrimidines): thymine and cytosine. Two are double-ring groups (purines): adenine and guanine. It is the order of these bases along the molecule that specifies the genetic code.

The two strands of the double helix are held together by hydrogen bonding between the bases. These bonds are formed between thymine and adenine, and between cytosine and guanine; the bases are paired in this way along the length of the DNA molecule. During the S phase of the cell cycle, DNA synthesis takes place (the process of *replication*) in which every base pair is accurately duplicated.

The first stage in the manufacture of proteins is the construction by the process of *transcription* of a messenger RNA (i.e. mRNA) that has a similar structure to a single strand of DNA except that the sugar groups are ribose in place of deoxyribose, and thymine is replaced by uracil. The decoding is based on the pairing of bases: A-U, C-G, G-C, T-A. Transcription is performed by RNA polymerases, which bind to DNA and generate the corresponding mRNA. The control of transcription is increasingly being elucidated and involves specific DNA sequences at the beginning and ends of genes that signal the initiation and end of transcription. Within the *coding region* of the gene there may be several stretches of DNA that are not required for mRNA. These are called *introns* (the required regions are *exons*) and they need to be removed at some point prior to the translation of the mRNA into protein. Protein production occurs at ribosomes where transfer RNA (tRNA) with an amino acid attached recognizes groups of three bases in the mRNA (*codons*) and in this way the amino acids are lined up in the correct sequence for the protein.

The very long DNA double-helix molecule, together with nuclear proteins, is organized within the cell through a number of levels of supercoiling. The DNA double helix (about 2.5 nm in diameter) is first coiled around protein cores made of histone proteins to form a bead-like string of nucleosomes, then coiled into a 25 nm fibre, which is further spiralized and becomes visible in the condensed form of a chromosome at mitosis. During interphase and in chromatin that has been gently extracted from cell nuclei, DNA shows a series of loops or *domains* that are attached to the nuclear matrix. A human chromosome may have around 2600 looped domains, each formed from about 0.4 mm of the 25 nm DNA fibre and containing 20 000–80 000 base pairs.

Radiation damage to DNA

Early experiments showed that irradiation leads to a loss of viscosity in DNA solutions. Subsequently this has been shown to result from DNA strand breaks. There are two categories of DNA strand breaks; single-strand (SSB) and double-strand breaks (DSB). The detection of these depends on a study of the size distribution of fragments of DNA after extraction from irradiated cells (see below). As shown in Figure 8.3, there is a variety of other types of DNA lesion that may have a role in cellular responses to radiation or chemical damage.

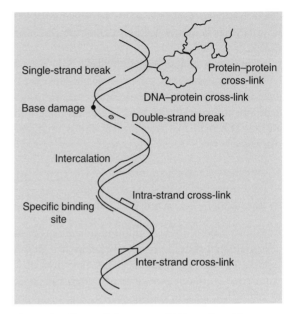

Figure 8.3 *Types of damage to DNA produced by radiation and chemical agents.*

Why do we believe that DNA damage is the critical event in radiation cell killing and mutation?

There are many sources of evidence, including the following:

- Micro-irradiation studies show that to kill cells by irradiation of only the cytoplasm requires far higher radiation dose than irradiation of the nucleus.
- Isotopes with short-range emission (such as ^{3}H, ^{125}I) when incorporated into cellular DNA efficiently produce radiation cell killing and DNA damage (Table 8.1).
- The incidence of chromosomal aberrations following irradiation is closely linked to cell killing.
- Thymidine analogues such as IUdR or BrUdR when specifically incorporated into chromatin modify radiosensitivity.

The number of lesions induced by radiation in DNA is far greater than those that eventually lead to cell killing. A dose of radiation that induces on average 1 lethal event per cell will kill 63% and leave 37% still viable (this results from Poisson statistics) and we call this the D_0 dose (see Section 7.3). D_0 values for oxic mammalian cells are usually in the region of

Table 8.1 *Toxicity of radioisotopes depends upon their subcellular distribution*

	Radiation dose to part of the cell* (Gy)		
	to nucleus	to cytoplasm	to membranes
x-Ray	3.3	3.3	3.3
[³H]Thymidine	3.8	0.27	0.01
[¹²⁵I]Concanavalin	4.1	24.7	516.7

* For each of these three treatments a dose has been chosen that gives 50% cell killing in CHO cells. The absorbed radiation doses to the nucleus, cytoplasm or membranes have then been calculated. [³H]Thymidine is bound to DNA, [¹²⁵I]concanavalin to cell membranes. It is the *nuclear* dose that is constant and thus correlates with cell killing, not the cytoplasmic or membrane doses. From Warters *et al.* (1977).

Table 8.2 *Double-strand DNA breaks correlate best with cell killing*

Modifier	Cell kill	DSB	SSB	Base	DNA-protein cross-links
High-LET radiation	↑	↑	↓	↓	–
Hypoxia	↓	↓	↓	0	↑
Thiols	↓	↓	↓	0	↓
Hyperthermia	↑	↑	0	0	0
Hydrogen peroxide	0	0	↑	↑	–

↑, Increased; ↓, decreased; 0, little or no effect; –, not known.
See Frankenburg-Schwager (1989) for further information on these relationships.

1–2 Gy. The numbers of DNA lesions per cell that are detected immediately after such a dose have been estimated to be approximately:

Events per D_0	
Base damage	>1000
Single-strand breaks	~1000
Double-strand breaks	~40

In addition, cross-links between DNA strands and between DNA and nuclear proteins are formed (Figure 8.3). Irradiation at clinically used doses thus induces a vast amount of DNA damage, most of which is successfully repaired by the cell. In a variety of experimental situations it has been found that the incidence of cell killing fails to correlate with the number of SSB induced, but relates better to the incidence of DSB (Table 8.2). Significantly, a dose of hydrogen peroxide that induces many SSB produces little cell killing and few DSB unless the number of SSB produced is so large that they are close enough to form DSB. On this basis it is generally believed that DSB are the critical lesions for radiation cell killing in most cell types, although as the next paragraph indicates it may be only some DSB that are important.

The realization that low-LET radiation produces 'hotspots' in which clusters of ionizations may occur within a diameter of a few nanometres (Section 8.1) has led to the notion that such an event may produce a particularly severe lesion if it impinges on the DNA molecule. This lesion might consist of one or more DSB together with a number of SSB, and also DNA base damage, etc. Ward (1986) has termed this a local multiply-damaged site (LMDS, Figure 8.1B). The importance of these hypothetical lesions derives from the fact mentioned above that the great majority of DNA lesions are repaired. Any difference in repair among DSB will lead to lethality being associated with the rare lesion that fails to repair, which may inherently be difficult to repair. An LMDS, which will be recognized by a strand-break assay as merely one DSB, may have a low repair probability and high probability of leading to cell death.

The importance of the initial slope of cell survival curves for clinical radiotherapy is described in Sections 17.5 and 18.2. The concept of a linear component of cell killing is also essential to the linear-quadratic and LPL models of cell killing (see Sections 7.5 and 7.6). LMDS are a type of radiation-induced lesion that could cause single-hit cell killing and therefore conceivably could give rise to the linear component.

Even strand breaks induced by single events may be heterogeneous. Over 20 products of thymine have been detected using gas chromatography and mass spectrometry. It is therefore highly likely that the chemical residues on the edges of a strand break vary markedly and the biological consequences of this are not yet known.

Radiation-induced mutations

Some damage induced by radiation may be insufficient to abolish the colony-forming ability of a cell but may still lead to an alteration in the base sequence in DNA. These are mutations; they result in the expression of an altered protein or in increase or decrease in the level of a normal protein. The frequency of radiation-induced mutations usually increases in a dose-dependent manner in the range of doses per fraction commonly used in clinical radiotherapy. At higher radiation doses, lethal events may predominate and the frequency of surviving mutant cells will fall.

The molecular analysis of non-lethal mutations has allowed a detailed examination of the sequelae of radiation-induced DNA damage. A wide spectrum of types of damage has been detected and an interesting observation is that ionizing radiation tends to produce a higher proportion of large deletions relative to simple base changes when compared with mutations that have arisen spontaneously (Yandell et al., 1990).

8.3 METHODS FOR DETECTING DNA DAMAGE

Since it is widely believed that strand breaks are the critical lesion produced by ionizing radiation, considerable effort has gone into producing methods by which they can be measured. These include the following.

Sucrose gradient sedimentation

Sucrose solutions are prepared within plastic centrifuge tubes with a sucrose concentration that varies continuously from around 30% at the bottom to 5% at the top. Cells are exposed to [^{14}C]thymidine for a sufficient period to label most of the DNA. They are then mixed with a solution that induces cell lysis and releases the DNA. Some solutions (such as 0.2 M NaOH) release DNA in a single-stranded form whereas at lower pH (i.e. less strongly alkaline) the double-stranded structure is retained. The mixture is floated on the top of the gradient. When the tubes are spun in a high-speed centrifuge at around 30 000 r.p.m., the large DNA fragments travel further and the profile of ^{14}C concentration down the gradient reflects the amount of DNA damage. This is detected by piercing the bottom of the centrifuge tube, collecting fractions of the fluid, and assaying for ^{14}C. The strand-break frequency is then deduced from the distribution of fragment sizes.

Neutral filter elution

Cells whose DNA has been made radioactive are lysed on the top of a filter whose pore size is about 2 mm (remember that the DNA fibre has a diameter of ~25 nm, 100 times smaller). A flow of elution buffer washes DNA fragments through the membrane and the rate of elution of DNA is related to the size of the DNA molecules on the membrane. To measure DSB, the elution buffer is at pH 7.4 or 9.6. The use of pH 9.6 increases the sensitivity of the technique but also allows the detection of alkali-labile sites that are not actual DSB at physiological pH. Comparison of the two buffers has sometimes led to different answers to biological questions. Increasing pH even further to 12.3 leads to denaturation of the two strands of the DNA and allows the measurement of SSB.

Nucleoid sedimentation technique

The lysis of cells at neutral pH in the presence of high salt concentration and a non-ionic detergent allows the interphase nucleus to open up and reveal the tangled mass of chromatin. The resulting structures, often called *nucleoids*, consist of supercoiled DNA still retaining attachment to residual protein structures. The sedimentation of these structures in a sucrose gradient is influenced by the induction of SSB, which allow the domains to relax and therefore enlarge. One adaptation of this technique, the *halo* method, assesses the expansion of nucleoids by incorporating a fluorescent dye (usually ethidium bromide) into the DNA and measuring the size of halos by microscopy. The concentration of the intercalating dye greatly influences the degree of unwinding of the domains, and the relationship between halo size and dye concentration gives information about the chromatin structure in the nucleoid.

Pulsed-field gel electrophoresis

Fragments of DNA carry a net negative charge and when incorporated into an agarose gel they generally migrate under an electric field at a speed that is inversely related to their size. In order to detect the movement of the DNA, this is either made radioactive (in the live cells prior to lysis) or is stained with a DNA-specific fluorescent dye after electrophoresis. With careful choice of parameters, constant-field gel electrophoresis can demonstrate sensitivity to modest doses of radiation. However, the separation of fragments is improved by pulsing the electric field and alternating it, for instance between directions at 60 degrees to the axis of migration. This technique overcomes problems of anomalous movement of large DNA molecules in an electric field, so that their separation can be translated into a measure of strand breakage produced by small radiation doses. DNA of known molecular weight (for instance intact yeast chromosomes) is used to calibrate the movement of irradiated DNA in the gels.

Single-cell gel electrophoresis

Cells are embedded in low-density agarose on a microscope slide and then lysed to release DNA. The domain structures unwind and when the preparations are subjected to electrophoresis the broken DNA migrates away from the general mass of DNA in the nucleus. The shape of the structure formed by this migration has led to this assay commonly being referred to as the 'comet' assay. Variations in the lysis conditions allow the measurement of different lesions (e.g. alkaline conditions assess SSB while neutral conditions allow the assessment of DSB) and the effect of chromatin structure can also be manipulated to some degree in a manner similar to nucleoid sedimentation. This assay has the advantages of high sensitivity to SSB (though not to DSB) and a requirement for only small numbers of cells.

8.4 CHROMOSOME ABERRATIONS

One of the most obvious cytological effects of irradiation is the production of damage to chromosomes. Irradiation induces a dose-dependent delay in the entry of cells into mitosis due to the activation of cell-cycle checkpoints (see Section 9.3), and when cells that were irradiated while in interphase begin to divide, some of them reveal chromosome aberrations. Whilst the most serious of these will lead to early cell death ('unstable' aberrations), some ('stable' aberrations) can be carried through many divisions. Some types of aberration are illustrated in Figure 8.4. They consist of a variety of exchanges and deletions: fragments may be exchanged between chromosomes, between the arms of a single chromosome, or even within a single arm. This can lead to chromosomes in which arm lengths are abnormal, and also to chromosomes sticking together and forming X or O structures, or to dicentric chromosomes containing two centromeres plus a chromosome fragment. It is now clear that even small doses of radiation can induce highly complex chromosomal rearrangements involving several chromosome sites.

Aberrations may also be classified as chroma*tid* or chromo*some* aberrations. The irradiation of cells in the G2 phase leads mainly to chromatid damage; radiation damage in G1, if unrepaired, will lead to defects involving both chromatids and thus to chromosome aberrations. Irradiation of cells in the S phase can lead to either type, depending on whether the affected chromosome sites had themselves undergone replication.

What is the relationship between chromosome aberrations and cell viability? Cells do seem to be able to tolerate a variety of structural chromosomal changes and in irradiated individuals some changes persist throughout life. Tumours are characterized by chromosomal instability (both in terms of chromosome structure and the number of chromosomes) and irradiation increases the extent of this. But some chromosome changes tend to be lethal. In general terms, the lethal events are those that eventually lead to the loss of a substantial part of the genome. Any rearrangement that leads to a portion of a chromosome lacking a centromere (an *acentric fragment*) will usually lead to its eventual loss from the cell. This may be seen in a subsequent interphase as a micronucleus. In diploid cells, the formation of

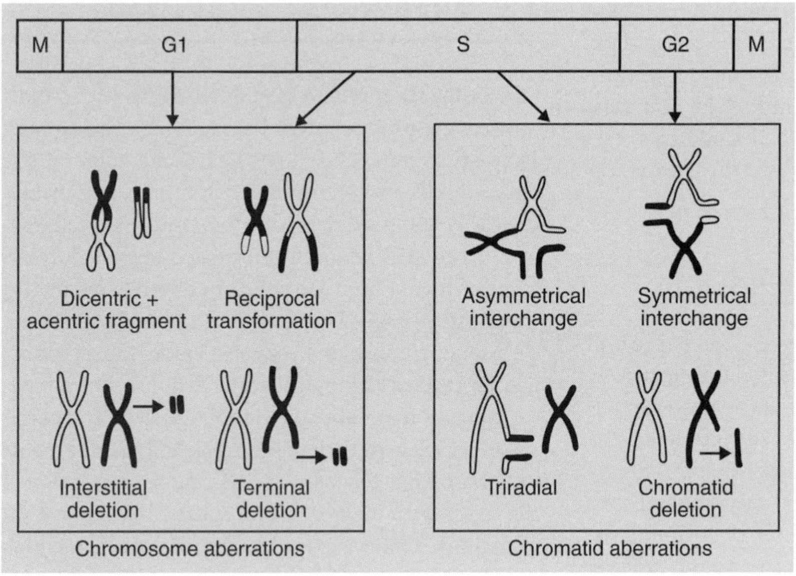

Figure 8.4 *Significant types of radiation-induced chromosome aberration. The cartoons show some of the products of damage to a chromosome, or interaction between two chromosomes (one shown black, the other white). Redrawn from Bedford (1991), with permission.*

a micronucleus signals cell death; in polyploid cells, the presence of multiple copies of chromosomes makes such genetic loss less serious. The significance of this manifestation of chromosomal damage has been exploited in the micronucleus assay for cell survival (see Section 6.4).

The technique of premature chromosome condensation

The morphological signs of chromosome damage are only visible when cells undergo mitosis. Cells irradiated early in the cell cycle take some hours to enter mitosis and therefore the chromosome breaks that are observed are those that have failed to rejoin during this period. However, if an interphase cell is fused with a mitotic cell, it is found that the interphase chromatin undergoes a process of premature chromosome condensation (PCC) in which its chromosomes become visible. The mitotic cell can be of a different cell type and its chromatin can be labelled with BrUdR so that within the binucleate fusion product it is possible to identify the chromosomes of the target cell. This technique enables breaks in chromatin to be scored within 10–15 minutes of irradiation and the speed of their rejoining can also be determined (Cornforth and Bedford, 1983; Bedford, 1991).

Fluorescence *in situ* hybridization (FISH)

The analysis of both chromosome aberrations and PCC has been greatly facilitated by the development of chromosome-specific lengths of DNA (i.e. *probes*) that can be used to identify specific gene sequences. In this technique the chromosomes are spread and fixed on microscope slides, then heated so that much of their DNA becomes single-stranded. The specimens are incubated with labelled probe DNA and the probe binds to those regions of the chromosomal DNA with which it is homologous. The bound probe is detected with a fluorescent ligand that binds to the probe and may be seen under fluorescence microscopy.

The use of FISH has made the individual chromosomes and translocations between chromosomes much easier to identify. It has enabled simple chromosomal rearrangements to be easily recognized and has also led to the identification of highly complex aberrations that were not previously detectable (Sachs *et al.*, 2000b).

When FISH staining for whole chromosomes is applied to *interphase* nuclei, it is found that each chromosome appears as a patch occupying a defined, though irregular, 'domain' within the nucleus (Sachs *et al.*, 2000a). As pointed out above, it is recognized that radiation cell death is closely associated with the loss of large fragments of the genome, in particular with the formation of micronuclei. Micronucleus formation is closely linked to unrejoined or incorrectly rejoined chromosome aberrations. Whether a particular particle traversal through an interphase nucleus can lead to the formation of an aberration joining (say) chromosome N to chromosome M will depend on whether the domains for these two chromosomes overlap at the time of the particle traversal: if they are far apart, the probability will be low; if they are contiguous then such an aberration may result. This area of radiation cytogenetics thus promises to throw new light on the processes leading to cell death.

8.5 MECHANISMS BY WHICH DNA DAMAGE IS 'PROCESSED'

The use of the word 'processed' reflects the current view that damage induced in DNA is modified by a series of enzymatic processes that may lead either to successful repair or to fixation of damage (i.e. *misrepair*). The outcome depends not only on the speed and efficiency of repair but also on the competition between these two processes. The nature of repair processes depends to a large degree on the type of lesion that is being repaired. Where damage involves simply a change in one of the DNA bases, it can be removed by a simple excision-repair process. This involves the nicking of the DNA on either side of the lesion, the removal of a few bases around the point of damage, synthesis of new DNA within the damaged region, and finally ligation of the newly synthesized DNA to the original DNA strand (Figure 8.5). One of these processes, namely nucleotide excision repair, has been well characterized in the repair of damage induced by ultraviolet light. Repair of lesions produced by other agents is based essentially on this scenario but with some variations, as described in Section 9.4.

8.6 CELL DEATH

The amount of chromosome damage observed at the first mitosis after irradiation is perhaps the subcellular end-point that correlates best with cell killing for most cell types. This has encouraged the view that the major cause of cell death after irradiation is physically

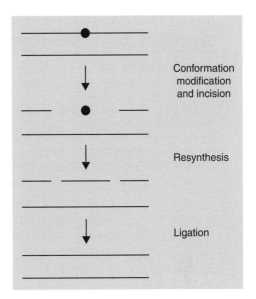

Figure 8.5 *Excision repair of damage in a single strand of DNA. The damage is recognized, the DNA unwound and the DNA strand nicked around the damage site. Following removal of the damaged bases, DNA is resynthesized using the opposite strand as a template and finally the new piece is ligated back into the DNA molecule.*

aberrant mitosis leading to uneven distribution of chromosomes or loss of chromosome fragments. Such large-scale loss of DNA probably leads to metabolic imbalance that is incompatible with further proliferation.

It has been recognized for many years that some irradiated cells do not enter mitosis before they begin to degenerate. Normal and leukaemic lymphocytes die rapidly in what has been called *interphase death* and this leads to the clinical consequences of a rapid fall in cell numbers after drug or radiation treatment. Some instances of interphase cell death are likely to be attributable to the process of *apoptosis*. This is characterized by distinctive morphological features that differ from necrosis (Table 8.3). Apoptosis is important in the embryological development of tissues, where it can truly be described as being a 'programmed' process. In recent years apoptosis has been described and studied in a wide range of normal and neoplastic tissues of adult organisms and it has been hypothesized that here, too, this process may be programmed and therefore potentially controllable for the benefit of cancer therapy. A large number of genes influence the incidence of apoptosis and the associated morphological changes

Table 8.3 *Characteristic features of necrosis and apoptosis*

Necrosis	Apoptosis
Increase in cell volume	Cell shrinkage
Less stainable nucleus	Condensation of chromatin
General DNA degradation	'Laddering' in electrophoresis gels*
Increased plasma membrane permeability	Plasma membrane blebbing
Decline in protein synthesis	Compaction of organelles and nuclear pores

*i.e. endonuclease-mediated DNA digestion producing fragments whose lengths are multiples of a regular unit, derived from cutting in inter-nucleosomal regions.

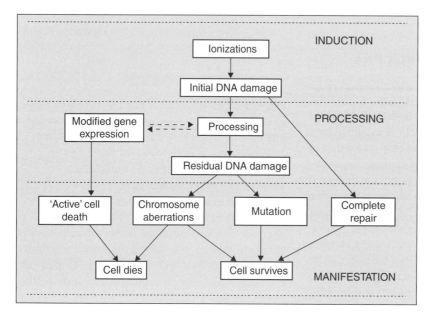

Figure 8.6 *The sequence of processes that take place in cells following exposure to ionizing radiation and which may lead eventually to cell death.*

have been identified in cells that have been treated with a number of different cytotoxic agents. However, the link between the incidence of apoptosis and tumour response is somewhat controversial as it is still not clear whether induction of apoptosis significantly affects the reproductive integrity of cells that otherwise would survive radiation treatment (Steel, 2001).

8.7 THE SEQUENCE OF EVENTS THAT DETERMINES RADIOSENSITIVITY

The complex sequence of processes that follows the initial induction of free-radical damage to DNA and may eventually lead to cell death or mutation are illustrated in Figure 8.6. This sequence may be divided

into three main sections: *induction*, *processing* and *manifestation*, each of which has been described in the foregoing sections of this chapter.

At what point in this sequence is radiosensitivity determined? There is no single answer to this question. Mammalian cells that are more than usually sensitive to ionizing radiation fall into a number of different categories, including:

1. stem cells of certain radiosensitive normal tissues (e.g. lymphocytes, spermatocytes);
2. cells from patients with inherited hypersensitive syndromes (e.g. ataxia telangiectasia, A-T);
3. radiosensitive tumour types (e.g. lymphomas, neuroblastomas);
4. radiosensitive mutants of established cell lines (e.g. *xrs* mutants, L5178Y-S).

There have been great advances in our understanding of the genetic and biochemical basis of some of these sensitivities (see Section 9.5). It is important to recognize that the mechanisms of sensitivity differ both within and between these categories.

Initial DNA damage

The radiosensitivity of mammalian cells may to a considerable extent be determined during the induction phase (Figure 8.6). Radford (1985, 1986) measured initial DNA damage in V79 and other cell lines irradiated under a variety of conditions; the cells were irradiated at 4°C and assayed immediately for DSB, thus preventing enzymatic processing. He found a good correlation between initial damage and cellular radiosensitivity. Whitaker *et al.* (1995) performed a similar study on a range of human tumour cell lines (category 3 above) and the level of damage induction, as detected by pulsed-field gel electrophoresis, was found to relate well to radiosensitivity.

The rate, extent, and fidelity of repair

Many studies have detected a correlation between the rejoining of DNA strand breaks and cell survival. In some cases it is the *speed* of rejoining that appears to be important (Schwartz *et al.*, 1988), in others it is the *residual level* of unrepaired DNA damage. These two parameters may of course be linked. It has also been appreciated that the rejoining of a DSB does not necessarily mean that the function of damaged genes has been restored. Using endonuclease-induced strand breaks in plasmid DNA, it has been possible to probe for the ability of mammalian cells to restore gene function and thus to gain a measure of the *fidelity of repair* of these lesions (Powell and McMillan, 1994). There was evidence that repair fidelity was lower in more radiosensitive human tumour cell lines.

8.8 RECENT DEVELOPMENTS IN THE UNDERSTANDING OF RADIATION CELL KILLING

A number of remarkable developments in radiation biology are adding new dimensions to the long-standing idea that cells die simply because of DSB produced by particle traversals through the cell nucleus.

Chromatin structure

DNA in the cell is associated with a variety of proteins, together making up the chromatin. The nature of DNA–protein interactions may influence both the enzymatic repair of DNA lesions and the chemical modification of the radiation-induced free radicals which do the damage. This has been well characterized following UV irradiation where it has been shown that transcribing regions of DNA are repaired more readily than non-transcribing regions. Indeed, it has also been shown that the transcribing strand may be more repairable than its opposite DNA strand. With ionizing radiation, the primary influence of chromatin structure seems to be at the level of damage induction, where DNA-associated histone proteins have been demonstrated to have a dramatic protective effect against radiation-induced strand breaks.

Membrane structure

It was suggested many years ago by Dr Tikvah Alper that not all the effects of radiation can be explained by a simple direct action on DNA itself. She and others have postulated that damage to cell membranes, perhaps at the point of attachment between DNA and the nuclear membrane, may also be important in some situations. There is also evidence to suggest that radiation-induced effects in the cell membrane can trigger the process of apoptosis.

Inducible responses to irradiation

Bacteria sometimes respond to DNA-damaging agents by increasing the expression of proteins that subsequently promote DNA repair. In mammalian cells there is also evidence for this process of inducible repair. For example, if a mammalian cell is irradiated and then exposed to irradiated virus, the virus may be repaired to a greater degree than if the mammalian cell had not been pre-irradiated (Jeeves and Rainbow, 1979): pre-irradiation appears to have induced the repair of the viral DNA damage. There is increasing evidence for gene activation by exposure to low doses of ionizing radiation. The genes that are switched on are diverse and include those for growth factors such as the fibroblast growth factor (FGF), nuclear signal transducers and natural cytotoxins like tumour necrosis factor (TNF-α). These genes are potentially involved in many biological responses to radiation, including repopulation, fibrosis, repair and, indeed, cell killing (Chapter 9). The process of apoptosis may also be classed as an inducible response.

The significance of these observations for radiation therapy is currently a matter of considerable research interest. It may be that the extraordinary HRS phenomenon seen in some cell systems is associated with repair induction processes (see Section 7.8).

Genomic instability

The principal effects of radiation on cells are seen soon after irradiation as mitotic delay, loss of colony-forming ability and cell death. Recently recognized is the tendency for cells that survive radiation exposure to have a persistently raised level of chromosomal aberrations (Kadhim *et al.*, 1992), which indicates that radiation can produce long-lasting sublethal effects that are manifested as 'genomic instability'. This phenomenon is predominantly seen after high-LET irradiation and it has important implications for the long-term effects of environmental radiation exposure. It may also be linked to the observation that cells irradiated *in vitro* often exhibit a low plating efficiency for many cell generations after irradiation, well beyond the time of initial cell death (Seymour and Mothersill, 1989).

'Bystander' effects

A development that perhaps challenges long-standing dogma more than any other is the suggestion that cells may die or suffer mutation as a result of radiation damage to other adjacent cells, without themselves receiving a particle traversal. This has been called the 'bystander' effect (Mothersill and Seymour, 1988). This idea was originally controversial but in recent years has received considerable support. Nagasawa and Little (1999) irradiated CHO cells with doses of α-particles below 5 cGy and studied the incidence of HPRT mutations. At these doses the number of particle traversals per cell was low (0.05–0.3) and most cells would not be hit directly; the number of cells that suffered mutations was greater that the number of cells that were traversed, and at a dose of around 1 cGy it was greater by a factor of roughly 5. Belyakov *et al.* (2001) employed a charged particle microbeam to irradiate individual primary human fibroblasts with 1–15 helium ions; for every targeted cell they

observed typically 80–100 damaged cells within the culture dish.

These and other similar observations show that radiation biology continues to produce surprises that challenge established dogma.

KEY POINTS

1. Ionizing radiation generates damaging free-radicals throughout the cell. The most significant damage is to DNA, either through direct effects on the molecule itself or indirectly by radicals produced in nearby water molecules.
2. At therapeutic doses of ionizing radiation, free-radical damage produces large numbers of single-strand and double-strand breaks; the vast majority of these are usually repaired satisfactorily. Less repairable are local multiply damaged sites, often known as 'complex lesions'.
3. Three stages of DNA damage: induction, processing, manifestation.
4. DNA damage leads to a variety of chromosome aberrations. Some are 'stable' and are tolerated by the cell; others are 'unstable' and tend to be lethal. Aberrations that lead to the loss at mitosis of a chromosome fragment are particularly lethal.
5. Most cells lethally damaged by radiation die at or around mitosis; some cells die in interphase, perhaps by the process of apoptosis.

BIBLIOGRAPHY

Bedford JS (1991). Sublethal damage, potentially lethal damage, and chromosomal aberrations in mammalian cells exposed to ionising radiations. *Int J Radiat Oncol Biol Phys* 21: 1457–69.

Belyakov OV, Malcolmson AM, Folkard M, Prise KM, Michael BD (2001). Direct evidence for a bystander effect of ionizing radiation in primary human fibroblasts. *Br J Cancer* 84: 674–9.

Chapman JD, Gillespie CJ (1981). Radiation-induced events and their time-scale in mammalian cells. *Adv Radiat Biol* 9: 143–98.

Cornforth MN, Bedford JS (1983). High-resolution measurement of breaks in prematurely condensed chromosomes by differential staining. *Chromosoma (Berlin)* **88**: 315–18.

Frankenburg-Schwager M (1989). Review of repair kinetics for DNA damage induced in eukaryotic cells in vitro by ionising radiation. *Radiother Oncol* **14**: 307–20.

Jeeves WP, Rainbow AJ (1979). Gamma-ray enhanced reactivation of gamma-irradiated adenovirus in human cells. *Biochem Biophys Res Commun* **90**: 567–74.

Kadhim MA, MacDonald DA, Goodhead DT *et al.* (1992). Transmission of chromosomal instability after plutonium α-particle irradiation. *Nature* **355**: 738–40.

Mothersill C, Seymour CB (1988). Cell-cell contact during gamma irradiation is not required to induce a bystander effect in normal human keratinocytes: evidence for release during irradiation of a signal controlling survival into the medium. *Radiat Res* **149**: 256–62.

Nagasawa H, Little JB (1999). Unexpected sensitivity to the induction of mutations by very low doses of alpha-particle irradiation: evidence for a bystander effect. *Radiat Res* **152**: 552–7.

Powell SN, McMillan TJ (1994). The repair fidelity of restriction-enzyme-induced double strand breaks in plasmid DNA correlates with radioresistance in human tumor cell lines. *Int J Rad Oncol Biol Phys* **29**: 1035–40.

Radford IR (1985). The level of induced DNA double-strand breakage correlates with cell killing after X-irradiation. *Int J Radiat Biol* **48**: 45–54.

Radford IR (1986). Evidence for a general relationship between the induced level of DNA double-strand breakage and cell killing after X-irradiation of mammalian cells. *Int J Radiat Biol* **49**: 611–20.

Sachs RK, Levy D, Chen AM *et al.* (2000a). Random breakage and reunion chromosome aberration formation model; an interaction-distance version based on chromosome geometry. *Int J Radiat Biol* **76**: 1579–88.

Sachs RK, Rogoff A, Chen AM *et al.* (2000b). Underprediction of visibly complex chromosome aberrations by a recombinational-repair ('one-hit') model. *Int J Radiat Biol* **76**: 129–48.

Schwartz JL, Rotmensch J, Giovanazzi S *et al.* (1988). Faster repair of DNA double-strand breaks in radioresistant human tumor cells. *Int J Rad Oncol Biol Phys* **15**: 907–12.

Seymour CB, Mothersill C (1989). Lethal mutations, the survival curve shoulder and split-dose recovery. *Int J Radiat Biol* **56**: 999–1010.

Steel GG (2001). The case against apoptosis. *Acta Oncol* **40**: 968–75.

Ward JF (1986). Mechanisms of DNA repair and their potential modification for radiotherapy. *Int J Radiat Oncol Biol Phys* **12**: 1027–32.

Warters RL, Hofer KG, Harris CR, Smith JM (1977). Radionuclide toxicity in cultured mammalian cells: elucidation of the primary site of radiation damage. *Curr Top Radiat Res Q* **12**: 389–407.

Whitaker SJ, Ung YC, McMillan TJ (1995). DNA double strand break induction and rejoining as determinants of human tumour cell radiosensitivity. A pulsed field gel electrophoresis study. *Int J Radiat Biol* **67**: 7–18.

Yandell DW, Dryja TP, Little JB (1990). Molecular genetic analysis of recessive mutations at a heterozygous autosomal locus in human cells. *Mutat Res* **229**: 89–102.

Genetic control of the cellular response to ionizing radiation

TREVOR J McMILLAN AND ADRIAN C BEGG

9.1 INTRODUCTION

Understanding of the pathways that are important in the processing of radiation damage and the genes involved has expanded greatly in recent years. There is great excitement at the depth of knowledge available, in particular on DNA repair and apoptosis, and these areas will undoubtedly have an important role in the future of radiotherapy. The scheme of processes that are known to influence radiosensitivity (see Figure 8.6) points us towards genes that are important to consider in this context. Each stage is controlled by several genes so that the total number of genes that can have an impact on the radiation response is large, although some will have a more significant impact than others.

9.2 DAMAGE INDUCTION

The amount of DNA damage induced by irradiation is markedly influenced by the ability of cells to scavenge the reactive molecules that are produced by free radical processes (see Section 8.1). This in turn is dictated by the activity of a series of enzymes that can catalyse the conversion of reactive species (e.g. glutathione-S-transferases, superoxide dismutases, glutathione peroxidase) and by the presence of thiol-containing compounds that can neutralize these reactive species. Of the enzymes involved, the glutathione-S-transferases are among the most significant since they facilitate the activity of glutathione, which is the most abundant non-protein thiol compound in the cell. Chemical manipulation of glutathione has been shown to alter the extent of DNA damage and also cell survival after irradiation, especially under hypoxic conditions. It is also now clear that the proteins that are intimately associated with DNA, including histones, play a major part in protecting DNA against radiation damage. There is some evidence to suggest that the degree of protection afforded by these proteins can differ between cells but the significance of this is not known.

9.3 CELL-CYCLE CONTROL

Treatment of mammalian cells with ionizing radiation causes delays in the movement of cells through the G1, S and G2 phases of the cell cycle. Early theories suggested that these cell-cycle delays allow time for cells to repair DNA damage, thus making them more resistant than they otherwise would be. While this may still be true to some degree, the relationship between cell-cycle delay and radiosensitivity now appears to be more complex as knowledge about the control of the cell cycle increases.

G1 arrest

The G1 cell-cycle delay depends strongly on the normal function of the tumour suppressor protein p53. This has been most clearly demonstrated with p53-null mice, which lack a G1 delay. These mice are more prone to radiation-induced carcinogenesis than mice with an active *TP53* gene but, as mentioned above, data regarding effects on radiosensitivity are equivocal. At the molecular level, irradiated cells appear to block in G1 because of a damage-induced increase in p53 protein levels, leading to the activation of downstream cell-cycle control proteins, principally the cyclin-dependent kinase inhibitor (CDKI) p21 (alternatively known as sdi-1, CIP-1 or WAF-1). CDKI p21 then interacts with cyclins and cyclin-dependent kinases to block replication. In particular, p21 inhibits the cyclin E/cdk2 complex which has as an important function the phosphorylation of the retinoblastoma protein (Rb). In its unphosphorylated state, Rb binds to the transcription factor E2F, thus preventing it from switching on genes essential for passage into the DNA synthesis phase of the cell cycle. Phosphorylation of Rb releases E2F and this allows S phase to begin so that the inhibition of this by p21 causes the arrest at the G1/S checkpoint (Figure 9.1).

G2 arrest

In yeast cells, the importance of the G2 delay is demonstrated by the isolation of mutants, such as *rad9*, that are defective in their ionizing-radiation-induced G2 delay. Such mutants are radiosensitive and have been shown to be defective in gene products

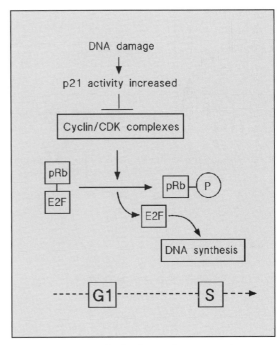

Figure 9.1 *The G1 checkpoint pathway. DNA damage blocks entry into S by preventing release of the transcription factor E2F from pRb. This is mediated by the tumour suppressor protein p53. P denotes a phosphate group.*

involved in the monitoring of DNA damage prior to mitosis. There have been recent advances in our understanding of the G2 delay in mammalian cells. It has been shown that the addition of low levels of caffeine to cells can increase mRNA levels of cyclin-B1 (the coenzyme regulating cdk1 activity), reduce the G2 delay, and sensitize cells to radiation, but the direct relationship between these end-points is unclear. What is clear, however, is that activation of the cyclin-dependent kinase cdk1 by cdc25c triggers the transition to mitosis. Radiation leads to inhibition of cdc25c, blocking cells in G2. Cdc25c inhibition in turn occurs by activating the *chk1* and *chk2* genes by *ATR* and *ATM* respectively (Figure 9.2). The cascade of phosphorylation events caused by the initial DNA damage thus prevents cells entering mitosis.

A noteworthy example of the modification of a G2 delay is the transformation of cells with the oncogenes *H-ras* and *V-myc* (McKenna *et al.*, 1992). Transformation with both oncogenes produces cells that are significantly more radioresistant than their parental cell lines and they show a greater G2 delay

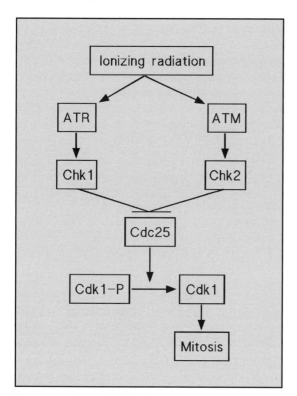

Figure 9.2 *The G2 checkpoint pathway. DNA damage blocks entry into M by preventing activation of* cdk1 *(cdc2). The protein products of the related genes* ATR *and* ATM *phosphorylate the chk1 and chk2 proteins, which in turn inactivate cdc25c, an activating kinase necessary for the G2/M transition.*

after ionizing radiation. The protein products of these oncogenes are important components of signal transduction pathways that control cell growth, and pharmacological manipulation of these pathways (for example, with agents that prevent the critical attachment of Ras protein to the cell membrane) is under investigation. Exactly how such pathways are initiated in response to DNA damage remains to be determined.

Cell-cycle arrest and radiosensitivity

Data in the literature on the relationship between check-points and radiosensitivity are conflicting, but a few conclusions can be drawn. There are several studies reporting either no change or an increased resistance in cell lines in which wild-type *TP53* has

been knocked out or mutated, and in which as a consequence the G1 block has been abolished. This is not consistent with the theory that G1 blocks allow more time to repair, since abolition would then lead to increased sensitivity. Normal human fibroblasts can also become non-clonogenic after irradiation by being permanently arrested in G1, again inconsistent with the 'time for repair' hypothesis. For G2, however, abolishing the block is indeed usually associated with increased sensitivity, and so repair time may therefore play a role here. The link with radiosensitivity thus may differ from one cell-cycle block to another.

9.4 DNA REPAIR

Each of the types of DNA damage induced by radiation is subject to reversal by one of several DNA repair pathways and the major ones are listed in Table 9.1. Of particular significance in determining the toxicity of ionizing radiation are those involved in the repair of DNA double-strand breaks, namely non-homologous end-joining (NHEJ) and homologous recombination repair (HRR). NHEJ has been characterized largely through the study of radiosensitive hamster and mouse cells. As an example, Figure 9.3 shows data on the murine xrs-6 cells; the defect in these cells leads to their being much more radiosensitive than the parent CHO cell line, and the right-hand panel in the figure shows slower and less successful rejoining of double-strand breaks.

Through a combination of gene mapping and gene-transfer methods, the gene defective in xrs-6 cells has been identified as the one encoding the Ku80 subunit of a DNA-dependent kinase (DNA-PK) that binds to the free DNA ends at the site of a DSB (Taccioli *et al.*, 1994). This is illustrated in Figure 9.4, which compares two distinct processes: homologous recombination and non-homologous end joining. In the non-homologous case, defects in two other components of this complex, ku70 and DNA-PKcs, also lead to greatly increased sensitivity to ionizing radiation (Jackson and Jeggo, 1995).

The catalytic subunit of the DNA-PK (DNA-PKcs) only becomes an active kinase, capable of further transmitting the damage signal, after it binds to the ku70/80 complex, which has attached to DNA ends. This kinase subunit is of particular interest

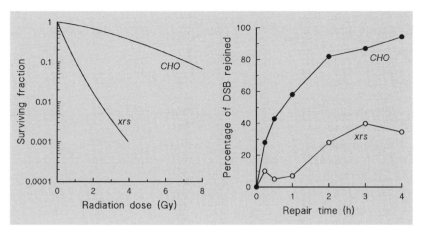

Figure 9.3 *Illustrating the importance of non-homologous end joining. xrs cells deficient in ku80, which forms part of the DNA-PK complex, are highly radiosensitive (left). This is probably caused by their slower and less complete DSB rejoining (right). From Whitaker and McMillan (1992), with permission.*

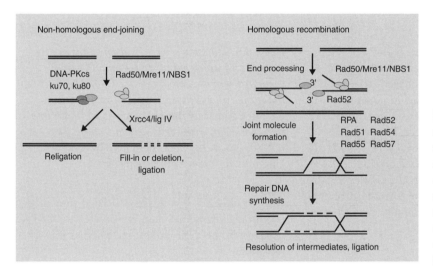

Figure 9.4 *DNA double-strand break repair. Schematic of the two major pathways used in mammalian cells: NHEJ (left) and homologous recombination (right). NHEJ is error-prone, whilst HRR uses a non-damaged homologous template and is therefore error-free.*

because it is the protein that is defective in mice with the 'severe combined immune deficiency' syndrome (SCID). These mice had been recognized as being sensitive to radiation and having a defect in their ability to rejoin radiation-induced DSB. The mode of action of the proteins in the DNA-PK complex is not yet fully elucidated but it is likely that the Ku proteins have an important role in protecting broken DNA ends from attack by nucleases and bringing them physically together for repair. The whole complex may initiate a signal transduction pathway that activates other key enzymes while inhibiting those that would interfere with DNA repair. Another important gene involved in this pathway is *XRCC4*, encoding a protein whose function is to bind to DNA ligase IV and recruit it to the site of the break, enabling ligation

and the completion of repair (Figure 9.4). As with genes involved in the DNA-PK complex, mutation in either *XRCC4* or ligase IV leads to a marked increase in radiosensitivity.

Homologous recombination

Homologous recombination has been recognized in yeast for some time as the most important pathway for repair of double-strand breaks in that organism. However, until recently it has been dismissed as relatively unimportant in mammalian cells. It is now clear that this process, by which a length of DNA of comparable sequence to the damaged molecule can be used as a template for the repair process (Figure 9.4), is also active in mammalian cells. Evidence for this comes from the finding that deficiency in this repair pathway is the basis for increased radiosensitivity in a group of radiosensitive mutant hamster cell lines. In particular, two radiosensitive cell lines, irs-1 and irs-1SF have been shown to be defective in genes *XRCC2* and *XRCC3* respectively, which are members of a family of genes (*recA/rad51*) previously identified as being important in recombination repair in bacteria and yeast. *XRCC3* interacts with the RAD51 protein, aiding pairing and strand transfer with the non-damaged homologous DNA partner. The formation of RAD51 foci in irradiated human nuclei has provided additional evidence for the activity and importance of homologous recombination in the repair of DSB in mammalian cells. The need for an identical DNA template in order for homologous recombination to be accurate means that this repair function is only significant in the S phase of the cell cycle when the replicated strand can provide an intact copy against which the damaged strand can be repaired. This is clearly seen in *XRCC2* and *XRRC3* mutants, which lose the characteristic radioresistance in S phase seen in wild-type cells. Figure 9.5 shows the results of experiments in which the sensitivity of cells through the cell cycle (see Section 6.8) was studied in irs-1 cells and the parent cell line V79; the mutant cells were distinctly more radiosensitive during the period from 3 to 7 hours into the cell cycle that corresponded to the S phase.

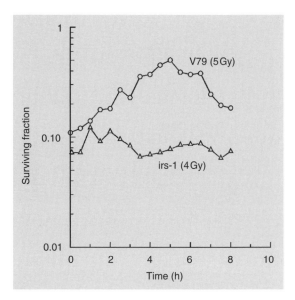

Figure 9.5 *Radiation sensitivity through the cell cycle in irs-1 cells, which have a defective* XRCC2 *gene, compared with the parent cell line (V79). The abscissa shows time after cells were synchronized in mitosis. Increased sensitivity is mainly seen at 3–7 hours into the experiment, where cells were in S phase. XRCC2 is a rad51-helper protein, necessary for HRR. Redrawn from Cheong* et al. *(1994), with permission.*

Base-excision repair

As described in Section 8.2, in addition to double-strand breaks, ionizing radiation also causes single-strand breaks in DNA, either directly or secondarily from oxidative attack. It also induces modification of the DNA bases and loss of bases, producing apurinic or apyrimidinic (AP) sites. Base damage and SSB are thought to be repaired largely by the base-excision repair (BER) pathway. This pathway consists of two sub-pathways called short-patch and long-patch, referring to the number of nucleotides that are replaced during the repair process (1, and up to 10, respectively). Each sub-pathway involves a different set of genes. BER is normally highly efficient and if one pathway or enzyme fails, then others can take over. However, defects in crucial proteins in these pathways can lead to an increase in radiosensitivity. For

example, XRCC1 is a ligase-associated protein that is centrally involved in base-excision repair and cells defective in this gene exhibit increased sensitivity to radiation.

Nucleotide-excision repair

Another major DNA repair pathway is nucleotide-excision repair (NER) (Table 9.1). This is mainly involved in removing bulky lesions from DNA; examples are pyrimidine dimers induced by UV-C irradiation and DNA adducts induced by chemotherapeutic agents such as cisplatin. It does not seem to be involved in repairing damage after ionizing radiation, however, since cells with mutations in genes involved in this pathway are not more radiosensitive. Similar conclusions can be drawn for transcription-coupled repair, a pathway involving efficient removal of lesions such as those caused by UV irradiation, and which does not appear to be involved in ionizing-radiation sensitivity. Mismatch repair is an important pathway for eliminating mutations from base

Table 9.1 *Pathways involved in the repair of DNA damage*

Repair pathway	Type of lesion	Involved in IR sensitivity?
Base excision repair (BER)	Base damage, AP sites, SSB	Yes
Homologous recombination repair (HRR)	DSB	Yes
Non-homologous end rejoining (NHEJ)	DSB	Yes
Nucleotide excision repair (NER)	Dimers, bulky adducts	No?
Transcription-coupled repair (TCR)	Dimers, bulky adducts	No?
Mismatch repair (MMR)	Base mismatches	No?

AP, apurinic/apyrimidinic; DSB, double-strand breaks; IR, ionizing radiation; SSB, single-strand breaks.

mismatches arising from faulty replication or repair, or from chemical base modification. There is little evidence, however, that it plays a significant role in ionizing-radiation damage. It should be noted that most studies have been done in cells that tend not to die by apoptosis, and so in more apoptosis-prone cells the importance of these additional damage types, and hence their associated repair pathways, may be greater.

Overall, research so far emphasizes the importance of the efficiency of DNA repair, in its various forms, in determining whether a cell lives or dies after ionizing radiation.

9.5 RADIOSENSITIVE SYNDROMES

Abnormally severe normal-tissue reactions to radiotherapy are not only a practical problem to the radiotherapist but in those cases where this has a genetic basis they are also of great interest from the point of view of the molecular nature of the underlying genetic abnormality (see Section 22.2).

Ataxia telangiectasia (A-T)

Some patients who show such a response have been identified as exhibiting the traits of specific inherited syndromes. In the case of ataxia telangiectasia (A-T), cells taken from the patient have frequently been found to be more radiosensitive than normal, although there are examples of clinically diagnosed A-T patients whose cells show little or no increased chromosomal damage following treatment with ionizing radiation. A-T is an autosomal recessive syndrome, which presents clinically as oculocutaneous telangiectasia and progressive cerebellar ataxia. Immunodeficiency and a high frequency of

neoplasia are also associated with this disease. A very severe normal-tissue reaction following radiotherapy was the first indication that these patients may have an increased sensitivity to ionizing radiation. This has been confirmed subsequently in the laboratory through experiments on lymphocytes and fibroblasts from A-T patients.

The gene mutated in A-T was found to lie on chromosome 11 (Savitsky *et al.*, 1995). This gene has been called the *ATM* (A-T mutated) gene and it appears to be mutated in members of all A-T complementation groups previously identified on the basis of the abnormal suppression of DNA synthesis. Thus there appears to be only a single A-T gene rather than four as previously thought. Considerable similarity has been found between the predicted amino acid sequence of the ATM protein and a number of other proteins involved, for example, in DNA repair, cell-cycle control and chromosome stability. The picture is thus emerging that the ATM protein is part of signal transduction pathways involved in many physiological processes. Of particular relevance to radiosensitivity are the similarities to cell-cycle-controlling genes, to a gene that can influence apoptosis, and to the catalytic subunit of the DNA-dependent protein kinases (DNA-PKcs), which is part of a protein complex that binds to double-strand breaks in DNA (Section 9.3).

In spite of these valuable clues, the process by which the genetic defect in A-T cells leads to increased radiosensitivity has yet to be identified conclusively. It is known that ATM is a kinase capable of phosphorylating a number of proteins involved in checkpoint responses (p53, MDM2, CHK2, hRAD17), DNA repair (BRCA1, NBS) and others (c-ABL, 53BP1). Consequently, disturbance of cell-cycle checkpoints and DNA repair are both observed in cells that have a defective *ATM* gene. Impaired DSB rejoining, a reduced fidelity of repair leading to an increased incidence of misrepair of DSB, and absence of the usual radiation-induced delay in the entry of cells into and through the S phase of the cell cycle are therefore all believed to play a role in the increased sensitivity of *ATM* mutants.

Nijmegen breakage syndrome (NBS)

This syndrome shows a similar radiosensitive phenotype to A-T. As with *ATM* mutants, cells deficient in the NBS1 protein (also called nibrin) are markedly more sensitive to ionizing radiation. They show checkpoint defects, particularly in G1 and S, and show a diminished and delayed p53 up-regulation after radiation. The NBS1 protein forms a complex with the MRE11 and RAD50 proteins and in doing so it functions to transport the complex to the nucleus. The three-protein complex binds to and processes DNA breaks, probably using the exonuclease activity of MRE11 to 'clean' the ends of DNA breaks in preparation for ligation. It may also have a structural function, stabilizing the DNA ends. The complex is involved in both of the key repair processes for ionizing-radiation damage: NHEJ and HRR (Section 9.4). Although the A-T and NBS syndromes are distinct, the underlying molecular pathways overlap. The ATM kinase can phosphorylate NBS1, apparently a crucial step in DNA repair and radioresistance.

9.6 EPIGENETIC MODULATION OF RADIATION SENSITIVITY

Epigenetic processes are those that alter gene expression without modifying the sequence of bases in DNA. Differentiation, for example, is largely an epigenetic process because it involves the switching on and off of specific genes at given times during cellular development. Within an individual not all cells have the same sensitivity. Bone marrow stem cells, for example, are more radiosensitive than fibroblasts or the stem cells of some epithelia. Little is known about what determines these differences but epigenetic processes no doubt play an important role. Some of the determinants of radiosensitivity in normal cells probably carry over into the neoplastic cells that derive from them, as evidenced by the radiosensitivity of leukaemias and some lymphomas (see Section 17.5).

9.7 INHERITED PREDISPOSITION TO CANCER AND THE CELLULAR RESPONSE TO IONIZING RADIATION

It has been recognized for some years that human syndromes that exhibit abnormal sensitivity to cytotoxic agents sometimes have a predisposition to certain types of cancer. For example, patients with xeroderma pigmentosum, who carry a severe sensitivity to UV light, have a high susceptibility to skin cancers. A-T homozygotes have an increased susceptibility to lymphomas and A-T heterozygotes are also believed to have an increased cancer susceptibility, especially to breast cancer. In some cases a sensitivity to ionizing radiation may be the direct cause of the tumours (Swift, 1994) but it is more likely that the biochemical defect leading to the increased cancer incidence also alters the sensitivity to other exogenous or endogenous carcinogens. Intriguing data relevant to this problem have come from the study of ionizing-radiation-induced chromosome aberrations in cells irradiated in the G2 phase of the cell cycle. It has been reported that even when no abnormal sensitivity to the killing effects of ionizing radiation is known, a large number of cancer-prone syndromes can be detected by this so-called G2 assay (Parshad *et al.*, 1983). These syndromes include xeroderma pigmentosum, Gardner's syndrome and ataxia telangiectasia. Thus the possibility of a close relationship between chromosomal sensitivity to ionizing radiation and cancer predisposition is raised and this deserves considerable experimental attention.

An additional dimension to this topic is the discovery that the two genes primarily associated with familial breast cancer, *BRCA1* and *BRCA2*, have been shown to be associated with key DNA repair pathways. Mouse cells with no functional *BRCA2* are highly radiosensitive, although there is currently only limited evidence of an increased radiosensitivity in cells with only one functional *BRCA1* or *BRCA2* gene. Thus the relevance of these gene mutations for radiotherapy is not yet clear.

9.8 APOPTOSIS

Apoptosis is a mode of radiation-induced cell death which is highly cell-type dependent (see Section 8.6). Cells from the haemopoietic and lymphoid systems are particularly prone to rapid radiation-induced apoptotic cell death. In most tumour cells, mitotic cell death and necrosis are observed at least as frequently as apoptosis. For many radiosensitive normal-tissue cells (e.g. stem cells at the base of the crypts of the small intestine) apoptosis appears to be a major mechanism of cell death whilst other cells, such as the differentiated cells higher in the crypt, do not appear to undergo radiation-induced apoptosis. The high sensitivity of crypt stem cells to apoptosis may be part of an efficient self-screening mechanism against carcinogenesis.

The apoptotic pathway has now been characterized in some detail (Figure 9.6) and there has been much research into its role in the cellular response to DNA damage. Of particular interest is the gene *TP53*, which encodes the tumour suppressor protein, p53. Thymocytes from p53-deficient mice (whose cells have no functional copy of *TP53*) do not undergo apoptosis after treatment with ionizing radiation, unlike those from mice with normal p53. Thus apoptosis after ionizing radiation seems commonly to be a p53-dependent process. Consistent with this is a small increase in radioresistance in fibroblasts in which the p53 protein has been made non-functional; however, this is not a totally general finding and the

association between p53 status, apoptosis and radiosensitivity still requires clarification. Whilst it is clear that apoptosis is an important mode of cell death after irradiation of some cell types, there is still debate as to whether in other systems it may simply be a description of the way a cell dies rather than a significant determinant of whether it dies. Evidence from mouse tumour systems suggests that in contrast to other forms of rapid apoptosis, apoptosis after ionizing radiation can be delayed, occurring beyond 24–48 hours. In some cases apoptosis can even be a post-mitotic event (i.e. occurring in the next cell cycle) and this makes the distinction between apoptotic and mitotic cell death conceptually difficult. In some experimental cell systems it has been suggested that it is the timing of apoptosis that is the critical factor in radiosensitivity, with sensitive cells showing earlier evidence of apoptosis than resistant cells. Genetic manipulation of the susceptibility of cells to undergo apoptosis may not necessarily affect the ultimate clonogenic potential of the cells (Aldridge *et al.*, 1995). A review by Brown and Wouters (1999) demonstrated in mouse tumours *in vivo* that the level of apoptosis can affect the level of initial tumour regression but that the long-term effect on tumour growth may be unaffected. This review also cited data on pairs of genetically identical cell lines, one of which was transfected with a gene (*p21*) which markedly altered apoptosis induction; the two cell lines showed almost identical sensitivity to radiation, etoposide, or tirapazamine, as detected by a clonogenic assay (Figure 9.7).

The impact of apoptosis on tumour response is complex and needs careful evaluation. It should be noted that poor correlation between apoptosis and clonogenic cell survival amongst different cell lines does not necessarily invalidate attempts to increase clonogenic kill by increasing apoptosis for a particular cell type. So far, however, such attempts have met with mixed success, and whether this proves to be therapeutically useful remains to be seen.

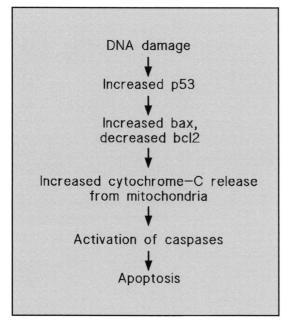

Figure 9.6 *Schematic of an apoptotic pathway after DNA damage, showing involvement of mitochondria and caspases.*

9.9 THERAPEUTIC EXPLOITATION

Knowledge of the molecular basis of sensitivity to ionizing radiation is not only of theoretical interest: it can and probably will lead to the identification of critical targets for designing drugs or other interventions

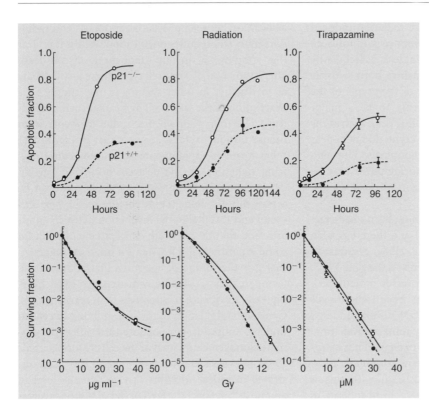

Figure 9.7 *Comparison of apoptosis induction and colony formation in p21^WAF1 knockout and wild-type murine fibroblasts. Lack of p21^WAF1 leads to increased apoptosis induction by three different cytotoxic agents (top row), but little or no difference in colony-forming ability (bottom row). From Brown and Wouters (1999).*

for increasing the radiosensitivity of tumour cells or for reducing the sensitivity of critical normal tissues. This will require detailed knowledge of pathways that are defective in the various cancer types, and preferably in individual tumours, in order to design optimum intervention schedules.

KEY POINTS

1. Genetic factors determine radiosensitivity through effects on damage induction, cell-cycle checkpoints and DNA repair.
2. Cells respond to ionizing radiation by interrupting cell-cycle progression at one or more checkpoints. These can occur in all phases of the cell cycle; when they occur they allow increased time for repair but if repair is insufficient, permanent blocks can also result. Abolishing the G1 block has different effects

in different cell types, but is often associated with increased radioresistance, while abolishing the G2 block often leads to increased radiosensitivity.

3. G1/S checkpoint genes include *TP53*, *p21* cyclins D1 and E, and *Rb*. G2/M checkpoint genes include cyclin B1, *cdk1*, *chk1*, *chk2*, *cdc25c*.
4. Several DNA repair pathways exist for handling the various types of damage that occur. For ionizing-radiation-induced damage, important pathways are those for repairing base damage and single-strand breaks (BER), and double-strand breaks (HRR, NHEJ). Defects in the NHEJ pathway lead to the greatest increases in radiosensitivity. HRR is important for repair occurring mainly in the S and G2 phases and is a primary cause of late-S resistance, whereas NHEJ is important in all cell-cycle phases.
5. Cells from patients with the A-T and NBS syndromes are highly radiosensitive and have

led to the discovery of the *ATM* and *NBS1/nibrin* genes, which operate in overlapping pathways. Mutations in either gene leads to defects in both checkpoints and DNA repair, although the DNA repair defects are the most likely cause of the increased radiosensitivity.

6. Cells can die by apoptosis after irradiation but apoptosis is only one of several modes of cell death. The correlation between apoptosis and clonogenic survival is generally poor, except for a few cell types including those of lymphoid origin.

7. Greater knowledge of the genes and pathways that determine radiosensitivity should lead to the identification of targets for therapeutic exploitation.

BIBLIOGRAPHY

Aldridge DR, Arends MJ, Radford IR (1995). Increasing the susceptibility of the rat 208F fibroblast cell line to radiation-induced apoptosis does not alter its clonogenic survival dose-response. *Br J Cancer* **71**: 571–7.

Brown JM, Wouters BG (1999). Apoptosis, p53 and tumour cell sensitivity to anticancer agents. *Cancer Res* **59**: 1391–9.

Cheong N, Wang X, Wang Y, Iliakis G (1994). Loss of S-phase-dependent radioresistance in irs-1 cells exposed to X-rays. *Mutat Res* **314**: 77–85.

Jackson SP, Jeggo PA (1995). DNA double-strand break repair and V(D)J recombination: involvement of DNA-PK. *TIBS* **20**: 412–15.

McKenna WG, Iliakis G, Muschel RJ (1992). Mechanism of radioresistance in oncogene transfected cell lines. In: *Radiation Research: A Twentieth Century Perspective* (eds Dewey WC, Eddington M, Fry RJM, Hall EJ, Whitmore GF), pp. 392–7. Academic Press, San Diego.

Parshad R, Sanford KK, Jones CM (1983). Chromatid damage after G2 phase X-irradiation of cells from cancer prone individuals implicates deficiency in DNA repair. *Proc Natl Acad Sci USA* **80**: 5612–16.

Savitsky K, Bar-Shira A, Gilad S *et al.* (1995). A single ataxia telangiectasia gene with a product similar to PI-3 kinase. *Science* **268**: 1749–53.

Swift M (1994). Ionizing radiation, breast cancer and ataxia-telangiectasia. *J Natl Cancer Inst* **21**: 1571–2.

Taccioli CE, Cottlieb TM, Blunt T *et al.* (1994). Ku8O: product of the XRCCS gene and its role in DNA repair and V(D)J recombination. *Science* **265**: 1442–5.

Whitaker SJ, McMillan TJ (1992). Pulsed-field gel electrophoresis in the measurement of DNA double-strand break repair in xrs-6 and CHO cell lines: DNA degradation under some conditions interferes with the assessment of double-strand break rejoining. *Radiat Res* **130**: 389–92.

FURTHER READING

Friedberg EC (1995). *DNA Repair and Mutagenesis.* ASM Press, Washington.

10

Dose–response relationships in radiotherapy

SØREN M BENTZEN

10.1 INTRODUCTION

Clinical radiobiology is concerned with the relationship between a given physical absorbed dose and the resulting biological response, also with factors that influence this relationship. The term tolerance is frequently misused when discussing radiotherapy toxicity and it is important to realize that there is no dose below which the complication rate is zero: there is no clear-cut limit of tolerance. What is seen in clinical practice is a broad range of doses where the risk of a specific type of radiation reaction increases from 0% towards 100% with increasing dose, i.e. a dose–response relationship.

An *end-point* is a specific event that may or may not have occurred at a given time after irradiation. The idea of dose–response is almost built into our definition of a radiation end-point: to classify a specific biological phenomenon as a radiation effect we would require that this phenomenon be never or rarely seen after zero dose and seen in nearly all cases

after very high doses. The concept of dose–response relationships was introduced in Section 1.5 and various ways to characterize normal-tissue end-points are discussed in Chapter 11.

With increasing radiation dose, radiation effects may increase in severity (i.e. grade), in frequency (i.e. incidence) or both. A plot of, say, stimulated growth hormone secretion after graded doses of cranial irradiation in children may reveal dose-dependence: an example of *severity* increasing with dose. Here we concentrate on the other type of dose–response relationship: a *dose–incidence* curve. In that example we can obtain a dose–incidence curve by plotting the proportion of children with growth hormone secretion below a certain threshold as a function of dose. Thus, the dependent variable in a dose–response plot is an *incidence* or a probability of response as a function of dose (Figure 10.1).

This chapter introduces some key concepts in the quantitative description of dose–response relationships. Many of these ideas are important in

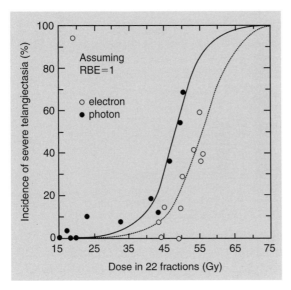

Figure 10.1 *Examples of dose–response relationships in clinical radiotherapy. Data are shown on the incidence of severe telangiectasia following electron or photon irradiation. From Bentzen and Overgaard (1991), with permission.*

understanding the general principles of radiotherapy. Furthermore, they form the basis of most of the more theoretical considerations in radiotherapy. Mathematics will be kept to a minimum but a few formulae are needed to substantiate the presentation.

Empirical attempts to establish dose–response relationships in the clinic date back to the first decade of radiotherapy. In 1936, the great clinical scientist Holthusen was the first to present a theoretical analysis of dose–response relationships and this had a major impact on the conceptual development of radiotherapy optimization (see Section 11.1). Holthusen demonstrated the sigmoid shape of dose–response curves both for normal-tissue reactions (i.e. skin telangiectasia) and local control of skin cancer. He noted the resemblance between these curves and the cumulative distribution functions known from statistics, and this led him to the idea that the dose–response curve simply reflected the variability in clinical radioresponsiveness of individual patients. This remains one of the main hypotheses for the origin of dose–response relationships and this idea has had a renaissance in recent years with the growing interest in patient-to-patient variability in response to radiotherapy.

10.2 SHAPE OF THE DOSE–RESPONSE CURVE

Radiation dose–response curves have a sigmoid (i.e. S) shape, with the incidence of radiation effects tending to zero as dose tends to zero and tending to 100% at very large doses. Many mathematical functions could be devised with these properties, but three standard formulations are used: the *Poisson*, the *logistic* and the *probit* dose–response models (Bentzen and Tucker, 1997). The first two are the most frequently used and this chapter concentrates on these. In principle, it is an empirical problem to decide whether one model fits observed data better than another. In reality, both clinical and experimental dose–response data are too noisy to allow statistical discrimination between these models, and in most cases they will give very similar fits to a data set. The situation where major discrepancies may arise is when these models are used for extrapolation of experience over a wide range of dose (Bentzen and Tucker, 1997).

The Poisson dose–response model

Munro and Gilbert published a landmark paper in 1961 in which they formulated the target-cell hypothesis of tumour control: 'The object of treating a tumour by radiotherapy is to damage every single potentially malignant cell to such an extent that it cannot continue to proliferate.' From this idea and the random nature of cell killing by radiation they derived a mathematical formula for the probability of tumour cure after irradiation of 'a number of tumours each composed of N identical cells'. More precisely, they showed that this probability depends only on the *average* number of clonogens surviving per tumour.

Figure 10.2 shows a Monte Carlo (i.e. random number) simulation of the number of surviving clonogens per tumour in a hypothetical sample of 100 tumours with an average number of 0.5 surviving clonogens per tumour. In the left-hand panel each tumour is represented by one of the squares in which the value indicates the actual number of surviving clonogens, these numbers having been generated at random. The cured tumours are those with zero surviving clonogens. In this simulation, there were 62 cured tumours. The relative frequencies of

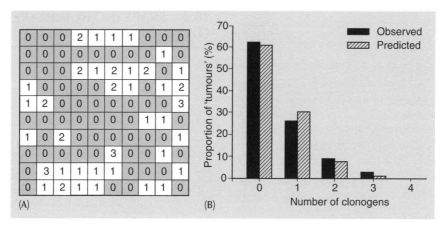

Figure 10.2 *Simulation of a Poisson distribution. (A) The number of clonogens surviving per tumour in a hypothetical sample of 100 tumours. The average number was 0.5 surviving clonogens/tumour. The histogram (B) shows the proportion of tumours with a given number of surviving clonogens (black bars) and this is compared with the prediction from a Poisson distribution with the same average number of surviving clonogens (hatched bars).*

tumours with 0, 1, 2, … surviving clonogens follow closely a statistical distribution known as the Poisson distribution, as shown in the right-hand panel. Many processes involving the counting of random events are (approximately) Poisson distributed: for example, the number of decaying atoms per second in a radioactive sample or the number of tumour cells forming colonies in a Petri dish.

When describing tumour cure probability (TCP), it is the probability of zero surviving clonogens in a tumour that is of interest. This is the zero-order term of the Poisson distribution and if λ denotes the average number of clonogens per tumour after irradiation this is simply

$$TCP = e^{-\lambda} \qquad (10.1)$$

Munro and Gilbert went one step further: they assumed that the average number of surviving clonogenic cells per tumour was a (negative) exponential function of dose. Under these assumptions they obtained the characteristic sigmoid dose–response curve (Figure 10.3). Thus the shape of this curve could be explained solely from the random nature of cell killing (or clonogen survival) after irradiation: there was no need to assume variability of sensitivity between tumours.

The Poisson dose–response model derived by Munro and Gilbert has had a strong influence on theoretical radiobiology. The simple exponential dose-survival curve was later replaced by the linear-quadratic model (see Section 7.5) and thus we arrive

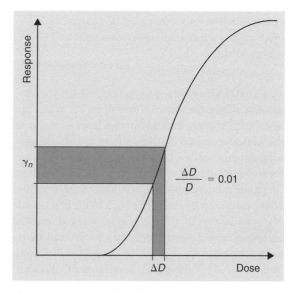

Figure 10.3 *Geometrical interpretation of γ. A 1% dose increment (ΔD) from a reference dose D yields an increase in response equal to γ percentage points. From Bentzen (1994), with permission.*

at what could be called the standard model of tumour control:

$$TCP = \exp[-N_0 \cdot \exp(-\alpha D - \beta dD)] \qquad (10.2)$$

Here, N_0 is the number of clonogens per tumour before irradiation and the second exponential is simply the surviving fraction after a dose D given with dose per fraction d according to the linear-quadratic model. Thus when we multiply these two quantities we obtain the (average) number of surviving clonogens per tumour and this is inserted into the Poisson expression in Eqn 10.1. N_0 can easily be expressed as a function of tumour volume and the clonogenic cell density (i.e. clonogens per cm^3 of tumour tissue) and similarly it is easy to introduce exponential growth into this model, with or without a lag time before accelerated repopulation begins (Bentzen *et al.*, 1991). The immediate attraction of the Poisson model is that the model parameters appear to have a biological or mechanistic interpretation. It turns out, however, that these parameter estimates will be influenced by biological and dosimetric heterogeneity and cannot usually be regarded as realistic measures of some intrinsic biological property of the tumour (Bentzen *et al.*, 1991; Bentzen, 1992).

The mechanistic interpretation of the Poisson model is most obvious when modelling tumour dose–response relationships. For most normal-tissue end-points, the biological interpretation of N_0 is not clear. Hendry and Thames (1986) have suggested that the Poisson dose–response model could describe the survival of some hypothetical tissue rescuing units (TRU) and N_0 would then be the initial number of TRU per volume of normal tissue. However, the biological reality of the TRU is questionable in many organs and tissues, and a mechanistic interpretation of the fitted dose–response parameters may therefore be misleading.

The logistic dose–response model

The logistic model is often introduced and used with more pragmatism than the Poisson model. This model has no simple mechanistic background and consequently the estimated parameters have no simple biological interpretation. Yet it is a convenient and flexible tool for estimating response probabilities after various exposures and is widely used in areas of biology other than radiobiology. The idea of the model is to write the probability of an event as:

$$P = \frac{\exp(u)}{1 + \exp(u)} \qquad (10.3)$$

where, when analysing data from fractionated radiotherapy, u has the form

$$u = a_0 + a_1 \cdot D + a_2 \cdot D \cdot d + \cdots \qquad (10.4)$$

Here, D is total dose and d is dose per fraction, and the representation of the effect of dose-fractionation in this way is of course reflecting the assumption of a linear-quadratic relationship between dose and effect. Additional terms, representing other patient or treatment characteristics, may be included in the model to see if they have a significant influence on the probability of effect. The coefficients $a_0, a_1, \ldots$ are estimated by *logistic regression*, a method that is available in many standard statistical software packages. The parameters a_1 and a_2 play a role similar to the coefficients α and β of the linear-quadratic model. But note that the mechanistic interpretation is not valid: a_1 is not an estimate of α and a_2 is not an estimate of β. What is preserved is the ratio a_1/a_2, which is an estimate of α/β.

Rearrangement of Eqn 10.3 yields the expression

$$u = \ln\left(\frac{P}{1 - P}\right) \qquad (10.5)$$

The ratio of P to $(1 - P)$ is called the *odds* of a response, and the natural logarithm of this is called the *logit* of P. Therefore, logistic regression is sometimes called logit analysis.

10.3 POSITION OF THE DOSE–RESPONSE CURVE

Several descriptors are used for the position of the dose–response curve on the radiation dose scale. They all have the unit of dose (Gy) and they specify the dose required for a given level of tumour control or normal-tissue complications. For tumours, the most frequently used position parameter is the TCD_{50}, i.e. the radiation dose for 50% tumour control. For normal-tissue reactions, the analogous parameter is the radiation dose for 50% response (RD_{50}) or in case of rare (severe) complications RD_5, that is the dose producing a 5% incidence of complications.

10.4 QUANTIFYING THE STEEPNESS OF DOSE–RESPONSE CURVES

The most convenient way to quantify the steepness of the dose–response curve is by means of the 'γ-value' or, more precisely, the *normalized dose–response gradient* (Brahme, 1984; Bentzen and Tucker, 1997). This measure has a very simple interpretation, namely the increase in response in percentage points for a 1% increase in dose. (Note: an increase in response from, say, 10% to 15% is an increase of 5 percentage points, but a 50% *relative* increase.) Figure 10.3 illustrates the definition of γ geometrically.

A more precise definition of γ requires a little mathematics. Let $P(D)$ denote the response as a function of dose, D, and ΔD a small increment in dose, then the 'loose definition' above may be written

$$\gamma \approx \frac{P(D + \Delta D) - P(D)}{(\Delta D/D) \cdot 100\%} \cdot 100\%$$

$$= D \cdot \frac{P(D + \Delta D) - P(D)}{\Delta D} = D \cdot \frac{\Delta P}{\Delta D} \quad (10.6)$$

The second term on the right-hand side is recognized as a difference-quotient, and in the limit where ΔD tends to zero we arrive at the formal definition of γ:

$$\gamma = D \cdot P'(D) \quad (10.7)$$

where $P'(D)$ is the derivative of $P(D)$ with respect to dose.

If we look at the right-hand side of Eqn 10.6, we arrive at the approximate relationship

$$\Delta P \approx \gamma \cdot \frac{\Delta D}{D} \quad (10.8)$$

In other words, γ is a multiplier that converts a *relative* change in dose into an (*absolute*) change in response probability. Most often we insert the relative change in dose in per cent and in that case P is the (approximate) change in response rate in percentage points. This relationship is very useful in practical calculations (see Section 13.9). For example, increasing the dose from 64 to 66 Gy in a schedule employing 2 Gy dose per fraction corresponds to a 3.1% increase in dose. If we assume that the γ-value is 1.8, this yields an estimated improvement in local control of $1.8 \times 3.1 \approx 5.6$ percentage points.

Mathematically, Eqn 10.8 corresponds to approximating the S-shaped dose–response curve by a straight line (actually the tangent of the dose–response curve). As discussed briefly below, this will only be a good approximation over a relatively narrow range of doses; exactly how narrow depends on the response level and the steepness of the dose-response curve.

Clearly, the value of γ depends on the response level at which it is evaluated: at the bottom or top of the dose-response curve a 1% increase in dose will produce a smaller increment in response than on the steep part of the curve. This local value of γ is typically written with an index indicating the response level, for example γ_{50} refers to the γ-value at a 50% response level. A compact and convenient way to report the steepness of a dose–response curve is by stating the γ-value at the level of response where the curve attains its maximum steepness: at the 37% response level for the Poisson curve and at the 50% response level for the logistic model. From this single value and a measure of the position of the dose–response curve, the whole mathematical form of the dose–response relationship is specified (Bentzen and Tucker, 1997). The steepness at any other dose or response level can then be calculated.

Table 10.1 shows how the γ-value varies with the response level for logistic dose–response curves of varying steepness. Using this table, it is possible to estimate the relevant γ-value at, say, a 20% response level for a curve where the γ_{50} is specified. The table also provides a useful impression of the range of response (or dose) where the simple linear approximation in Eqn 10.8 will be reasonably accurate. Clearly, if we

Table 10.1 *γ-values as a function of the response level for logistic dose–response curves of varying steepness*

γ_{50}	Response level (%)								
	10	20	30	40	50	60	70	80	90
1	0.2	0.4	0.7	0.9	1.0	1.1	1.0	0.9	0.6
2	0.5	1.1	1.5	1.8	2.0	2.0	1.9	1.5	0.9
3	0.9	1.7	2.3	2.8	3.0	3.0	2.7	2.1	1.3
4	1.2	2.3	3.2	3.7	4.0	3.9	3.5	2.8	1.6
5	1.6	3.0	4.0	4.7	5.0	4.9	4.4	3.4	2.0

Note how the γ-values decrease as we move away from a point close to the 50% response level.

extrapolate between two response levels where the γ-value has changed markedly, the approximation of assuming a fixed value for γ will not be very precise.

10.5 CLINICAL ESTIMATES OF THE STEEPNESS OF DOSE–RESPONSE CURVES

Several clinical studies have found evidence for a significant dose–response relationship and have provided data allowing an estimation of their steepness. Clinical dose–response curves generally originate from studies where the dose has been changed while keeping either the *dose per fraction* or the *number of fractions* fixed. A further advantage of tabulating the γ-value at the steepest point of the dose–response curve is that this value is independent of the dose-fractionation details in the case of a dose–response curve generated using a fixed dose per fraction (Bentzen, 1994; Brahme, 1984). Figure 10.4 shows estimates of γ_{37} for head and neck tumours estimated under the assumption of a fixed dose per fraction (Bentzen, 1994). Typical values range from 1.5 to 2.5. This means that around the midpoint of the dose–response curve, for each percentage increment in dose, the probability of controlling a head and neck tumour will increase by roughly two percentage points. Steepness estimates from dose–response curves for other tumour histologies have recently been reviewed (Okunieff *et al.*, 1995) but it should be noted that data for other histologies are generally more sparse than for the head and neck tumours. Also, some estimated values are obviously outliers that cannot be taken as a serious estimate of the steepness of the clinical dose–response curve. These extreme values may have arisen as a result of patient selection bias or errors in dosimetry.

In the absence of other sources of variation, the maximum steepness of a tumour control curve is determined by the Poisson statistics of survival of clonogenic cells (Figure 10.2); the Poisson process by itself gives a limiting steepness value of $\gamma_{37} \approx 7$ (Suit *et al.*, 1992). Even in transplantable mouse tumour models under highly controlled experimental conditions, values as high as this are not achieved (Khalil *et al.*, 1997). The principal reason why dose–response curves in the laboratory and in the clinic are shallower than this theoretical limit is dosimetric and biological heterogeneity. The tendency for vocal cord tumours to have γ_{37} values at the upper end of the interval seen for other head and neck subsites (Figure 10.4) probably reflects the relatively lower heterogeneity among laryngeal carcinomas treated with radiotherapy. Other patient and treatment characteristics will influence both the position and the steepness of the dose–response curve. It can be shown (Brahme, 1984) that the γ_{37} of a Poisson dose–response curve for a fixed dose per fraction depends only on the number of clonogens that have to be sterilized to cure the tumour. As mentioned in Section 10.2, many tumour and treatment variables, for example tumour volume and overall treatment time, are thought to affect the (effective) number of clonogens to be sterilized. Therefore, in a multivariate analysis, γ_{37} will depend on all the significant patient and treatment characteristics.

Figure 10.5 shows a selection of γ_{50} values for normal-tissue end-points. Estimates are given both for treatment with a fixed dose per fraction and, where possible, also for treatment in a fixed number of fractions, namely 22. The estimates in the latter situation are considerably higher, which is as expected from the linear-quadratic model. The explanation is that when treating with a fixed number of fractions, increasing the dose leads to a simultaneous increase in *dose per fraction*, and this is associated with an increased

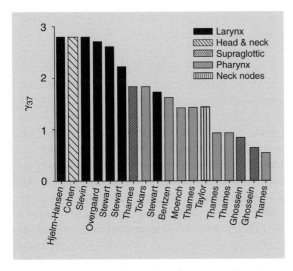

Figure 10.4 *Estimated γ_{37} values from a number of studies on dose–response relationships for squamous cell carcinoma in various sites of the head and neck. From Bentzen (1994), where the original references may be found.*

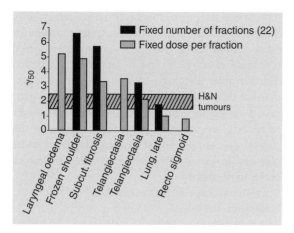

Figure 10.5 *Estimated γ_{50} values for various late normal-tissue end-points. Estimates are shown for treatment with a fixed dose per fraction and a fixed number of fractions. The shaded horizontal band corresponds to the typical γ-values at the point of maximum steepness for dose-response curves in head and neck tumours. Compare with Figure 10.4. Data from Bentzen (1994) and Bentzen and Overgaard (1996), where the original references may be found.*

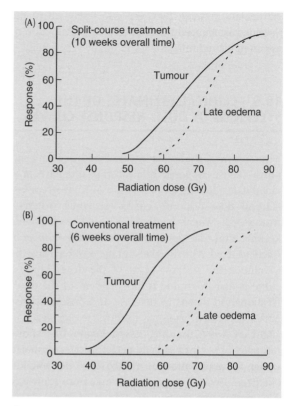

Figure 10.6 *Dose–response curves for local control of laryngeal carcinoma (full line) and late laryngeal oedema as estimated from the data by Overgaard et al. (1988). Protraction of overall treatment time narrowed the therapeutic window. From Bentzen and Overgaard (1996), with permission.*

biological effect per Gy. This is a manifestation of the '*double trouble*' phenomenon discussed in Section 13.10.

Figure 10.5 shows a spectrum of γ_{50} values for the various normal-tissue end-points. The dose–response curves for many late end-points are steeper than for head and neck cancer. An exception is rectosigmoid complications after combined external-beam and intracavitary brachytherapy where considerable dose–volume heterogeneity is present due to the steep gradients in the dose-distribution from the intracavitary sources. Also, the lung data arise from a treatment technique where the dose to the lung tissue was heterogeneous. Thus it is likely that dosimetric rather than intrinsic biological factors are the main cause of the relatively low steepness seen for these end-points.

10.6   THE THERAPEUTIC WINDOW

As with any other medical procedure, prescription of a course of radiotherapy must represent a balance between risks and benefits (see Section 1.6). The relative position and shape of the dose–response

curves for tumour control and a given radiotherapy complication determine the possibility of delivering a sufficient dose with an acceptable level of side-effects. This was nicely illustrated by Holthusen, who plotted dose–response curves for tumour control and complications in the same co-ordinate system for two hypothetical situations: one favourable, that is with a wide therapeutic window between the two curves, and the other one less favourable. Figure 10.6 shows an example of how changing treatment parameters may affect the therapeutic window. For split-course treatment (panel A) the tumour and oedema curves are closer together than for conventional treatment, and the therapeutic window is therefore narrower than in the absence of a gap. In practice, there will be several sequelae of clinical concern and each of these will have its characteristic dose–response curve and will respond differently to treatment modifications. This complicates the simple strategy for optimization suggested by Figure 10.6.

Several parameters are found in the literature for quantifying the effect of treatment modifications on the therapeutic window. Holthusen's proposal was to calculate the probability of uncomplicated cure, and this is still used frequently in the literature. The difficulty with this measure is that it gives equal weight to the complication in question and to tumour recurrence, which may often be fatal, and this is against common sense. A simple alternative, which is easy to interpret, is to specify the tumour control probability at isotoxicity with respect to a specific end-point, as illustrated in Figure 1.3.

10.7 METHODOLOGICAL PROBLEMS IN ESTIMATING DOSE–RESPONSE RELATIONSHIPS FROM CLINICAL DATA

An increasing number of publications are concerned with the quantitative analysis of clinical radiobiological data. Many methodological problems must be addressed in such a study and these may roughly be grouped as clinical, dosimetric and statistical.

Clinical aspects include the evaluation of well-defined end-points for tumour and normal-tissue effects. End-points requiring prolonged observation of the patients, such as local tumour control or late complications, should be analysed using actuarial statistical methods. Special concerns exist for evaluation, grading and reporting of normal-tissue injury and these are discussed in some detail in Chapter 11. For dose–response data obtained from non-randomized studies, the reasons for variability in dose should be carefully considered. Subsets of patients treated with low/high doses may not be comparable in terms of other patient characteristics influencing the outcome. An example is where patients receive a lower total dose than prescribed because of their poor general condition, severe early reactions, or because of progressive disease during treatment.

Dosimetric aspects involve a detailed account of treatment technique and the quality assurance procedures employed. Furthermore, the identification of biologically relevant dosimetric reference points and a proper evaluation of the doses to these points are required.

Statistical aspects include the choice of valid statistical methods that are appropriate for the data type in question and which use the available information in an optimal way. Statistical tests for significance or, preferably, confidence limits on estimated parameters should be specified. When negative findings are reported, an assessment of the statistical power of the study should be given. Finally, the censoring (i.e. incomplete follow-up) and latency should be allowed for.

For an overview of the quantitative analysis of clinical data, see Bentzen *et al.* (1988).

10.8 CLINICAL IMPLICATIONS: MODIFYING THE STEEPNESS OF DOSE–RESPONSE CURVES

The γ-value is not only useful as a multiplier in converting from a dose change to a change in response but may also be used as a multiplier for converting an *uncertainty* in dose into an *uncertainty* in response. If the standard deviation of the absorbed-dose distribution in a population of patients is $\pm 5\%$, a γ-value of 3 would yield an estimated $\pm 15\%$ standard deviation on the response-probability distribution. Note that in this situation it is generally the γ for a fixed *number of fractions* that applies. Figure 10.5 shows that the high γ-values at the maximum steepness of the dose–response curve for normal tissues would yield a large variability in response probability for a $\pm 5\%$ variability in absorbed dose. This provides an indication of the precision required in treatment planning and delivery in radiotherapy.

Another field where the steepness of the dose–response curves for tumours and normal-tissue reactions plays a crucial role is in the design of clinical trials. For a discussion of this topic see Bentzen (1994).

A final issue in this chapter is the prospect for modifying the steepness of the clinical dose–response curve. Several authors have shown that patient-to-patient variability in tumour biological parameters could strongly affect the steepness of the dose–response curve (Bentzen *et al.*, 1990; Bentzen, 1992; Suit *et al.*, 1992; Webb and Nahum, 1993). Compelling support for this idea also comes from experimental studies (Khalil *et al.*, 1997). A direct illustration of the effect of interpatient variability is obtained from an analysis of local tumour control in patients with oropharyngeal cancers (Bentzen, 1992). Analysing the data with the Poisson model yielded $\gamma_{37} = 1.8$. An analysis taking an assumed variability in tumour cell radiosensitivity into account allowed the dose–response curve to be broken down into a series of very steep curves, each of which would apply to a subpopulation of patients stratified according to intrinsic radiosensitivity (Figure 10.7).

This interpatient variability also has a major influence on the parameter estimates in the Poisson model (Bentzen, 1992). Fenwick (1998) has proposed a closed form expression of the Poisson dose–response model that takes patient-to-patient variability explicitly into account, but this approach has so far only been used in few analyses.

Viewing the curves of Figure 10.7 in relation to Figure 10.6, it is clear that some of these subgroups could be expected to have a greater therapeutic window than others. If, by means of a reliable predictive assay, the subgroups could be identified prior to starting therapy, a substantial therapeutic benefit could be realized.

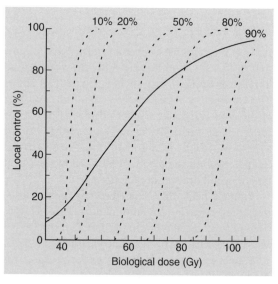

Figure 10.7 *Local control of oropharyngeal carcinoma as a function of the biological dose in 2 Gy fractions. Dotted lines are theoretical dose–response curves after stratification for intrinsic radiosensitivity. These represent dose–response relationships from five homogeneous patient populations with radiosensitivity equal to selected percentiles of the radiosensitivity distribution in the total population. From Bentzen (1994), with permission.*

10.9 NTCP MODELS

Several dose–volume models for normal tissues have been proposed in the literature and these are relevant to a consideration of volume effects in radiation therapy (see Section 5.4). The most widely used model is that of Lyman (1985). This model gives the normal-tissue complication probability, NTCP, as a function of the absorbed dose, D, in a partial organ volume, V:

$$\text{NTCP}(D,V) = \frac{1}{\sqrt{2\pi}} \cdot \int_{-\infty}^{u(D,V)} \exp\left(-\tfrac{1}{2} \cdot x^2\right) dx \quad (10.9)$$

where the dependence of dose and volume is in the upper limit of the integral:

$$u(D,V) = \frac{D - D_{50}(V)}{m \cdot D_{50}(V)} \quad (10.10)$$

The volume dependence of the D_{50} is assumed to follow the relationship

$$D_{50}(V) = \frac{D_{50}(1)}{V^n} \quad (10.11)$$

Note that many publications citing these equations contain at least one typographical error. A closer inspection of these three equations shows that there are two independent variables, D and V, and three model parameters: m, $D_{50}(1)$ and n. $D_{50}(1)$ is the uniform total dose producing a 50% incidence of the specific end-point if the whole organ is receiving this dose. The volume exponent, n, is always between zero and 1.0 and the larger the value, the more pronounced is the volume effect. The third parameter, m, is inversely related to the steepness of the dose–response curve, i.e. smaller values of m correspond to steeper dose–response curves. The Lyman model has no simple mechanistic background but should be seen as an empirical model for fitting dose–volume data sets. More mechanistic models have been developed but none of these has so far found wider use.

Lyman's model only applies to fractional volumes receiving uniform doses. In practice, this is rarely (never) the case. The most common way of summarizing information on a non-uniform dose distribution in an organ is the dose–volume histogram (DVH). In order to estimate NTCP from a DVH using the Lyman model, it is necessary to reduce the DVH into a single point in the dose–volume space. Perhaps the two most frequently used methods for doing this are the interpolation method (Lyman, 1985) and the effective-volume method (Kutcher and Burman, 1989). In the former, the DVH is transformed into an equivalent dose given to the whole organ, in the latter, the DVH is transformed into a fractional volume that received the maximum dose in the DVH. The basic assumption in the effective-volume method is that each fractional volume will follow the same dose–volume relationship (described by the Lyman model) as the whole organ. The partial volume in a specific bin on the dose axis is then converted into a (smaller) volume placed at the bin corresponding to the maximum absorbed dose in the DVH.

The ability of the Lyman model to correctly predict tissue complication probabilities in patients has been questioned (Boersma *et al.*, 1998) and even the DVH as a summary measure of a dose distribution has been criticized because the spatial distribution of voxels in the organ or tissue is lost (Travis *et al.*, 1997). The use of NTCP models in clinical decision-making and in dose planning is therefore highly controversial and should at present not be done outside a research setting.

KEY POINTS

1. There is no well-defined 'tolerance dose' for radiation complications or 'tumoricidal dose' for local tumour control: rather, the probability of a biological effect rises from 0% to 100% over a range of doses.
2. The steepness of a dose–response curve at a response level of n% may be quantified by the value γ_n, that is the increase in response in percentage points for a 1% increase in dose.
3. Dose–response curves for late normal-tissue end-points tend to be steeper (typical γ_{50} between 2 and 6) than the dose–response curves for local control of squamous cell carcinoma of the head and neck (typical γ_{50} between 1.5 and 2.5).
4. The steepness of a dose–response curve is greater if the data are generated by varying the dose while keeping the number of fractions constant ('double trouble') than if the dose per fraction is fixed.

5. Dosimetric and biological heterogeneity cause the population dose–response curve to be more shallow.
6. Normal-tissue complication probability (NTCP) models, incorporating dose fractionation as well as irradiated volume, have not been validated in any clinical setting and should not be routinely used outside a research protocol.

BIBLIOGRAPHY

Bentzen SM (1992). Steepness of the clinical dose–control curve and variation in the in vitro radiosensitivity of head and neck squamous cell carcinoma. *Int J Radiat Biol* **61**: 417–23.

Bentzen SM (1994). Radiobiological considerations in the design of clinical trials. *Radiother Oncol* **32**: 1–11.

Bentzen SM, Overgaard M (1991). Relationship between early and late normal-tissue injury after postmastectomy radiotherapy. *Radiother Oncol* **20**: 159–65.

Bentzen SM, Overgaard J (1996). Clinical normal-tissue radiobiology. In: *Current Radiation Oncology* (eds Tobias JS, Thomas PRM), pp. 37–67. Arnold, London.

Bentzen SM, Tucker SL (1997). Quantifying the position and steepness of radiation dose-response curves. *Int J Radiat Biol* **71**: 531–42.

Bentzen SM, Christensen JJ, Overgaard J, Overgaard M (1988). Some methodological problems in estimating radiobiological parameters from clinical data. Alpha/beta ratios and electron RBE for cutaneous reactions in patients treated with postmastectomy radiotherapy. *Acta Oncol* **27**: 105–16.

Bentzen SM, Thames HD, Overgaard J (1990). Does variation in the in vitro cellular radiosensitivity explain the shallow clinical dose–control curve for malignant melanoma? *Int J Radiat Biol* **57**: 117–26.

Bentzen SM, Johansen LV, Overgaard J, Thames HD (1991). Clinical radiobiology of squamous cell carcinoma of the oropharynx. *Int J Radiat Oncol Biol Phys* **20**: 1197–206.

Boersma LJ, van den Brink M, Bruce AM *et al.* (1998). Estimation of the incidence of late bladder and rectum complications after high-dose (70–78 Gy) conformal radiotherapy for prostate cancer, using dose-volume histograms. *Int J Radiat Oncol Biol Phys* **41**: 83–92.

Brahme A (1984). Dosimetric precision requirements in radiation therapy. *Acta Radiol Oncol* **23**: 379–91.

Fenwick JD (1998). Predicting the radiation control probability of heterogeneous tumour ensembles: data analysis and parameter estimation using a closed-form expression. *Phys Med Biol* **43**: 2159–78.

Hendry JH, Thames HD (1986). The tissue-rescuing unit. *Br J Radiol* **59**: 628–30.

Holthusen H (1936). Erfahrungen über die Verträglichkeitsgrenze für Röntgenstrahlen und deren Nutzanwendung zur Verhütung von Schäden. *Strahlentherapie* **57**: 254–69.

Khalil AA, Bentzen SM, Overgaard J (1997). Steepness of the dose–response curve as a function of volume in an experimental tumor irradiated under ambient or hypoxic conditions. *Int J Radiat Oncol Biol Phys* **39**: 797–802.

Kutcher GJ, Burman C (1989). Calculation of complication probability factors for non-uniform normal-tissue irradiation: the effective volume method. *Int J Radiat Oncol Biol Phys* **16**: 1623–30.

Lyman JT (1985). Complication probability as assessed from dose-volume histograms. *Radiat Res* **104**: S13–19.

Munro TR, Gilbert CW (1961). The relation between tumour lethal doses and the radiosensitivity of tumour cells. *Br J Radiol* **34**: 246–51.

Okunieff P, Morgan D, Niemierko A, Suit HD (1995). Radiation dose–response of human tumors. *Int J Radiat Oncol Biol Phys* **32**: 1227–37.

Overgaard J, Hjelm-Hansen M, Johansen LV, Andersen AP (1988). Comparison of conventional and split-course radiotherapy as primary treatment in carcinoma of the larynx. *Acta Oncol* **27**: 147–52.

Suit HD, Skates S, Taghian A, Okunieff P, Efird JT (1992). Clinical implications of heterogeneity of tumor response to radiation therapy. *Radiother Oncol* **25**: 251–60.

Travis EL, Liao ZX, Tucker SL (1997). Spatial heterogeneity of the volume effect for radiation pneumonitis in mouse lung. *Int J Radiat Oncol Biol Phys* **38**: 1045–54.

Webb S, Nahum AE (1993). A model for calculating tumour control probability in radiotherapy including the effects of inhomogeneous distributions of dose and clonogenic cell density. *Phys Med Biol* **38**: 653–66.

FURTHER READING

Bentzen SM (1993). Quantitative clinical radiobiology. *Acta Oncol* **32**: 259–75.

Bentzen SM (1994). Radiobiological considerations in the design of clinical trials. *Radiother Oncol* **32**: 1–11.

Bentzen SM, Overgaard J (1996). Clinical normal-tissue radiobiology. In: *Current Radiation Oncology* (eds Tobias JS, Thomas PRM), pp. 37–67. Arnold, London.

Withers HR (1992). Biologic basis of radiation therapy. In: *Principles and Practice of Radiation Oncology* (eds Perez CA, Brady LW), pp. 64–96. Lippincott, Philadelphia.

11

Clinical manifestations of normal-tissue damage

MICHAEL BAUMANN AND SØREN M BENTZEN

11.1 DOCUMENTATION OF NORMAL-TISSUE INJURY IS AN ESSENTIAL COMPONENT OF RADIOTHERAPY

Even the most advanced radiotherapy technique will inevitably result in irradiation of normal tissues, and the volume of normal tissue within the planning target volume that receives the prescribed dose often exceeds the gross tumour volume. Even larger volumes of normal tissues are irradiated with less than the prescribed dose. As a consequence, radiotherapy is associated with a broad spectrum of normal-tissue reactions and it is impossible to cure a tumour by radiotherapy without the risk of complications. The aim of radiotherapy research is to optimize the probability of uncomplicated tumour control, i.e. tumour control in the absence of unacceptable normal-tissue damage. This was clearly realized in 1936 by Holthusen and is illustrated in Figure 14.1. From the concepts of uncomplicated tumour control and therapeutic index (Section 1.6), it is obvious that documentation of tumour response without thorough documentation of the normal-tissue reactions is inadequate when evaluating treatment outcome. This principle applies equally in routine clinical practice and in clinical research where new treatment strategies are developed. The importance of late side-effects increases as long-term survival after cancer therapy improves.

The trade-off between tumour control and treatment-related morbidity becomes particularly clear when the morbidity is potentially fatal to the patient. An example of this is the long-standing discussion about the role of adjuvant radiotherapy in patients with early breast cancer. A large meta-analysis including nearly 20 000 patients in 40 randomized studies showed that while postoperative radiotherapy significantly improved locoregional tumour control, it had no significant effect on survival (Early Breast Cancer Trialists' Collaborative Group, 1995, 2000). Remarkably, radiotherapy significantly decreased the number of cancer-related deaths, whereas deaths from other causes were significantly increased. This observation is consistent with the excess cardiac mortality after radiotherapy seen in studies comparing death rates from ischaemic heart disease in patients treated for left-sided versus right-sided breast cancer (Rutqvist and Johansson, 1990). More recent studies have used improved radiotherapy techniques to minimize radiation dose to the heart and the incidence of ischaemic heart disease was no higher in patients with left-sided rather than right-sided breast cancer and also no higher than in non-irradiated patients (Figure 11.1). More recent

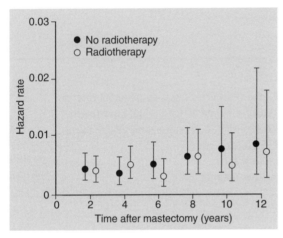

Figure 11.1 *The hazard rates of morbidity from ischaemic heart disease after postoperative radiotherapy for breast cancer in the Danish randomized breast cancer trials. Postoperative radiotherapy in these trials did not increase the risk of ischaemic heart disease over a follow-up period of 12 years. Error bars show 95% confidence intervals. From Højris et al. (1999), with permission.*

trials have found that the improved locoregional tumour control by postoperative radiotherapy did translate into a survival advantage for pre- and post-menopausal patients with breast cancer (Overgaard *et al.*, 1997, 1999; Ragaz *et al.*, 1997).

11.2 CLASSIFICATION OF NORMAL-TISSUE DAMAGE

There are several established ways to classify normal-tissue reactions in clinical practice. These classification systems are not mutually exclusive and there are situations where more than one may be employed.

Early versus late responses

The distinction between early and late normal-tissue reactions is described in Section 4.2 and their clinical manifestations are summarized in Table 11.1. Early reactions occur during or shortly after a course of radiotherapy. There is a convention to define any treatment-related morbidity that occurs within 90 days after the start of radiotherapy as an early reaction (Cox *et al.*, 1995). Typical examples of early reactions include mucositis, dermatitis and depletion of the cellular compartments of the bone marrow with a consequent decline in the blood cell count. Early reactions are usually transient. Figure 11.2 shows as an example the time-course of mucositis of the oral cavity, as seen in a CHART trial (Bentzen *et al.*, 2001): mucositis appeared after the first week of radiotherapy, it increased in severity to reach a peak

Table 11.1 *Clinical and biological characteristics of early and late radiation reactions*

	Early reactions	Late reactions
Latency	<90 days, typically 3–9 weeks. No strong dependence on extent of damage, but greater damage may lead to slower healing of injury	>90 days, typically 0.5–5 years. Greater damage leads to shorter latent period
Fractionation sensitivity	Low ($\alpha/\beta \approx 10$ Gy)	High ($\alpha/\beta \approx 1$–5 Gy)
Influence of overall treatment time	Shorter overall time leads to greater injury	No significant influence
Clinical course	Transient, but consequential late reactions may occur	Irreversible. Compensatory mechanisms may occur; rehabilitation or treatment for complications may relieve

From Bentzen and Overgaard, 1996.

around weeks 5–6 (after conventional fractionation). The reaction then gradually resolved as a consequence of the regenerative response of the mucosal epithelium. Figure 11.2 also shows that shortening of the overall treatment time by accelerated radiotherapy leads to more severe early reactions that peak earlier. The duration of confluent mucositis was similar after accelerated and conventional radiotherapy (Bentzen et al., 2001). As described in Section 12.5, the α/β ratio for early reactions tends to be high (~8–12 Gy, see Table 13.1) and there is less influence of dose per fraction on the severity of early as compared with late reactions.

Late reactions occur several months or even years after radiotherapy. Typical examples of late reactions are chronic myelopathy, lung or subcutaneous fibrosis, telangiectasia, bone necrosis and radiation nephropathy. The pathogenesis of these sequelae is described in Sections 4.3 and 4.4. By convention, any treatment-related morbidity that occurs later than 90 days after the start of radiotherapy is defined as a late reaction. This definition is not absolute, however, as the time necessary for complete disappearance of early reactions may be longer than 90 days and slowly healing early effects may incorrectly be scored as late effects. Consequential late reactions (see below) are of special concern when early reactions are severe, for instance

after accelerated radiotherapy or after combined radio-chemotherapy. Another problem in the distinction between early and late effects is that some reactions, such as radiation pneumonitis, often occur around day 90. Depending on whether these reactions are reported before or after the cut-off point, the same biological reaction could be categorized as either early or late, which obviously makes no sense. It is therefore important to judge all symptoms and signs as well as the time-course of a given reaction for correct categorization. Holthusen had already recognized in 1936 that typical late reactions are irreversible. The severity of late reactions progresses with time and although some adaptation and compensatory mechanisms may occur, most late reactions fail to resolve. An example of the long latent times and progressive nature of late reactions is shown in Figure 11.3. This shows skin telangiectasia scores in breast cancer patients who had been irradiated with five fractions of 1.8 Gy per week to a total of 35 fractions after surgery, and who were followed up for over 10 years (Turesson, 1990). The percentage of patients who showed skin telangiectasia increased progressively and another striking finding in this study was that the individual variation in progression rate was very large for the same treatment. For

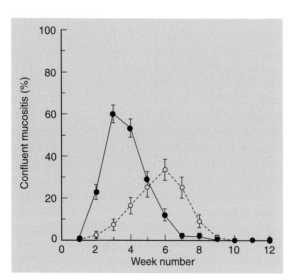

Figure 11.2 *Prevalence of confluent mucositis as a function of time after the start of radiotherapy using the CHART regime (●) or conventional radiotherapy (○). From Bentzen* et al. *(2001), with permission.*

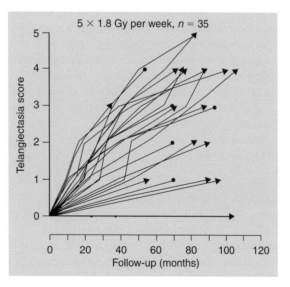

Figure 11.3 *Progression of skin telangiectasia in individual patients treated with five fractions of 1.8 Gy per week to a total of 35 fractions. Note the pronounced differences between patients and the continuous increase in severity even up to 8 years. From Turesson (1990), with permission.*

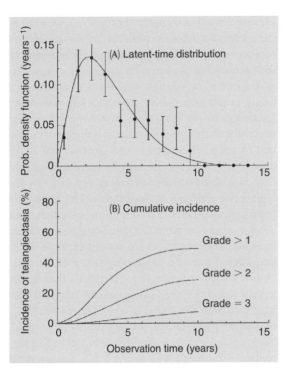

Figure 11.4 *(A) The latent-time distribution for any grade of telangiectasia as observed in 174 treatment fields with an intermediate probability of developing this reaction (grade ≥ 1). The probability density function may be interpreted as the fraction of patients who expressed the radiation reaction within a specific year after treatment. Even 9 years after treatment, about 2% of the patients showed the mildest grade of telangiectasia for the first time. (B) The cumulative incidence of telangiectasia as a function of time for various grades of reaction following 44.4 Gy in 25 fractions. Model calculation based on observation in a total of 401 treatment fields. From Bentzen* et al. *(1990), with permission.*

example, the latency for grade 2 telangiectasia ranged from 17 to 90 months. Possible reasons for the large individual variation in progression rate after the same treatment are dealt with in Section 11.5. An alternative representation of data on telangiectasia following breast radiotherapy is shown in Figure 11.4. This shows the progressive increase in the development over 10 years of the incidence of grade 1, 2 or 3 telangiectasia.

In comparison with early reactions, dose per fraction has more influence on the severity and incidence of late reactions (see Section 12.5). The α/β ratio is usually low, around 1–5 Gy (see Table 13.1). Also in

contrast to early reactions, the overall treatment time has little or no impact on late reactions, although the results of recent clinical trials have shown that late reactions may be more severe after accelerated fractionation. Possible reasons for this finding are discussed in Section 14.7.

Genuine versus consequential late reactions

Late complications of radiotherapy may occur without more than usual early effects, and severe early effects may resolve completely without the development of any late effects. Thus, in general there is little correlation between the expression of early and late normal-tissue injury in individual patients. However, evidence is accumulating that late reactions in some tissues and organs may occur as a consequence of severe early reactions (see Sections 4.2 and 4.3; Dörr and Hendry, 2001). Clinical examples of consequential late reactions are the occurrence of bone and soft-tissue necrosis after severe mucosal denudation or the increased risk of developing telangiectasia after moist desquamation. The first carefully documented application of radiotherapy was by Freund who in 1897 treated a large hairy naevus in a little girl and observed late effects (telangiectasia and fibrous scarring) in an area of the skin that showed severe early reactions with ulceration and delayed healing (described by Kogelnik, 1997). An important problem in the clinical evaluation of consequential late effects is that the incidence of both early and late effects increases steeply with total dose. Thus, heterogeneous dose distributions with hotspots in individual patients or variable dose prescriptions in a cohort of patients may artificially suggest a causal relationship between early and late reactions. Furthermore, several co-factors such as genetic hypersensitivity and interactions with other treatment modalities may increase early as well as late reactions (Section 11.5). Deciding whether a specific late reaction is or is not consequential is generally not possible in individual patients. Some of these problems can be overcome in experiments on animals that so far have provided evidence of consequential late effects for the bladder, the rectum and the small intestine.

Consequential late reactions may 'inherit' some of the characteristics of early reactions, for example a sensitivity to changed overall treatment time. Similarly,

Table 11.2 *Severity of impaired shoulder movement compared with frequency of subjective symptoms*

Grade	Pain at movement (%)	Pain* at rest (%)	Reduced working ability (%)
0	6	6	8
1	9	4	28
2	27**	16***	62
3	31**	20***	99

* Defined as moderate or severe (grade 3 only) pain on a scale including no pain and slight pain.
** 5% had severe pain.
*** 1.5% had severe pain.
From Bentzen *et al.* (1989a).

sparing of late reactions through the use of low dose per fraction may be offset in situations where late reactions are consequential. Consequential late reactions are of special concern when early reactions are severe, for instance after accelerated radiotherapy or after combined radio-chemotherapy.

Subjective versus objective end-points

Objective end-points are usually preferable in clinical science but they do not provide a complete picture of the patient's situation after therapy. Table 11.2 shows an example where the physician's evaluation of impairment of shoulder movement was compared with the patient's perception of pain. Whether or not a given grade of objective reaction limits the patient's ability to live a normal life is very important in evaluating treatment-related morbidity. For example, the fact that 27% of patients with a 'moderate' (i.e. grade 2) impairment of shoulder movement had pain associated with movement of the shoulder is important information characterizing the patient's condition.

Quality-of-life measures have been used in a few studies as a surrogate end-point for treatment toxicity. This cannot be justified: quality of life is not toxicity and toxicity is not quality of life. Obviously, quality of life end-points are important in the characterization of the patient's perception of his or her own situation but such measures are not necessarily related in any simple way with objective clinicobiological changes. How the patient actually copes with treatment sequelae is influenced by several cultural and psychosocial factors. Minimization of treatment-related morbidity will always be a goal even if the patient can cope with the sequelae.

The objective evaluation of normal-tissue damage may depend to a considerable extent on the observer. Physical measurements often have minimal observer or operator dependency and should usually be preferred, but the results of such measurements may not be superior to an overall judgement by the physician, taking into account many different aspects of response to radiotherapy.

Cosmetic versus functional end-points

Cosmetic changes constitute a major problem in many irradiated patients and must therefore be a concern of the radiotherapist as well. Serious cosmetic changes after radiotherapy may arise from retardation of the growth of muscle and bone in children and adolescents, or visible skin changes on the face or hands. Changes in body image may also lead to secondary problems such as sexual dysfunction. Some cosmetic effects rarely trouble the patient, and this may be the case with telangiectasia on parts of the body normally covered by clothes. In contrast, functional end-points of injury almost inevitably influence the patient's quality of life.

Mild versus severe reactions

Patients as well as physicians may describe a given normal-tissue injury as mild or severe. The problem with these apparently simple descriptors is they may have a completely different meaning for different persons. For example, an erythema with patchy moist desquamation in a skin fold might be categorized as mild to moderate by a radiation oncologist but as a severe 'burn' by the patient or the family practitioner. It is therefore necessary to use unequivocal definitions of end-points and grades for the quantification of normal-tissue reactions after radiotherapy (Section 11.3).

Treatable versus untreatable sequelae

Some interventions may modify the time-course or the severity of radiation damage to normal tissue and they can be very successful. A good example is hormone replacement after irradiation of the thyroid, where side-effects can be satisfactorily corrected (Hancock *et al.*, 1995). Other examples of interventions that may ameliorate the sequelae of radiotherapy

Table 11.3 *Three types of clinical toxicity data*

Type of end-point	Statistical data type	Scoring system	Examples
Binary	Categorical; all-or-nothing response	Yes/no	Radiation-induced second tumours
Graded	Ordinal; ranking of severity	e.g. None/mild/moderate/severe	Telangiectasia; subcutaneous fibrosis
Continuous	Continuous	'Laboratory value'	Kidney $[^{51}Cr]$EDTA clearance; CT density of pulmonary fibrosis

are microsurgical transplantation of skin for chronic ulcerations, lymphatic drainage in case of lymphoedema, training for contracture of joints, and rectal installation of corticoids or sucralfate for chronic proctitis. There is currently much interest in the treatment of a variety of late sequelae by the use of hyperbaric oxygen. The effectiveness of these interventions has often not been rigorously tested in adequately sized randomized clinical trials, but their value does need to be carefully considered. Much more preclinical and clinical research is needed in this important area to define evidence-based strategies of intervention and modification. Treatment of radiation damage, whether or not it is objectively successful, frequently reduces the patient's perception of its severity and this is a further reason why clinical research must be based on objective scoring procedures.

Deterministic versus stochastic damage

The preceding discussion has mainly dealt with normal-tissue responses that are deterministic in nature, i.e. their severity increases with increasing dose. By contrast, the induction of secondary tumours by radiotherapy or chemotherapy is a stochastic or all-or-nothing event: with increasing dose it is the frequency of induced tumours that increases with dose rather than the intensity of the response. The occurrence of second tumours can also be described as a binary end-point (Table 11.3). Binary end-points are all-or-nothing events, and no grading is possible for these. A further example is radiation myelopathy (Withers *et al.*, 1988) where damage beyond a critical limit results in an all-or-nothing response.

By contrast, many functional tests produce a continuum of responses and these are sometimes called non-stochastic responses. In between are the graded response end-points where different outcomes can

be ranked in order of increasing severity. However, no numerical relationship can be assumed between the various grades and the reporting of average scores should be avoided as this practice mixes up the severity and the incidence of reactions.

By a process of data reduction it is possible to convert a continuous response into a graded or even a binary response. Continuous responses may be divided into grades, either on the basis of fixed levels of measured response or (as in the case of skin reactions) on the basis of a qualitative judgement of severity. Graded responses may be converted to an all-or-nothing end-point by defining a binary variable as a response that is above or below a specific threshold value. This is illustrated in Figure 11.5 and an example is shown in Figure 11.4.

11.3 SYSTEMS FOR RECORDING AND REPORTING NORMAL-TISSUE INJURY

Several attempts have been made to devise a comprehensive system for the grading and reporting of normal-tissue complications. None of these has so far gained general acceptance, although the RTOG/EORTC Late Morbidity Scoring Criteria and Acute Radiation Morbidity Scoring Criteria have been used in quite a few studies (Cox *et al.*, 1995). In 1995, the RTOG/EORTC working groups on late effects of normal tissues have jointly proposed the LENT/SOMA system for assessment and recording of radiotherapy-related morbidity (Pavy *et al.*, 1995; Rubin *et al.*, 1995). Parts of this system have now been tested systematically and compared with already established scoring systems. The general impression from these studies is that the scoring of reactions using the LENT/SOMA system is feasible and that concordance with other scoring systems is generally good. The

Figuxre 11.5 *The proportion of patients with a reaction above a certain threshold may be treated as a binary variable. The lower panel shows continuous dose–response curves corresponding to three different degrees of sensitivity. We can then calculate the frequency of responses above or below a defined threshold (upper panel). If tissue sensitivity varies among a group of patients, this will lead to a cumulative frequency response that is sigmoid in shape. From Field and Upton (1985), with permission.*

use of this system is, however, time-consuming, which may hamper its wide implementation in clinical practice. Scoring systems are under continual evolution with the aim of improving them further.

For early morbidity the National Cancer Institute in the USA has revised and expanded the Common Toxicity Criteria (CTC) into a comprehensive and standardized system applicable to radiotherapy, systemic therapy and surgery (Trotti *et al.*, 2000). The CTC v. 2.0 replaces the previous NCI CTC and the RTOG Acute Radiation Morbidity Scoring.

The ideal system should be complete, reproducible and sensitive. Complete means that it should be possible to record and score any relevant adverse effect of radiotherapy. Reproducible means that the inter- and intra-observer variability should be low

compared with the variation between patients, i.e. that the system can be applied with a reasonable agreement between different observers and that individuals can reasonably reproduce their own scoring. Sensitive means that the system should be able to detect changes in treatment intensity, for example in detecting the change in toxicity resulting from dose escalation. Once these aspects of the system are established, the ideal system would be easy to use, clinically relevant and would ensure that as much information as possible is available for radiobiological analysis. The RTOG/ EORTC system, for example, is clinically rather than radiobiologically oriented. The grading of late skin reactions pools data on hair loss, telangiectasia and atrophy/ulceration, which biologically are three different end-points, most likely resulting from the depletion of different target-cell populations. An example of part of the LENT/ SOMA system which differentiates these biologically different end-points is given in Table 11.4.

In spite of the problems of the currently available scoring protocols, the use of a standard system of reporting is strongly encouraged (Overgaard and Bartelink, 1995). It is to be hoped that the current efforts in developing improved reporting of toxicity will lead to the realization of a comprehensive system that is widely acceptable to both radiotherapists and biologists.

11.4 PRACTICAL ASPECTS OF NORMAL-TISSUE MORBIDITY RECORDING, DATA ANALYSIS AND REPORTING

What data need to be recorded?

For any given treatment site a list of normal tissues at risk should be compiled. As a minimum, any occurrence of adverse effects of radiotherapy in these tissues, the patient performance status, and any secondary tumours should be documented during each follow-up examination. It is strongly encouraged to use a validated standard system for recording of early and late normal-tissue reactions. All data requested by this specific system must be recorded, including grade 0 scores. Standardized protocol sheets are preferable to free notes. As the complexity and therefore the time necessary for recording of the data

Table 11.4 *LENT/SOMA scoring system for late effects of radiotherapy in skin and subcutaneous tissue at rest*

	Grade 1	Grade 2	Grade 3	Grade 4
Subjective				
Scaliness/roughness	Present/ asymptomatic	Symptomatic	Requires constant attention	
Sensation	Hypersensitivity, pruritus	Intermittent pain	Persistent pain	Debilitating dysfunction
Objective				
Oedema	Present/ asymptomatic	Symptomatic	Secondary dysfunction	Total dysfunction
Alopecia (scalp)	Thinning	Patchy, permanent	Complete, permanent	
Pigmentation change	Transitory, slight	Permanent, marked		
Ulcer/necrosis	Epidermal only	Dermal	Subcutaneous	Bone exposed
Telangiectasia	Minor	Moderate <50%	Gross ≥50%	
Fibrosis/scar	Present/ asymptomatic	Symptomatic	Secondary dysfunction	Total dysfunction
Atrophy/contraction	Present/ asymptomatic	Symptomatic/ <10%	Secondary dysfunction/ (10–30%)	Total dysfunction/ >30%
Management				
Dryness			Medical intervention	
Sensation		Intermittent medical intervention	Continuous medical intervention	
Ulcer			Medical intervention	Surgical intervention/ amputation
Oedema			Medical intervention	Surgical intervention/ amputation
Fibrosis/scar			Medical intervention	Surgical intervention/ amputation
Analytic				
Colour photograph	Assessment of changes in appearance			

From Pavy *et al.* (1995).
Grade 0 indicates absence of toxicity.

varies considerably between different systems, the feasibility of using a given recording system must be based on workload and on the specific question to be addressed. After a decision has been made, the recording system must not be changed until the study is completed. Before initiation of a multi-centre trial, it is import to ensure that all participating centres will have the capacity and the expertise to use the intended recording system. A well established and easy system that focuses on the main end-points

of the given trial may be more robust and yield higher quality data than incorrectly or incompletely filled forms of a very comprehensive and time-consuming scoring system.

One very important aspect for the use of any recording system is that baseline scores before the initiation of radiotherapy must be documented. For example, patients irradiated for lung cancer often have considerable restriction in lung capacity before the start of treatment and patients postoperatively treated for soft-tissue sarcomas may have a functional deficit resulting from surgery. If such pre-existing conditions are not documented, the adverse effects of radiotherapy on normal tissues will, of course, be overestimated.

As discussed in Section 11.5, many treatment- and patient-related factors have an important influence on the development of radiation injury to normal tissues. It is therefore important to explore and document such co-factors, for instance smoking habits or medication, especially with cytotoxic agents. In view of the dose-dependence of normal-tissue reactions, it is necessary to document as precisely as possible the location of a normal-tissue reaction to enable comparison with the radiation-dose distribution.

It is important to ask the patients directly whether they have experienced specific symptoms. General questions, such as 'do you feel well?' often lead to an underestimation of normal-tissue effects, especially of minor or moderate degree. Even when asked directly, many patients feel uncomfortable about giving information on sexual function.

Another important practical problem is that many recording systems such as the RTOG/EORTC system include different biological end-points in a single grade of reaction in a specific organ. This problem can be diminished by the separate recording of each end-point and by reporting supplementary information on toxicity whenever possible. A strong warning is needed here regarding the LENT/SOMA system. The original publications suggested scoring several specific toxicity items for an organ and afterwards calculating the average score as an overall measure of toxicity. This is a very misleading procedure as it may dilute the score of very serious complications.

Follow-up: how long?

Late radiation responses in humans occur after latent periods of between 3 months and many years. To obtain a reliable estimate of the incidence of late complications therefore requires an extended period of follow-up (Figures 11.1, 11.3 and 11.4). A 5-year follow-up is widely used for reporting the outcome of cancer therapy but it must be stressed that this period may not be sufficient to give reliable estimates on very late-occurring sequelae such as damage to the central nervous system and peripheral nerves. Furthermore, it has been established that higher grades of late reaction are on average seen at later times than lower grades,

and that increased treatment toxicity may considerably shorten the latent period. Thus, follow-up at a fixed time after treatment is usually not sufficient and a complete description of the latent-time distribution should be the objective. Good examples of the variable time-courses for a variety of late sequelae are given by Svoboda et al. (1999) who summarized treatment-related side-effects in a group of patients treated for rectal cancer with an unconventional sandwich-radiotherapy, and by Jung et al. (2001) who further analysed these data and a large number of data sets from the literature (see also the commentary by Bentzen and Dische, 2001).

Analysis of data on early normal-tissue reactions

In a group of patients, the time-course of normal-tissue damage can be shown as a plot of prevalence as a function of time. Figure 11.2 is an example, showing the prevalence of confluent mucositis as a function of time in the CHART head and neck trial (Bentzen et al., 2001). The prevalence of this reaction at a specific time, say week 3, is simply the number of patients experiencing confluent mucositis at week 3 divided by the total number of patients scored at that time. The peak prevalence is the maximum prevalence of mucositis at any point in time. As not all patients will reach the peak grade of reaction at the same time, the *incidence* will be larger than or equal to the peak prevalence. The incidence of confluent mucositis is the fraction of patients reaching this grade of reaction at any point during the follow-up period.

Analysis of early reactions does not require actuarial statistics but may be analysed using standard methods for binary or ordinal data (e.g. Fisher's exact test or Spearman's rank correlation coefficient), depending on the actual question of interest. Multivariate analysis is typically performed using logistic regression or generalizations of that method (Bentzen et al., 2001).

Analysis of data on late normal-tissue reactions

Patients who die of their disease or from an unrelated cause early after therapy are clearly less likely to have developed late normal-tissue damage than patients who live longer. Similarly, some patients may have incomplete follow-up because they were entered late into the study and only a short period before the data analysis. Such data are said to be *censored*, because the status of the patients after a certain time is unknown. To restrict the analysis to patients who have completed a specified minimum observation time, say 2 years or 5 years, may involve considerable loss of information. Even more seriously, such a procedure may lead to selection bias, as it is not necessarily a random subset of all patients who would be included in the analysis. In statistical terminology, data of this type are called *failure-time data*: for each patient we record the time of reaching the end-point or, for patients who were alive without complications when last seen, the time of their last follow-up.

There is an extensive statistical literature on the analysis of failure-time data. Popularly, these methods are often referred to as *survival statistics*, analysed by actuarial methods. To provide a full description of this field is far beyond the scope of this chapter but a few key methods should be mentioned. Estimates of the complication rate at a given time may be obtained by the life-table method or the Kaplan–Meier estimate (Machin and Gardner, 1989). In statistical literature the latter is called the product-limit estimate. From these estimates the median latent time can be estimated (Bentzen *et al.*, 1990). Testing for a statistically significant difference between the time-course of complications in two groups may be done by one of the versions of the log-rank test. Finally, multivariate methods have been used for analysing failure-time data in radiobiology: the Cox Proportional Hazards Model (Taylor *et al.*, 1987) and the Mixture Model

(Bentzen *et al.*, 1989c). The former has become very popular in the analysis of survival data and is readily available in many standard statistical computer programs. It has been shown that these methods provide virtually identical estimates of the incidence of radiation reactions (Taylor and Kim, 1993). However, the mixture model provides an attractive framework for more biologically oriented analyses. For an (admittedly technical!) discussion see Bentzen *et al.* (1989c).

Clinical importance of correct analysis and reporting of normal-tissue damage

Even if normal-tissue reactions are recorded, many studies fail to use proper statistical methods for reporting the data. This is not just a statistical technicality, as two reports using different statistical methods cannot be compared in any meaningful way. Toxicity data are often given in terms of the crude proportion of patients with complications, i.e. the number of patients with a specific type and grade of complication divided by the total number of patients treated. As indicated above, this is not a useful characterization of toxicity as it is influenced not only by treatment intensity but also by the life expectancy of the group of patients under study. Table 11.5 shows the difference between crude and actuarial estimates in selected clinical examples. If life expectancy is short, as with the lung cancer study by Hatlevoll *et al.* (1983), a treatment regimen may look safe even when it produces a high risk of severe complications among the long-term survivors. Similarly,

Table 11.5 *Crude and actuarial estimates of complication frequencies*

End-point	Primary tumour	Crude estimate	Actuarial	Remarks	Reference
Radiation myelopathy	Lung	4 ± 1% at 3 years	30 ± 15%	Median survival 9 months	Hatlevoll *et al.* (1983)
Marked telangiectasia	Breast	39 ± 6%	62%	Follow-up 1.5–6 years; long latent period	Bentzen *et al.* (1995)
Severe* rectosigmoid complications	Uterine cervix:			Patients with IIIb and IVa disease received a higher dose but had fewer complications	Unpublished
	FIGO IIb	9 ± 5%	10 ± 6% at 5 years		
	FIGO IIIb + IVa	15 ± 3%	39 ± 8% at 5 years		

Frequencies given with ±1 standard error of the estimate.
* Requiring treatment.
From Bentzen *et al.* (1995), where original references may be found.

an increase in treatment intensity may be overlooked if two groups differ in the number of person-years at risk because of different follow-up or a difference in prognosis. Actuarial methods are required to get round these problems. Some authors have advocated the use of alternative statistical methods for the estimation of late effects of cancer treatment. For a discussion of these see Bentzen *et al.* (1995) and references in that paper. It is strongly recommended that any report on late treatment-related toxicity should include actuarial estimates as a minimum requirement. Any other statistics may be given as a supplement to this.

Another example of the clinical importance of correct analysis of normal-tissue damage is the use of so-called tolerance doses for prescription of radiotherapy (see Section 4.1). The tolerance dose represents an estimate of the total dose at which for a given treatment a certain percentage of all patients will develop a specified normal-tissue reaction of a specified grade in a specified period (Rubin and Casarett, 1968; Emami *et al.*, 1991). For severe late normal-tissue damage, many radiation oncologists consider that the maximum dose that can be delivered is defined by a risk of 5% at 5 years; the tolerance dose is thus termed $TD_{5/5}$. For especially debilitating sequelae such as radiation myelitis, the radiation dose may be chosen to limit the risk to below 1% (Baumann, 1995; Dische, 1999).

If the principle of treatment to tolerance, as just described, were widely followed one would expect that the incidence of severe late normal-tissue morbidity in long-term survivors after radiotherapy should generally be less than 5%. However, a host of well-documented clinical studies report higher figures even after standard treatments. One important reason for this discrepancy is that conventional tolerance doses have often not been obtained from actuarial analysis of reliable clinical data but rather reflect the best guess of experienced radiation oncologists based on weak evidence.

Use of surrogate markers for normal-tissue damage

The term surrogate marker is used to denote a laboratory assay that can predict the likelihood of late radiation damage to normal tissues long before it becomes clinically relevant. This is a theoretically attractive idea that might enable intervention to reduce the risk of damage in individual patients and that, in a clinical trial, might also give an early indication of the likely outcome. Despite intense research effort, currently no surrogate markers for late normal-tissue damage are available for routine clinical practice; the current status of this field is outlined in Section 22.5.

11.5 FACTORS INFLUENCING NORMAL-TISSUE DAMAGE

Factors influencing the incidence and severity of normal-tissue damage can broadly be characterized as treatment-related, and patient-related. These factors need to be recorded, analysed and reported as precisely as possible for a better understanding of the biological effects of radiotherapy.

Treatment-related factors

The most important factors in the radiotherapy prescription are total dose, dose per fraction, dose rate, time interval between fractions, overall treatment time and dose–volume parameters. These factors are dealt with in Chapters 5, 10, 14 and 18. In addition, concomitant treatment with other modalities such as chemotherapy and surgery, even treatments that are not in themselves associated with significant morbidity, may 'top up' the radiation-induced damage and make it clinically overt. This phenomenon may seriously confound the radiation dose–response relationships for development of normal-tissue damage after radiotherapy.

Figure 11.6 illustrates the influence of adjuvant chemotherapy on the development of subcutaneous fibrosis following post-mastectomy radiotherapy. The data have been corrected for latency, and error bars show binomial standard errors on the frequency of responders. Radiotherapy and the first cycles of chemotherapy were given concomitantly. After 44 Gy in 22 fractions, the risk of ultimately developing marked subcutaneous fibrosis increased from 19% to 50% when the CMF combination (cyclophosphamide, methotrexate and 5-fluorouracil) was given as an adjuvant to radiotherapy. No such change was seen with cyclophosphamide as a single agent.

A study by Bentzen *et al.* (1996) showed that treatment with tamoxifen during post-mastectomy radiotherapy significantly enhanced the risk of

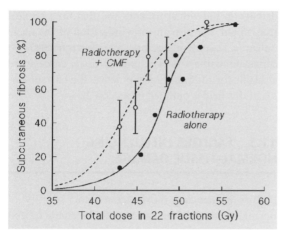

Figure 11.6 *Effect of adjuvant chemotherapy on the incidence of radiation-induced subcutaneous fibrosis.* ●, *Post-mastectomy radiotherapy alone;* ○, *radiotherapy plus adjuvant CMF (cyclophosphamide + methotrexate + 5-fluorouracil). From Bentzen* et al. *(1989b), with permission.*

radiation-induced lung fibrosis compared with patients receiving radiotherapy alone. The odds ratio for the development of lung fibrosis was 2.9 with a 95% confidence interval of 1.3–6.3. Whereas interactions between cytotoxic agents and radiation are well described, this finding is remarkable in so far as tamoxifen is usually considered to be non-toxic. A possible mechanism for this effect is that tamoxifen has been shown to induce TGF-β and this cytokine has been implicated in the pathogenesis of radiation-induced lung fibrosis (see Section 4.3).

An example illustrating the influence of transurethral resection of the prostate on the development of urethral strictures after 3D conformal radiotherapy is shown in Figure 11.7 (Sandhu *et al.*, 2000). The 5-year actuarial likelihood of developing a stricture was 4% (5 out 120) compared with 1% for patients ($n = 980$) who did not undergo a prior resection ($P = 0.01$).

Patient-related factors

Several patient characteristics and in particular various coexisting diseases have been claimed to influence normal-tissue damage after radiation therapy and thus perhaps to contribute to inter-patient variability in response (Bentzen and Overgaard, 1994; Baumann,

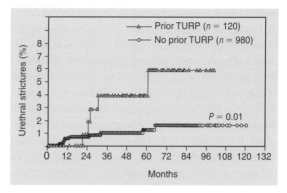

Figure 11.7 *Actuarial incidence of urethral stricture after 3D conformal radiotherapy for prostate cancer among patients with and without a prior history of transurethral resection of the prostate. From Sandhu* et al. *(2000), with permission.*

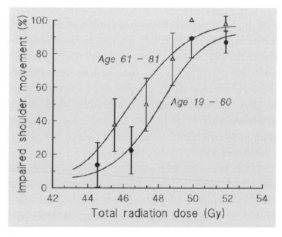

Figure 11.8 *Dose–response relationships for moderate and severe impairment of shoulder movement after post-mastectomy radiotherapy in relation to the age of the patient.* Δ, *Patients 61–81 years of age;* ●, *patients 19–60 years of age. All patients received 12 dose fractions. The effect of age is significant (P = 0.005). From Bentzen* et al. *(1989a), with permission.*

1995). However, a critical review of the literature gives only weak support for the importance of many of these proposed risk factors. Table 11.6 summarizes some of these factors with a rough evaluation of whether the literature at the time of writing provides adequate support for their importance. This is definitely a field where more clinical research is needed.

As an example of such studies, Figure 11.8 shows the influence of the age of the patient on the dose–response

Table 11.6 *Some patient-related factors that have been proposed to affect normal-tissue reactions after radiotherapy*

Factor	Remarks
Young age	Growth retardation is an additional complication Deficient development of cognitive functions following brain irradiation
Old age	Reduced tissue reserve capacity Less exercise leads to reduced compensation for normal-tissue deficits
Smoking	Enhances a number of early and late reactions; decreases pneumonitis
Diet	Suggestion from animal experiments of protective effect of some diets on rectal damage; clinical data less clear
Diabetes mellitus	Risk factor for retinopathy and radiation sequelae of the rectum, influence on other reactions doubtful
Haemoglobin level	Low haemoglobin appears to be protective for early and late normal-tissue reactions, further confirmation needed
Hypertension	Doubtful effect on radiation reactions
Infections/immunosuppression	Infections may add to radiation effects, especially in immunosuppressed individuals
Rheumatoid arthritis	No influence
Non-rheumatoid arthritis collagen vascular disease	Risk factor for a variety of late sequelae
Regional enteritis and colitis	Risk factor for intestinal complications
Pre-existing functional deficit in irradiated organs	Risk factor for a variety of late sequelae, e.g. lung damage
Skin pigmentation and hair colour	No influence
Genetic syndromes	Several of these are associated with clinical over-reaction to radiotherapy*

*See Section 9.1.
Adapted from Bentzen and Overgaard (1994); Baumann (1995).

relationship for moderate and severe impairment of shoulder movement after post-mastectomy radiotherapy. In the clinical examination of these patients, a relative measure of impaired shoulder movement was used and the ability to move the treated and the untreated shoulders was compared in individual patients. There was a significant tendency for the older patients to experience greater impairment.

KEY POINTS

1. Documentation of radiation damage to normal tissues is an essential component of radiotherapy.
2. 'Early' and 'late' manifestations of radiation damage differ significantly in pathogenesis and in their implications for management.
3. Consequential late reactions retain some of the characteristics of early reactions, and therefore need to be distinguished.
4. It is strongly recommended to record radiation-induced damage by means of an established scoring system. However, a well-completed simple system is preferable to a comprehensive system that is less satisfactorily carried out.
5. The statistical analysis of clinical data has many pitfalls and should be carried out by an experienced statistician.

BIBLIOGRAPHY

Baumann M (1995). Impact of endogenous and exogenous factors on radiation sequelae.

In: *Late Sequelae in Oncology* (eds Dunst J, Sauer R). Springer-Verlag, Berlin.

Bentzen SM, Dische S (2001). Late morbidity: the Damocles sword of radiotherapy? *Radiother Oncol* **61**: 219–221.

Bentzen SM, Overgaard J (1994). Patient-to-patient variability in the expression of radiation-induced normal tissue injury. *Semin Radiat Oncol* **4**: 68–80.

Bentzen SM, Overgaard J (1996). Clinical normal-tissue radiobiology. In: *Current Radiation Oncology*, Vol. 2 (eds Tobias JS, Thomas PRM). Arnold, London.

Bentzen SM, Overgaard M, Thames HD (1989a). Fractionation sensitivity of a clinical end-point: impaired shoulder movement after post-mastectomy radiotherapy. *Int J Radiat Oncol Biol Phys* **17**: 531–7.

Bentzen SM, Overgaard M, Thames HD *et al.* (1989b). Early and late normal-tissue injury after postmastectomy radiotherapy alone or combined with chemotherapy. *Int J Radiat Biol* **56**: 711–15.

Bentzen SM, Thames HD, Travis EL *et al.* (1989c). Direct estimation of latent time for radiation injury in late-responding normal tissues: gut, lung and spinal cord. *Int J Radiat Biol* **55**: 27–43.

Bentzen SM, Turesson I, Thames HD (1990). Fractionation sensitivity and latency of telangiectasia after postmastectomy radiotherapy. A graded response analysis. *Radiother Oncol* **18**: 95–106.

Bentzen SM, Vaeth M, Pedersen DE, Overgaard J (1995). Why actuarial estimates should be used in reporting late normal-tissue effects of cancer treatment … NOW. *Int J Radiat Oncol Biol Phys* **32**: 1531–4.

Bentzen SM, Skoczylas JZ, Overgaard M, Overgaard J (1996). Radiotherapy-related lung fibrosis enhanced by tamoxifen. *J Natl Cancer Inst* **88**: 918–22.

Bentzen SM, Saunders MI, Dische S, Bond SJ (2001). Radiotherapy-related early morbidity in head and neck cancer: quantitative clinical radiobiology as deduced from the CHART trial. *Radiother Oncol* **60**: 123–35.

Cox JD, Stetz J, Pajak TF (1995). Toxicity criteria of the Radiation Therapy Oncology Group (RTOG) and the European Organization for Research and Treatment of Cancer (EORTC). *Int J Radiat Oncol Biol Phys* **31**(5): 1341–6.

Dische S (1999). Revealing morbidity. *Radiother Oncol* **53**: 173–5.

Dörr W, Hendry J (2001). Consequential late effects in normal tissue. *Radiother Oncol* **61**: 223–31.

Early Breast Cancer Trialists' Collaborative Group (1995). Effects of radiotherapy and surgery in early breast cancer: an overview of the randomized trials. *N Engl J Med* **333**: 1444–55.

Early Breast Cancer Trialists' Collaborative Group (2000). Favourable and unfavourable effects on long-term survival of radiotherapy for early breast cancer: an overview of the randomised trials. *Lancet* **355**: 1757–70.

Emami B, Lyman J, Brown A *et al.* (1991). Tolerance of normal tissue to therapeutic irradiation. *Int J Radiat Oncol Biol Phys* **21**: 109–22.

Field SB, Upton AC (1985). Non-stochastic effects: compatibility with present ICRP recommendations. *Int J Radiat Biol* **48**: 81–94.

Hancock SL, McDougall IR, Constine LS (1995). Thyroid abnormalities after therapeutic external radiation. *Int J Radiat Oncol Biol Phys* **31**: 1165–70.

Hatlevoll R, Host H, Kaalhus O (1983). Myelopathy following radiotherapy of bronchial carcinoma with large single fractions: a retrospective study. *Int J Radiat Oncol Biol Phys* **9**: 41–4.

Holthusen H (1936). Erfahrungen über die Verträglichkeitsgrenze für Röntgenstrahlen und deren Nutzanwendung zur Verhütung von Schäden. *Strahlentherapie* **57**: 254–69.

Højris I, Overgaard M, Christensen JJ *et al.* (1999). Morbidity and mortality of ischaemic heart disease in high-risk breast-cancer patients after adjuvant postmastectomy systemic treatment with or without radiotherapy: analysis of DBCG 82b and 82c randomised trials. *Lancet* **354**: 1425–30.

Jung H, Beck-Bornholdt HP, Svoboda V, Alberti W, Herrmann T (2001). Quantification of late complications after radiation therapy. *Radiother Oncol* **61**: 233–46.

Kogelnik HD (1997). Inauguration of radiotherapy as a new scientific speciality by Leopold Freund 100 years ago. *Radiother Oncol* **42**: 203–11.

Machin D, Gardner MJ (1989). Calculating confidence intervals for survival time analyses. In: *Statistics with Confidence* (eds Gardner MJ, Altman DG), pp. 64–70. British Medical Journal, London.

Overgaard J, Bartelink H (1995). About tolerance and quality. An important notice to all radiation oncologists. *Radiother Oncol* **35**: 1–3.

Overgaard M, Hansen PS, Overgaard J *et al.* (1997). Postoperative radiotherapy in high-risk premenopausal women with breast cancer who receive adjuvant chemotherapy. *N Engl J Med* **337**: 949–55.

Overgaard M, Jensen MB, Overgaard J *et al.* (1999). Postoperative radiotherapy in high-risk postmenopausal breast cancer patients given adjuvant tamoxifen: Danish Breast Cancer Cooperative Group DBCG 82c trial. *Lancet* **353**: 1641–8.

Pavy J-J, Denekamp J, Letchert J *et al.* (1995). Late effects toxicity scoring: the SOMA scale. *Radiother Oncol* **35**: 11–60.

Ragaz J, Jackson SM, Le N *et al.* (1997). Adjuvant radiotherapy and chemotherapy in node-positive premenopausal women with breast cancer. *N Engl J Med* **337**: 956–62.

Rubin P, Casarett G (1968). *Clinical Radiation Pathology*. Saunders, Philadelphia.

Rubin P, Constine LS, Fajardo LF, Phillips TL, Wasserman TH (1995). Late effects of normal tissues (LENT) consensus conference. Special issue. *Int J Radiat Oncol Biol Phys* 31: 1035–364.

Rutqvist LE, Johansson H (1990). Mortality by laterality of the primary tumour among 55,000 breast cancer patients from the Swedish cancer registry. *Br J Cancer* 61: 866–8.

Sandhu AS, Zelefsky MJ, Lee HJ, Lombardi D, Fuks Z, Leibel SA (2000). Long-term urinary toxicity after 3-dimensional conformal radiotherapy for prostate cancer in patients with prior history of transurethral resections. *Int J Radiat Oncol Biol Phys* 48: 634–7.

Svoboda V, Beck-Bornholdt HP, Herrmann T, Alberti W, Jung H (1999). Late complications after a combined pre and postoperative (sandwich) radiotherapy for rectal cancer. *Radiother Oncol* 53: 177–87.

Taylor JMG, Kim DK (1993). Statistical models for analysing time-to-occurrence data in radiobiology and radiation oncology. *Int J Radiat Biol* 64: 627–40.

Taylor JMG, Withers HR, Vegesna V, Mason K (1987). Fitting the linear-quadratic model using time of occurrence as the end-point for quantal response multifraction experiments. *Int J Radiat Biol* 52: 459–68.

Trotti A, Byhardt R, Stetz J *et al.* (2000). Common toxicity criteria: version 2.0: an improved reference for grading the acute effects of cancer treatment: impact on radiotherapy. *Int J Radiat Oncol Biol Phys* 47: 13–47.

Turesson I (1990). Individual variation and dose dependency in the progression rate of skin telangiectasia. *Int J Radiat Oncol Biol Phys* 19: 1569–74.

Withers HR, Taylor JMG, Maciejewski B (1988). Treatment volume and tissue tolerance. *Int J Radiat Oncol Biol Phys* 14: 751–9.

FURTHER READING

Bentzen SM (1998). Towards evidence based radiation oncology: improving the design, analysis, and reporting of clinical outcome studies in radiotherapy. *Radiother Oncol* 46: 5–18.

Bentzen SM, Overgaard J (1994). Patient-to-patient variability in the expression of radiation-induced normal tissue injury. *Semin Radiat Oncol* 4: 68–80.

Bentzen SM, Overgaard J (1996). Clinical normal-tissue radiobiology. In: *Current Radiation Oncology*, Vol. 2 (eds Tobias JS, Thomas PRM). Arnold, London.

Dische S (1999). Revealing morbidity. *Radiother Oncol* 53: 173–5.

Dische S, Warburton MF, Jones D, Lartigau E (1989). The recording of morbidity related to radiotherapy. *Radiother Oncol* 16: 103–8.

Overgaard J, Bartelink H (1995). About tolerance and quality. An important notice to all radiation oncologists. *Radiother Oncol* 35: 1–3.

Trotti A (2000). Toxicity in head and neck cancer: a review of trends and issues. *Int J Radiat Oncol Biol Phys* 47: 1–12.

Time–dose relationships: the linear-quadratic approach

MICHAEL C JOINER AND SØREN M BENTZEN

12.1 INTRODUCTION

Major developments in radiotherapy fractionation have taken place during the past two decades and these have grown out of developments in radiation biology. The relationships between total dose and dose per fraction for late-responding tissues, acutely responding tissues and tumours provide the basic information required to optimize radiotherapy according to the dose per fraction and number of fractions.

A milestone in this subject was the publication by Thames *et al.* (1982) of a survey of isoeffect curves for various normal tissues, mainly in mice. Their summary is shown in Figure 12.1. Each of the investigations contributing to this chart was a study of the response of a normal tissue to fractionated radiation treatment using a range of doses per fraction. In order to minimize the effects of repopulation, the survey was restricted to experiments in which the overall time was kept short by the use of multiple treatments

per day, or 'where an effect of regeneration of target cells was shown to be unlikely'. This summary thus represents the influence of dose per fraction on response and excludes the influence of overall treatment time. It was possible in each study, and for each chosen dose per fraction, to determine the total radiation dose that produced some defined level of normal-tissue damage. These end-points of tolerance differed from one normal tissue or experimental study to another. Each line in Figure 12.1 is an isoeffect curve determined in this way. The dashed lines show isoeffect curves for acutely responding tissues and the full lines are for late-responding tissues. Note that fraction number increases from left to right along the abscissa and therefore the dose per fraction scale *decreases* from left to right. The results of this survey show that the isoeffective total dose increases more rapidly with decreasing dose per fraction for late effects than for acute effects. If the vertical axis is regarded as a tissue tolerance dose, it can be deduced immediately from this plot that using lower doses per fraction (towards the right-hand end of the abscissa) will tend to spare late reactions if the total dose is adjusted to keep the acute reactions constant.

The linear-quadratic (LQ) cell survival model, introduced in Chapter 7, can be used to describe this relationship between total isoeffective dose and the dose per fraction in fractionated radiotherapy. The LQ model can thus form a robust mathematical environment for considering the balance between acute and late reactions (and effect on the tumour) as dose per fraction and total dose are changed. This is one of the most important recent developments in radiobiology applied to therapy. This chapter presents the theoretical background and supporting data that have led to the wide adoption of the LQ approach to describing fractionation and shows the basic framework from which calculations can be made using this model. Examples of such calculations in a clinical setting are demonstrated practically in Chapter 13.

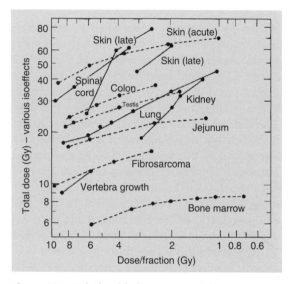

Figure 12.1 *Relationship between total dose and dose per fraction for a variety of normal tissues in experimental animals. The results for late-responding tissues (full lines) are systematically steeper than those for early-responding tissues (broken lines). From Thames et al. (1982), with permission.*

12.2   LINEAR-QUADRATIC VERSUS NOMINAL STANDARD DOSE

Two specific examples of isoeffect plots for radiation damage to normal tissues in the mouse are shown in Figure 12.2: skin is an early-responding tissue and kidney a late-responding tissue. In each case the total radiation dose to give a fixed level of damage is plotted against dose per fraction and fraction number. Note that the curve for kidney is steeper than that for skin.

The solid lines in Figure 12.2 are calculated by an equation based on the linear-quadratic (LQ) model:

$$\text{Total dose} = \frac{\text{constant}}{1 + d/(\alpha/\beta)} \qquad (12.1)$$

where d is the dose per fraction. See Section 12.4 for the derivation of this equation. The steepness and curvature of these lines are both determined by one parameter: the α/β ratio. For the skin data

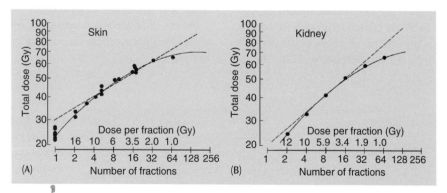

Figure 12.2 *Relationship between total dose to achieve an isoeffect and number of fractions. (A) Acute reactions in mouse skin (Douglas and Fowler, 1976). (B) Late injury in mouse kidney (Stewart et al., 1984). Note that the relationship for kidney is steeper than that for skin. The broken lines are NSD formulae fitted to the central part of each data set. The solid lines show the LQ model, from which the guide to the dose per fraction has been calculated. Reproduced with permission.*

(Figure 12.2A), α/β is about 10. The units of α/β are Gy, so the α/β ratio in this case is 10 Gy. For the kidney data, α/β is about 2 Gy.

The LQ model fits these data very well. Also shown in Figure 12.2 are broken lines showing the fit of Ellis's nominal standard dose (NSD) model (Ellis, 1969) to both data sets. The equation is:

$$\text{Total dose} = \text{NSD} \cdot N^{0.24} \cdot T^{0.11}$$

In these animal studies, the overall treatment time (T) was constant. The NSD model gives a straight line in this type of plot.

The NSD equation fits the skin data well from 4 to 32 fractions but the data points fall below the broken line both for small and large dose per fraction. The discrepancy for doses per fraction of 1–2 Gy is important in relation to hyperfractionation (see Section 14.3). For late reactions, as illustrated by the kidney data in Figure 12.2B, the NSD formula again does not fit as well as the LQ formula, even though the N exponent has been raised from 0.24 to 0.35 in order to allow for the greater slope. A similar modification, but not necessarily by the same amount, must be made for all late-responding tissues if the NSD formulation is to be even approximately correct.

A crucial therapeutic conclusion is illustrated by these two sets of data. At both ends of the scale, in the region of large and small dose per fraction, the NSD equation *overestimates* the actual tolerance dose (as shown by the experimental data). This means that the NSD equation is *unsafe* in these regions, a conclusion that is well supported by clinical experience (see Section 13.11). At the present time it is strongly recommended that the LQ model should be preferred, with a correctly chosen α/β ratio, to describe isoeffect dose relationships. This is especially so when considering doses per fraction below 2 Gy. The LQ

model is simple to use in clinical calculations and comparisons, and does not require the use of 'look-up tables'. Sections 12.4–12.6 and Chapter 13 provide a straightforward guide to LQ calculations.

12.3 CELL SURVIVAL BASIS OF THE LQ MODEL

What is the explanation for the difference between the fractionation response of early- and late-responding tissues that is shown in Figures 12.1 and 12.2? Figure 12.3 shows hypothetical single-dose (one-fraction) survival curves for the target cells in early- and late-responding tissues, drawn according to the LQ equation (see Figure 7.2B). E represents the reduction in cell survival that is equivalent to tissue tolerance. The total dose that would need to be given in two fractions is obtained by drawing a straight line from the origin through the survival curve at E/2 and measuring the intersection of this line with the dose axis. As shown by the dashed line labelled 2 in panel A, a dose of around 11 Gy takes us down to E/2 and (with assumed constant effect per fraction) a second 11 Gy gives the isoeffect E: the total isoeffect dose is ~22 Gy. This compares with a single dose of ~14 Gy to give the same isoeffect E, shown by the solid line. The total dose for three fractions is obtained in the same way by drawing a line through E/3 on the survival curve, and similarly for the other fraction numbers. Because the late-responding survival curve (Figure 12.3B) is more 'bendy' (it has a lower α/β ratio), the isoeffective total dose increases more rapidly with increasing number of fractions compared with the early-responding tissue where the survival curve bends less sharply.

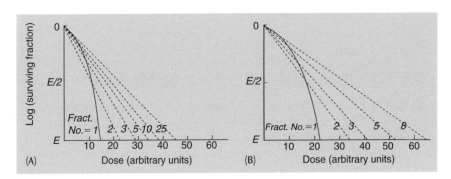

Figure 12.3 *Schematic survival curves for target cells in (A) acutely responding and (B) late-responding normal tissues. The abscissa is radiation dose on an arbitrary scale. From Thames and Hendry (1987), with permission.*

12.4   THE LQ MODEL IN DETAIL

The surviving fraction (SF_d) of target cells after a dose per fraction d is given in Section 7.5 as:

$$SF_d = \exp(-\alpha d - \beta d^2)$$

Radiobiological studies have shown that each successive fraction in a multi-dose schedule is equally effective, so the effect (E) of n fractions can be expressed as:

$$E = -\log_e(SF_d)^n = -n \log_e(SF_d)$$
$$= n(\alpha d + \beta d^2) = \alpha D + \beta dD$$

where the total radiation dose $D = nd$. This equation may be rearranged into the following forms:

$$1/D = (\alpha/E) + (\beta/E)d \qquad (12.2)$$

$$1/n = (\alpha/E)d + (\beta/E)d^2 \qquad (12.3)$$

$$D = (E/\alpha)/[1 + d/(\alpha/\beta)] \qquad (12.4)$$

The practical working of these equations may be illustrated by the results of careful fractionation experiments on the mouse kidney (Stewart *et al.*, 1984). Functional damage to the kidneys was measured by EDTA clearance up to 48 weeks after irradiation with 1–64 fractions. Figure 12.4 shows the response as a function of total radiation dose for each fraction number. To apply the LQ model to this example, we first measure off from the graph the total doses at a fixed level of effect (shown by the arrow) and then plot the reciprocal of these total doses against the corresponding dose per fraction. Equation 12.2 shows that this should give a straight line whose slope is β/E and whose intercept on the vertical axis is α/E. That this is true is shown in Figure 12.5A: the points fit a straight line well. This line cuts the x-axis at -3 Gy; it can be seen from Eqn 12.2 that this is equal to $-\alpha/\beta$,

thus providing a measure of the α/β ratio for these data. The relative contributions of α and β to the α/β ratio can be judged by comparing the reciprocal total dose intercept (α/E) and the slope of the line (β/E).

An alternative way of deriving parameter values from these data is to plot the reciprocal of the number of fractions against the dose per fraction as suggested by Eqn 12.3. Figure 12.5B shows that this gives the shape of the putative target-cell survival curve with the y-axis proportional to $-\log_e(SF_d)$. (Statistical note: this method combined with non-linear least-squares curve fitting is preferred over the linear-regression method shown in Figure 12.5A for determining α/β, because the $1/n$ and the dose-per-fraction axes are independent.) Equation 12.4 shows

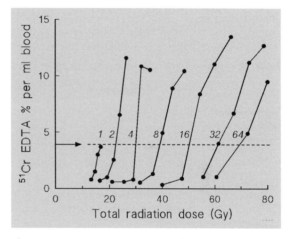

Figure 12.4 *Dose–response curves for late damage to the mouse kidney with fractionated radiation exposure. Damage is indicated by a reduction in EDTA clearance, curves determined for 1 to 64 dose fractions, illustrating the sparing effect of increased fractionation. From* Stewart et al. (1984), *with permission.*

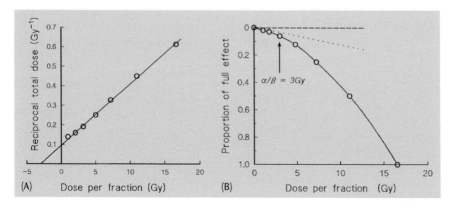

Figure 12.5 *The data of Figure 12.4 after two different transformations. (A) A reciprocal-dose plot according to Eqn 12.2. (B) Transformation according to Eqn 12.3 with the same data plotted as a proportion of full effect.*

the LQ model in the form used already to describe the relationship between total dose and dose per fraction (Figure 12.2).

A common clinical question is: 'What change in total radiation dose is required when we change the dose per fraction?' This can be dealt with very simply using the LQ approach. Rearranging Eqn 12.4:

$$E/\alpha = D \cdot [1 + d/(\alpha/\beta)]$$

For isoeffect in a selected tissue, E and α are constant. The first schedule employs a dose per fraction d_1 and the isoeffective total dose is D_1; we change to a dose per fraction d_2 and the new (unknown) total dose is D_2. D_2 is related to D_1 by the equation:

$$\frac{D_2}{D_1} = \frac{d_1 + (\alpha/\beta)}{d_2 + (\alpha/\beta)} \qquad (12.5)$$

This simple isoeffect equation was first proposed by Withers et al. (1983). It has widely been found to be successful in clinical calculations.

12.5 THE VALUE OF α/β

Many detailed fractionation studies of the type analysed in Figures 12.2 and 12.4 have been made in animals. Table 12.1 summarizes the α/β values obtained from many of these experiments. For acutely responding tissues which express their damage within a period of days to weeks after irradiation, the α/β ratio is in the range 7–20 Gy, while for late-responding tissues, which express their damage months to years after irradiation, α/β generally ranges from 0.5 to

Table 12.1 *Values for the α/β ratio for a variety of early- and late-responding normal tissues in experimental animals*

	α/β	References		α/β	References
Early reactions			**Late reactions**		
Skin			Spinal cord		
—Desquamation	9.1–12.5	Douglas and Fowler (1976)	—Cervical	1.8–2.7	van der Kogel (1979)
	8.6–10.6	Joiner et al. (1983)	—Cervical	1.6–1.9	White and Hornsey (1978)
	9–12	Moulder and Fischer (1976)	—Cervical	1.5–2.0	Ang et al. (1983)
Jejunum			—Cervical	2.2–3.0	Thames et al. (1988)
—Clones	6.0–8.3	Withers et al. (1976)	—Lumbar	3.7–4.5	van der Kogel (1979)
	6.6–10.7	Thames et al. (1981)	—Lumbar	4.1–4.9	White and Hornsey (1978)
Colon				3.8–4.1	Leith et al. (1981)
—Clones	8–9	Tucker et al. (1983)		2.3–2.9	Amols, Yuhas (quoted by Leith et al., 1981)
—Weight loss	9–13	Terry and Denekamp (1984)	Colon		
Testis			—Weight loss	3.1–5.0	Terry and Denekamp (1984)
—Clones	12–13	Thames and Withers (1980)	Kidney		
Mouse lethality			—Rabbit	1.7–2.0	Caldwell (1975)
—30d	7–10	Kaplan and Brown (1952)	—Pig	1.7–2.0	Hopewell and Wiernik (1977)
—30d	13–17	Mole (1957)	—Rats	0.5–3.8	van Rongen et al. (1988)
—30d	11–26	Paterson et al. (1952)	—Mouse	1.0–3.5	Williams and Denekamp (1984a, 1984b)
Tumour bed			—Mouse	0.9–1.8	Stewart et al. (1984a)
—45d	5.6–6.8	Begg and Terry (1984)	—Mouse	1.4–4.3	Thames et al. (1988)
			Lung		
			—LD$_{50}$	4.4–6.3	Wara et al. (1973)
			—LD$_{50}$	2.8–4.8	Field et al. (1976)
			—LD$_{50}$	2.0–4.2	Travis et al. (1983)
			—Breathing rate	1.9–3.1	Parkins and Fowler (1985)
			Bladder		
			—Frequency, capacity	5–10	Stewart et al. (1984b)

α/β values are in Gy.
From Fowler (1989); for references, see the original.

6 Gy. It is important to recognize that the α/β ratio is not constant and its value should be chosen carefully to match the specific tissue under consideration.

Values of the α/β ratio for human normal tissues and tumours are given in Table 13.1. The fractionation response of well-oxygenated tumours is thought to be similar to that of early-responding normal tissues, sometimes with an even higher α/β ratio. The values shown in Figure 12.6 were compiled by Williams *et al.* (1985). Values calculated from data obtained in experiments on rat and mouse tumours under fully radiosensitized conditions (marked 'miso' and 'oxic' in the figure) are plotted directly, and values calculated from fractionation responses under hypoxic conditions (marked 'clamp', 'anoxic' and 'hypoxic') are plotted after dividing by an assumed oxygen enhancement

ratio (OER) of 2.7, because the α/β ratios for cells and tissues under anoxic and oxic conditions are in the same proportion as the OER. Error bars are estimates of the 95% confidence range on each value. Such experiments assayed the effect of radiation either *in situ* by regrowth delay or local tumour control, or by excising the tumour from the animal and measuring the survival of cells *in vitro* (see Section 6.4).

12.6 HYPOFRACTIONATION AND HYPERFRACTIONATION

Figure 12.7A shows the form of Eqn 12.5. Curves are shown for two ranges of α/β values: 1–4 Gy and 8–15 Gy, which respectively apply to most late- and

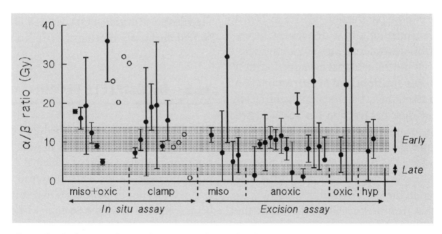

Figure 12.6 *Values of α/β for experimental tumours, determined under a variety of conditions of oxygenation (see text). The stippled areas indicate the range of values for early- and late-responding normal tissues. From Williams* et al. *(1985), with permission.*

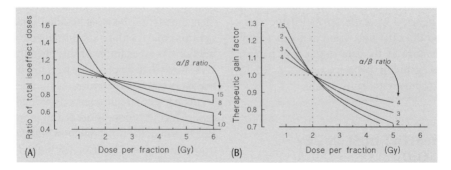

Figure 12.7 *(A) Theoretical isoeffect curves based on the LQ model for various α/β ratios. The outlined areas enclose curves corresponding to early-responding and late-responding normal tissues. (B) Therapeutic gain factors for various α/β ratios of normal tissue, assuming an α/β ratio of 10 Gy for tumours.*

acute-responding tissues. It can be seen that when dose per fraction is increased above a reference level of 2 Gy, the isoeffective dose falls more rapidly for the late-responding tissues than for the early responses. Similarly, when dose per fraction is reduced below 2 Gy, the isoeffective dose *increases* more rapidly in the late-responding tissues. Late-responding tissues are more sensitive to a change in dose per fraction and this can be thought to reflect the greater curvature of the underlying target-cell survival curve (Section 12.3).

Since the change in total dose is greater for the lower α/β values, so is the potential for error if a wrong α/β value is used. α/β values should therefore be selected carefully and always conservatively when doing calculations involving changing dose per fraction. Examples of the conservative choice of α/β values and other radiobiological parameters are given in Section 13.11 (case 7) and Section 13.12 (case 9).

An increase in dose per fraction relative to 2 Gy is termed *hypo*fractionation and a decrease is *hyper*fractionation (this use of terms may seem contradictory but it reflects the thought that *hypo*fractionation involves fewer dose fractions and *hyper*fractionation requires more fractions). A therapeutic gain factor (TGF) for a new dose per fraction can be calculated from the ratio of the relative isoeffect doses for tumour and normal tissue. An example is shown in Figure 12.7B where the tumour is taken to have an α/β ratio of 10 Gy. It is assumed here that the new regimen is given in the same overall time as the 2 Gy regimen and that treatment is always limited by the late reactions. It can be seen from the figure that hyperfractionation is predicted to give a therapeutic gain, and hypofractionation a therapeutic loss. Note, however, that this situation would be nullified, or even reversed, for specific tumours that have low α/β ratios (e.g. some melanomas and sarcomas). If an unacceptable increase in acute normal-tissue reactions prevented the total dose from being increased to the full tolerance of the late-responding tissues, the therapeutic gain for hyperfractionation would also be less than shown in Figure 12.7B.

12.7 EQUIVALENT DOSE IN 2 Gy FRACTIONS (EQD₂)

The LQ approach leads to various formulae for calculating isoeffect relationships for radiotherapy,

all based on similar underlying assumptions. These formulae seek to describe a range of fractionation schedules that are isoeffective. The simplest method of comparing the effectiveness of schedules consisting of different total doses and doses per fraction is to convert each schedule into an equivalent schedule in 2 Gy fractions which would give the same biological effect. This is the approach that we recommend as the method of choice and can be done using equation 12.5:

$$EQD_2 = D\frac{d + (\alpha/\beta)}{2 + (\alpha/\beta)} \qquad (12.6)$$

where EQD_2 is the dose in 2 Gy fractions that is biologically equivalent to a total dose D given with a fraction size of d Gy. Values of EQD_2 may be numerically added for separate parts of a treatment schedule. They have the advantage that since 2 Gy is a commonly used dose per fraction, EQD_2 values will be recognized by radiotherapists as being of a familiar size.

12.8 INCOMPLETE REPAIR

The simple LQ model described by Eqns 12.1–12.5 assumes that sufficient time is allowed between fractions for complete repair of sublethal damage to take place after each dose. This full-repair interval is at least 6 hours but in some cases (e.g. spinal cord) may be as long as 1 day (see Section 13.4). If the inter-fraction interval is reduced below this value, for example when multiple fractions per day are used, the overall damage from the whole treatment is increased because the repair (or more correctly, recovery) of damage due to one radiation dose may not be complete before the next fraction is given, and there is then interaction between residual unrepaired damage from one fraction and the damage from the next fraction. As an example of this phenomenon, Figure 12.8 shows data from mouse jejunum irradiated with five x-ray fractions in which the number of surviving crypts per gut circumference is plotted against total dose. Much less dose is needed to produce the same effects when the inter-fraction interval is reduced from 6 hours to 1 hour or 0.5 hour. This phenomenon is called *incomplete repair*.

The influence of incomplete repair is determined by the repair half-time ($T_{1/2}$) in the tissue. This is the time required between fractions, or during low-dose-rate treatment, for half the maximum possible repair to take place. Incomplete repair will tend to reduce the isoeffective dose and corrections have to be made for the consequent loss of tolerance. This can be accomplished by the use of the incomplete repair model as introduced by Thames (1985). In this model, the amount of unrepaired damage is expressed by a function H_m which depends upon the number of equally spaced fractions (m), the time interval between them and the repair half-time. For the purpose of tolerance

calculations the extra H_m term is added to the basic EQD_2 formula thus:

$$EQD_2 = D \frac{d(1 + H_m) + (\alpha/\beta)}{2 + (\alpha/\beta)} \qquad (12.7)$$

(for fractionated radiotherapy)

Once again, d is the dose per fraction and D the total dose. If repair from one day to the next is assumed to be complete, m is the number of fractions per day. Values of H_m are given in Table 12.2 for repair half-times up to 4 hours and for two or three fractions per day given with inter-fraction intervals down to 3 hours. Other values can be calculated using the formulae given in the Appendix to this chapter. Table 12.3 shows values of $T_{1/2}$ for some normal tissues in laboratory animals and the available values for human normal-tissue end-points are summarized in Table 13.2. [Advanced note: In several cases, experiments have indicated that repair has fast and slow components. The EQD_2 equation above (also BED and TE formulae) have to be reformulated in a more complex form to take account of these cases (Guttenberger et al., 1992; Millar and Canney, 1993).]

Figure 12.9 demonstrates the fit of the incomplete repair LQ model to data for pneumonitis in mice following fractionated thoracic irradiation with intervals of 3 hours between doses (Thames et al., 1984). The end-point was mortality, expressed as the LD_{50}. In these reciprocal-dose plots, incomplete repair makes the data bow upwards away from the straight line (dashed), which shows the pure LQ relationship obtained when there is complete repair between successive doses, as will be the case with long time intervals

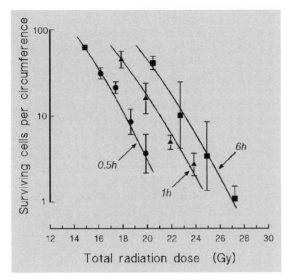

Figure 12.8 *Effect of inter-fraction interval on intestinal radiation damage in mice. The total dose required in five fractions for a given level of effect is less for short intervals, illustrating incomplete repair between fractions. From Thames* et al. *(1984), with permission.*

Table 12.2 *Incomplete repair factors: fractionated irradiation (*H_m *factors)*

Repair per day half-time (h)	Interval (h) for m = 2 fractions per day					Interval (h) for m = 3 fractions				
	3	4	5	6	8	3	4	5	6	8
0.5	0.0156	0.0039	0.0010	0.0002	0	0.0210	0.0052	0.0013	0.0003	0
0.75	0.0625	0.0248	0.0098	0.0039	0.0006	0.0859	0.0335	0.0132	0.0052	0.0008
1.0	0.1250	0.0625	0.0312	0.0156	0.0039	0.1771	0.0859	0.0423	0.0210	0.0052
1.25	0.1895	0.1088	0.0625	0.0359	0.0118	0.2766	0.1530	0.0859	0.0487	0.0159
1.5	0.2500	0.1575	0.0992	0.0625	0.0248	0.3750	0.2265	0.1388	0.0859	0.0335
2.0	0.3536	0.2500	0.1768	0.1250	0.0625	0.5547	0.3750	0.2565	0.1771	0.0859
2.5	0.4353	0.3299	0.2500	0.1895	0.1088	0.7067	0.5124	0.3750	0.2766	0.1530
3.0	0.5000	0.3969	0.3150	0.2500	0.1575	0.8333	0.6341	0.4861	0.3750	0.2265
4.0	0.5946	0.5000	0.4204	0.3536	0.2500	1.0285	0.8333	0.6784	0.5547	0.3750

Table 12.3 *Half-times for recovery from radiation damage in normal tissues of laboratory animals*

Tissue	Species	Dose delivery[#]	$T_{1/2}$ (hours)	Source
Haemopoietic	Mouse	CLDR	0.3	Thames *et al.* (1984)
Spermatogonia	Mouse	CLDR	0.3–0.4	Delic *et al.* (1987)
Jejunum	Mouse	F	0.45	Thames *et al.* (1984)
	Mouse	CLDR	0.2–0.7	Dale *et al.* (1988)
Colon (acute injury)	Mouse	F	0.8	Thames *et al.* (1984)
	Rat	F	1.5	Sassy *et al.* (1988)
Lip mucosa	Mouse	F	0.8	Ang *et al.* (1985)
	Mouse	CLDR	0.8	Scalliet *et al.* (1987)
	Mouse	FLDR	0.6	Stüben *et al.* (1991)
Tongue epithelium	Mouse	F	0.75	Dörr *et al.* (1993)
Skin (acute injury)	Mouse	F	1.5	Rojas *et al.* (1991)
	Mouse	CLDR	1.0	Joiner *et al.* (unpublished)
	Pig	F	0.4 + 1.2*	van den Aardweg and Hopewell (1992)
	Pig	F	0.2 + 6.6*	Millar *et al.* (1996)
Lung	Mouse	F	0.4 + 4.0*	van Rongen *et al.* (1993)
	Mouse	CLDR	0.85	Down *et al.* (1986)
	Rat	FLDR	1.0	van Rongen (1989)
Spinal cord	Rat	F	0.7 + 3.8*	Ang *et al.* (1992)
	Rat	CLDR	1.4	Scalliet *et al.* (1989)
	Rat	CLDR	1.43	Pop *et al.* (1996)
Kidney	Mouse	F	1.3	Joiner *et al.* (1993)
	Mouse	F	0.2 + 5.0	Millar *et al.* (1994)
	Rat	F	1.6–2.1	van Rongen *et al.* (1990)
Rectum (late injury)	Rat	CLDR	1.2	Kiszel *et al.* (1985)
Heart	Rat	F	>3	Schultz-Hector *et al.* (1992)

* Two components of repair with different half-times.
[#] CLDR, continuous low dose rate; F, acute dose fractions; FLDR, fractionated low dose rate.

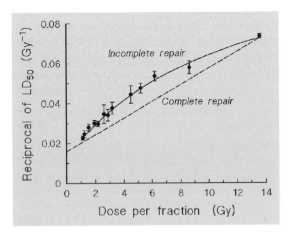

Figure 12.9 *Reciprocal dose plot (compare Figure 12.5A) of data for pneumonitis in mice produced by fractionated irradiation; the points derive from experiments with different dose per fraction (and therefore different fraction numbers), always with 3 hours between doses. The upward bend in the data illustrates lack of sparing due to incomplete repair. From Thames* et al. *(1984), with permission.*

between fractions. An estimate of the repair half-time can be found by fitting data of the type shown in Figures 12.8 and 12.9 using the incomplete repair LQ model and seeking the $T_{1/2}$ value that gives the best fit.

Continuous irradiation

Another common situation in which incomplete repair occurs in clinical radiotherapy is during continuous irradiation. As described in Sections 18.1–18.3, irradiation must be given at a very low dose rate (below about 5 cGy h^{-1}) for full repair to occur during irradiation. At the other extreme, a single irradiation at high dose rate may allow no significant repair to occur during exposure. As the dose rate is reduced below the range used in external-beam radiotherapy, the duration of irradiation becomes longer and the induction of damage is counteracted by repair, leading to an increase in the isoeffective dose. The corresponding EQD$_2$ formula for continuous irradiation

Table 12.4 *Incomplete repair factors: continuous irradiation (g factors)*

Repair half-time (h)	Exposure time (h)					
	1	2	3	4	8	12
0.5	0.6622	0.4774	0.3671	0.2959	0.1641	0.1130
0.75	0.7517	0.5888	0.4774	0.3983	0.2339	0.1641
1	0.8040	0.6622	0.5571	0.4774	0.2959	0.2115
1.25	0.8382	0.7137	0.6165	0.5394	0.3504	0.2555
1.5	0.8622	0.7517	0.6622	0.5888	0.3983	0.2959
2	0.8938	0.8040	0.7276	0.6622	0.4774	0.3671
2.5	0.9136	0.8382	0.7720	0.7137	0.5394	0.4269
3	0.9272	0.8622	0.8040	0.7517	0.5888	0.4774
4	0.9447	0.8938	0.8471	0.8040	0.6622	0.5571

Repair half-time (h)	Exposure time (days)						
	1	1.5	2	2.5	3	3.5	4
0.5	0.0583	0.0393	0.0296	0.0238	0.0198	0.0170	0.0149
0.75	0.0861	0.0583	0.0441	0.0354	0.0296	0.0254	0.0223
1	0.1130	0.0769	0.0583	0.0469	0.0393	0.0338	0.0296
1.25	0.1390	0.0952	0.0723	0.0583	0.0488	0.0420	0.0369
1.5	0.1641	0.1130	0.0861	0.0695	0.0583	0.0502	0.0441
2	0.2115	0.1475	0.1130	0.0916	0.0769	0.0663	0.0583
2.5	0.2555	0.1803	0.1390	0.1130	0.0952	0.0822	0.0723
3	0.2959	0.2115	0.1641	0.1339	0.1130	0.0977	0.0861
4	0.3671	0.2693	0.2115	0.1739	0.1475	0.1280	0.1130

incorporates the factor g to allow for incomplete repair:

$$EQD_2 = D\frac{dg + (\alpha/\beta)}{2 + (\alpha/\beta)} \quad (12.8)$$

(for continuous low-dose-rate radiotherapy)

where D is the total dose (= dose rate × time). The parameter d is retained, as in the equation for fractionated radiotherapy, in order to deal with fractionated low-dose-rate exposures. For a single continuous exposure $d = D$. This equation assumes that there is full recovery between the low-dose-rate exposures; if not, the H_m factor must be added (see Appendix). Table 12.4 gives values of the g factor for exposure times between 1 hour and 4 days.

12.9 SHOULD A TIME FACTOR BE INCLUDED?

If the overall duration of fractionated radiotherapy is increased there will usually be greater repopulation of the irradiated tissues, both in the tumour and in normal tissues. So far, the change in total dose necessary to compensate for changes in the overall duration of treatment has not been discussed. Overall time is included in the NSD model but not in the basic LQ approach described above. The reason is because the time factor in radiotherapy is now perceived to be more complex than was previously supposed. For example, Figure 12.10 shows that the extra dose needed to counteract proliferation in mouse skin does not become significant until about 2 weeks after the start of daily fractionation. For this situation the time factor in the NSD formula (broken line: total dose $\propto T^{0.11}$) gives a false picture because it predicts a large amount of sparing if the overall time was increased from 1 to 12 days. These wrong time factors have not led to major clinical disasters because they predict much less effect on total dose compared with changing the number of fractions. Thus the $T^{0.11}$ factor in the NSD model predicts only an 8% increase in total dose for a doubling of overall time, for example from 3½ to 7 weeks.

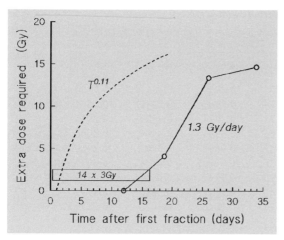

Figure 12.10 *Extra dose required to counteract proliferation in mouse skin. Test doses of radiation were given at various intervals after a priming treatment with fractionated radiation. Proliferation begins about 12 days after the start of irradiation and is then equivalent to an extra dose of approximately 1.3 Gy per day. The broken line shows the prediction of the NSD equation. Adapted from Denekamp (1973), with permission.*

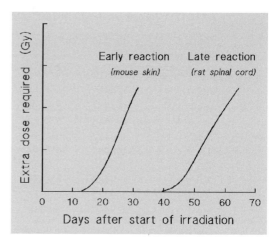

Figure 12.11 *Schematic diagram showing that the extra dose required to counteract proliferation does not become significant until much later for late-responding normal tissues such as spinal cord, beyond the 6-week duration of conventional radiotherapy. From Fowler (1984), with permission.*

Nevertheless, the $T^{0.11}$ factor is clearly misleading and should not be used. The use of the LQ model in clinical practice with no time factor at all is probably the best strategy for late-reacting tissues because any extra dose needed to counteract proliferation does not become significant until beyond the overall time of treatment, even up to 6 weeks. This is illustrated in Figure 12.11, which diagrammatically shows the different effects of overall time in early- and late-responding tissues. Attempts have been made to include time factors in the LQ model for early-responding normal tissues and tumours, but such factors depend in a complex way on the dose per fraction and inter-fraction interval as well as on the tissue type, and have to take account of any delay in onset of proliferation which may depend in some way on these factors also. We therefore recommend considering the influence of changing overall time on radiotherapy as a separate problem from the effect of changing the dose per fraction, which can be done in a straightforward way using the LQ model as described here. The practical approaches to handling changes in overall time are described in Section 13.6.

12.10 ALTERNATIVE ISOEFFECT FORMULAE BASED ON THE LQ MODEL

Two other formulations that can be used for comparing schedules with differing doses per fraction are the concepts of Extrapolated Tolerance Dose (ETD) introduced by Barendsen (1982) and Total Effect (TE) described by Thames and Hendry (1987). Both these methods are mathematically (and biologically) equivalent with the EQD_2 concept, but are mentioned here because they have found some use in the literature.

Extrapolated total dose (ETD) or biologically effective dose (BED)

ETD and BED are mathematically identical concepts. Fowler (1989) preferred the term biologically effective dose (BED), because it can logically be understood to refer to levels of effect that are below normal-tissue tolerance, whereas the term ETD implies the full tolerance effect. First, we must define a particular effect, or end-point. Although the validity of the LQ approach to fractionation depends principally on its ability to predict isoeffective schedules successfully, there is an implicit assumption that the isoeffect has a direct relationship with a certain level of cell inactivation (or final cell survival, $(SF_d)^n$). Generally, the fraction of surviving cells associated with an isoeffect is unknown and it is customary to work in terms of a level of tissue effect, which we denote as E. From Eqn 12.4:

$$E/\alpha = D[1 + d/(\alpha/\beta)] = \text{biologically effective dose (BED)}$$

BED is a measure of the effect (E) of a course of fractionated or continuous irradiation; when divided by α it has the units of dose and is usually expressed in Gy. Note that as the dose per fraction (d) is reduced towards zero, BED becomes $D = nd$ (i.e. the total radiation dose). Thus, BED is the theoretical total dose that would be required to produce the isoeffect E using an infinitely large number of infinitesimally small dose fractions. It is therefore also the total dose required for a single exposure at very low dose rate (see Section 18.5). As with the simpler concept of EQD_2, values of BED from separate parts of a course of treatment may be added in order to calculate the overall BED value. A disadvantage of BED as a measure of treatment intensity is that it is numerically much greater than any prescribable radiation dose of fractionated radiotherapy and is therefore difficult to relate to everyday clinical practice, which is the main reason why the use of EQD_2 is recommended in this book.

Total effect (TE)

The TE formulation is conceptually similar to BED and has also been used in the literature. In this case, we divide E by β rather than α, to get

$$E/\beta = D[(\alpha/\beta) + d] = \text{total effect (TE)}$$

The units of TE are $(Gy)^2$, which again means that the TE values have no simple interpretation. The TE isoeffect formulae are similar to the EQD_2 formulae except that the denominator $(2 + \alpha/\beta)$ is omitted. This has the computational advantage that division by this factor is done only for the final TE value and not for any intermediate calculations. However, it has the disadvantage that these intermediate results are not recognizable doses, and we prefer the EQD_2 method as a means of making it easier to detect numerical errors in the calculation process.

KEY POINTS

1. The LQ model satisfactorily describes the relationship between total isoeffective dose and dose per fraction over the range of dose per fraction from 1 Gy up to large single doses. By contrast, the NSD formulation can only be made to fit data over a limited range of dose per fraction.
2. The α/β ratio describes the *shape* of the fractionation response: a low α/β (0.5–6 Gy) is characteristic of late-responding normal tissues and indicates a rapid increase of total dose with decreasing dose per fraction and a survival curve for the putative target cells that is significantly curved.
3. A higher α/β ratio (7–20 Gy) is characteristic of early-responding normal tissues and tumours; it indicates a less rapid increase in total dose with decreasing dose per fraction and a less curved survival response for the putative target cells.
4. The EQD_2 formulae provide a simple and convenient way of calculating isoeffective radiotherapy schedules, based on the LQ model. Tolerance calculations require an estimate of the α/β ratio.
5. For short inter-fraction intervals, a correction may be necessary for incomplete repair. When using the EQD_2 formulae to calculate schedules with multiple fractions per day or continuous low dose rate, an estimate of the repair half-time is also needed.
6. The basic LQ model is appropriate for calculating the change in total dose for an altered dose per fraction, assuming the new and old treatments are given in the *same overall time*. For late reactions it is probably unnecessary to modify total dose in response to a change in overall time, but for early reactions (and for tumour response) the effect of overall time is complex. The effect of this should be considered separately from the LQ calculation.

BIBLIOGRAPHY

Barendsen GW (1982). Dose fractionation, dose rate, and isoeffect relationships for normal tissue responses. *Int J Radiat Oncol Biol Phys* **8**: 1981–97.

Denekamp J (1973). Changes in the rate of repopulation during multifraction irradiation of mouse skin. *Br J Radiol* **46**: 381.

Douglas BG, Fowler JF (1976). The effect of multiple small doses of *x*-rays on skin reactions in the mouse and a basic interpretation. *Radiat Res* **66**: 401–26.

Ellis F (1969). Dose, time and fractionation: a clinical hypothesis. *Clin Radiol* **20**: 1–7.

Fowler JF (1984). What next in fractionated radiotherapy? *Br J Cancer* **49**(Suppl VI): 285–300.

Guttenberger R, Thames HD, Ang KK (1992). Is the experience with CHART compatible with experimental data? A new model of repair kinetics and computer simulations. *Radiother Oncol* **25**: 280–6.

Fowler JF (1989). The linear-quadratic formula and progress in fractionated radiotherapy. *Br J Radiol* **62**: 679–94.

Millar WT, Canney PA (1993). Derivation and application of equations describing the effects of fractionated protracted irradiation, based on multiple and incomplete repair processes. Part 1. Derivation of equations. *Int J Radiat Biol* **64**: 275–91.

Nilsson P, Thames HD, Joiner MC (1990). A generalized formulation of the 'incomplete-repair' model for cell survival and tissue response to fractionated low dose-rate irradiation. *Int J Radiat Biol* **57**: 127–42.

Stewart FA, Soranson JA, Alpen EL, Williams MV, Denekamp J (1984). Radiation-induced renal damage: the effects of hyperfractionation. *Radiat Res* **98**: 407–20.

Thames HD (1985). An 'incomplete-repair' model for survival after fractionated and continuous irradiations. *Int J Radiat Biol* **47**: 319–39.

Thames HD, Hendry JH (1987). *Fractionation in Radiotherapy*. Taylor & Francis, London.

Thames HD, Withers HR, Peters LJ, Fletcher GH (1982). Changes in early and late radiation responses with altered dose fractionation: implications for dose survival relationships. *Int J Radiat Oncol Biol Phys* **8**: 219–26.

Thames HD, Withers HR, Peters LJ (1984). Tissue repair capacity and repair kinetics deduced from multifractionated or continuous irradiation regimens with incomplete repair. *Br J Cancer* **49**(Suppl VI): 263–9.

Williams MV, Denekamp J, Fowler JF (1985). A review of α/β ratios for experimental tumors: implications for clinical studies of altered fractionation. *Int J Radiat Oncol Biol Phys* **11**: 87–96.

Withers HR, Thames HD, Peters LJ (1983). A new isoeffect curve for change in dose per fraction. *Radiother Oncol* **1**: 187–91.

FURTHER READING

Fowler JF (1989). The linear-quadratic formula and progress in fractionated radiotherapy. *Br J Radiol* **62**: 679–94.

Joiner MC (1989). The dependence of radiation response on the dose per fraction. In: *The Scientific Basis for Modern Radiotherapy (BIR Report 19)* (ed. McNally NJ), pp. 20–6. British Institute of Radiology, London.

Thames HD, Hendry JH (1987). *Fractionation in Radiotherapy*. Taylor & Francis, London.

Thames HD, Bentzen SM, Turesson I, Overgaard J, van den Bogaert W (1990). Time-dose factors in radiotherapy: a review of the human data. *Radiother Oncol* **19**: 219–35.

APPENDIX: SUMMARY OF FORMULAE

Basic equations

$$E = n(\alpha d + \beta d^2) = D(\alpha + \beta d)$$
$$d = \text{dose per fraction}$$
$$D = \text{total dose}$$
$$n = \text{number of fractions}$$

$$SF = \exp(-E) = \exp[-(\alpha + \beta d)D]$$

For schedules having the same *E*, i.e. isoeffective schedules,

$$\frac{D}{D_{ref}} = \frac{d_{ref} + (\alpha/\beta)}{d + (\alpha/\beta)}$$

$$\text{hence: } EQD_2 = D\frac{d + (\alpha/\beta)}{2 + (\alpha/\beta)}$$

Low dose rate

$$\mu = \frac{\log_e 2}{T_{1/2}} \quad T_{1/2} = \text{repair half-time}$$

$$g = 2[\mu t - 1 + \exp(-\mu t)]/(\mu t)^2$$
$$t = \text{exposure duration}$$

$$EQD_2 = D\frac{dg + (\alpha/\beta)}{2 + (\alpha/\beta)}$$

Incomplete repair correction

$$\phi = \exp(-\mu \Delta T) \quad \Delta T = \text{interval between fractions}$$

$$H_m = \left(\frac{2}{m}\right) \cdot \left(\frac{\phi}{1 - \phi}\right) \cdot \left(m - \frac{1 - \phi^m}{1 - \phi}\right)$$

$$m = \text{number of fractions per day}$$

$$EQD_2 = D\frac{d(1 + H_m) + (\alpha/\beta)}{2 + (\alpha/\beta)}$$

Incomplete repair between low-dose-rate fractions

$$\phi = \exp[-\mu(t + \Delta T)]$$
$$\Delta T = \text{interval between fractions}$$
$$t = \text{exposure duration per fraction}$$

$$g = 2[\mu t - 1 + \exp(-\mu t)]/(\mu t)^2$$

$$H_m = \left(\frac{2}{m}\right) \cdot \left(\frac{\phi}{1 - \phi}\right) \cdot \left(m - \frac{1 - \phi^m}{1 - \phi}\right)$$

$$m = \text{number of fractions per day}$$

$$C = g + 2\frac{\cosh(\mu t) - 1}{(\mu t)^2} \cdot H_m$$

$$EQD_2 = D\frac{dC + (\alpha/\beta)}{2 + (\alpha/\beta)}$$

For a full derivation of these equations, see Nilsson *et al.* (1990).

13

The linear-quadratic model in clinical practice

SØREN M BENTZEN AND MICHAEL BAUMANN

13.1 INTRODUCTION: CAUTION IN USING ISOEFFECT CALCULATIONS

Several mathematically equivalent methods have been devised for performing isoeffect calculations with the linear-quadratic (LQ) model, as discussed in Chapter 12. An intuitively attractive, although perhaps not the most mathematically elegant, method is to convert all parts of a treatment into the isoeffective dose in 2 Gy fractions, the EQD_2 (see Section 12.7). This has the advantage that these doses are clinically relevant and they are measured on the scale where much of the clinical experience on dose–response relationships is available. The EQD_2 values from various parts of a fractionation schedule may be added directly.

It should be stressed at the outset that biological effect calculations should be used only as guidance for clinical decision-making. All of the formulae applied here have a limited field of applicability, the model

assumptions may be violated in some circumstances, relevant parameters may not be known for human tissues and tumours, and the uncertainty in parameter estimates, even when these are available, may give rise to considerable uncertainty in the biological effect estimates. A (self-)critical and cautious attitude is recommended and the health and safety of patients should not be compromised by reliance on the results of calculations of the type described in this chapter. Having said that, a numerical estimate is often very useful when considering various therapeutic options and it is often possible to get a simple impression of how reliable such an estimate is by doing a simple calculation as illustrated in this chapter.

13.2 THE α/β RATIO

Many fractionation studies in the laboratory, mainly in rodents, have shown the ability of the linear-quadratic model to provide a close quantitative relationship between dose per fraction and the isoeffective total dose. These studies have also produced a number of α/β estimates for various end-points in normal tissues and organs (see Table 12.1). In parallel with these experimental studies, a number of clinical studies have produced estimates for human end-points and these are summarized in Table 13.1.

Table 13.1 *α/β ratios for human normal tissues and tumours*

Tissue/organ	End-point	α/β (Gy)	95% conf. lim. (Gy)	Reference
Early reactions				
Skin	Erythema	8.8	[6.9; 11.6]	Turesson and Thames (1989)
	Erythema	12.3	[1.8; 22.8]	Bentzen et al. (1988)
	Desquamation	11.2	[8.5; 17.6]	Turesson and Thames (1989)
Oral mucosa	Mucositis	9.3	[5.8; 17.9]	Denham et al. (1995)
	Mucositis	15	[−15; 45]	Rezvani et al. (1991)
	Mucositis	~8	N/A	Chogule and Supe (1993)
Late reactions				
Skin/vasculature	Telangiectasia	2.8	[1.7; 3.8]	Turesson and Thames (1989)
	Telangiectasia	2.6	[2.2; 3.3]	Bentzen et al. (1990)
	Telangiectasia	2.8	[−0.1; 8.1]	Bentzen and Overgaard (1991)
Subcutis	Fibrosis	1.7	[0.6; 2.6]	Bentzen and Overgaard (1991)
Muscle/vasculature/ cartilage	Impaired shoulder movement	3.5	[0.7; 6.2]	Bentzen et al. (1989)
Nerve	Brachial plexopathy	<3.5*	N/A	Olsen et al. (1990)
	Brachial plexopathy	~2	N/A	Powell et al. (1990)
	Optic neuropathy	1.6	[−7; 10]	Jiang et al. (1994)
Spinal cord	Myelopathy	<3.3	N/A	Dische et al. (1981)
Eye	Corneal injury	2.9	[−4; 10]	Jiang et al. (1994)
Bowel	Stricture/perforation	3.9	[2.5; 5.3]	Deore et al. (1993)
	Various late effects	4.3	[2.2; 9.6]	Dische et al. (1999)
Lung	Pneumonitis	4.0	[2.2; 5.8]	Bentzen et al. (2000)
	Lung fibrosis (radiological)	3.1	[−0.2; 8.5]	Dubray et al. (1995)
Head and neck	Various late effects	3.5	[1.1; 5.9]	Rezvani et al. (1991)
	Various late effects	4.0	[3.3; 5.0]	Stuschke and Thames (1999)
Supraglottic larynx	Various late effects	3.8	[0.8; 14]	Maciejewski et al. (1986)
Oral cavity + oroph.	Various late effects	0.8	[−0.6; 2.5]	Maciejewski et al. (1990)
Tumours				
Head and neck				
—Larynx		14.5*	[4.9; 24]	Rezvani et al. (1993)
—Vocal cord		~13	Wide	Robertson et al. (1993)
—Oropharynx		~16*	N/A	Horiot et al. (1992)
—Buccal mucosa		6.6	[2.9; infinity]	Maciejewski et al. (1989)
—Tonsil		7.2	[3.6; infinity]	Maciejewski et al. (1989)
—Nasopharynx		16	[−11; 43]	Lee et al. (1995)
—Various		10.5	[6.5; 29]	Stuschke and Thames (1999)
Skin		8.5*	[4.5; 11.3]	Trott et al. (1984)
Prostate		Low?**		Brenner and Hall (1999)
Melanoma		0.6	[−1.1; 2.5]	Bentzen et al. (1989)
Liposarcoma		0.4	[−1.4; 5.4]	Thames and Suit (1986)

* Re-analysis of original published data. ** Data currently insufficient to quantify. Compiled by Bentzen and Thames (unpublished). See also Thames et al. (1990). Reference details are available from Søren Bentzen and Michael Baumann.

13.3 CHANGING THE DOSE PER FRACTION

The simplest case considered in this chapter is where the dose per fraction is changed without change in the overall treatment time and when fractions are far enough apart to make incomplete repair negligible. The Withers formula is used to convert a total dose D delivered with dose per fraction d into the isoeffective dose in 2 Gy fractions:

$$EQD_2 = D \frac{d + (\alpha/\beta)}{2 + (\alpha/\beta)} \qquad (12.6)$$

Note that the only parameter in this formula is the α/β ratio; this is a characteristic of the tissue and end-point of interest. Any biological dose calculation will therefore start with the identification of the tumour or normal-tissue end-point of concern in that particular clinical situation and a consideration of the appropriate α/β ratios for these end-points.

Example 1: how to convert a dose into the isoeffective dose in 2 Gy fractions

Problem

A patient with metastatic bone pain located to the 5th thoracic vertebra is considered for palliative radiotherapy using 4×5 Gy. We are concerned about possible radiation damage to the spinal cord. To evaluate this we need to calculate the isoeffective dose in 2 Gy fractions to the cord.

Solution

First we need to choose a value for the α/β ratio. From Table 13.1 it is seen that the upper bound on α/β from human data on myelopathy is 3.3 Gy. Experimental animal studies (see Table 12.1) have produced estimates that average around 2 Gy. We choose $\alpha/\beta = 2$ Gy, insert the values for total dose (20 Gy) and dose per fraction (5 Gy) into Eqn 12.6 and get:

$$EQD_2 = 20 \cdot \frac{5 + 2}{2 + 2} = 35\,Gy$$

Thus, 20 Gy delivered in 5 Gy fractions is biologically equivalent to 35 Gy in 2 Gy fractions in a tissue with $\alpha/\beta = 2.0$ Gy.

13.4 CHANGING THE TIME INTERVAL BETWEEN DOSE FRACTIONS

Radiotherapy schedules using multiple fractions per day are associated with an increased biological effect unless the interval between fractions is sufficiently long to allow full recovery between fractions. There are data to suggest (Table 13.2) that the characteristic half-time for repair is in the region of 4–5 h for some human late end-points (Bentzen et al., 1999) and possibly even longer for spinal cord and brain (Dische and Saunders, 1989; Lee et al., 1999). This means that repair will not be complete even with a 6–8 h interval between fractions. In this situation it is necessary to modify the simple LQ model as described in Section

Table 13.2 *Repair half-time for human normal-tissue end-points*

End-point	Dose delivery*	$T_{1/2}$ (hours)	95% CI (hours)	Source
Erythema, skin	MFD	0.35 and 1.2**	?	Turesson and Thames (1989)
Mucositis, head and neck	MFD	2–4	?	Bentzen et al. (1996)
	FLDR	0.3–0.7	?	Denham et al. (1995)
Laryngeal oedema	MFD	4.9	[3.2; 6.4]	Bentzen et al. (1999)
Radiation myelopathy	MFD	>5	?	Dische and Saunders (1989)
Skin telangiectasia	MFD	0.4 and 3.5**	?	Turesson and Thames (1989)
	MFD	3.8	[2.5; 4.6]	Bentzen et al. (1999)
Subcutaneous fibrosis	MFD	4.4	[3.8; 4.9]	Bentzen et al. (1999)
Temporal lobe necrosis	MFD	>4	?	Lee et al. (1999)
Various pelvic complications	HDR/LDR	1.5–2.5	?	Fowler (1997)

*MFD, multiple fractions per day; FLDR, fractionated low-dose-rate irradiation; HDR/LDR, high-dose-rate/low-dose-rate comparison. **Evidence of two components of repair with different half-times. Reference details are available from Søren Bentzen and Michael Baumann.

12.8. Equation 12.7 can be used under the assumption that repair is complete in the long overnight interval, i.e. between the last fraction delivered in one day and the first fraction on the following day. Even this assumption starts to be problematic with repair half-times of 4–5 hours. Guttenberger *et al.* (1992) have derived a formula in which unrepaired damage is allowed to accumulate throughout the fractionation course. Unfortunately, this formula is not easy to tabulate as it depends not only on the repair half-time and the dose per fraction but also on the exact arrangement of dose fractions over time, e.g. whether treatments are given on Saturdays and Sundays as well as on weekdays.

Example 2: incomplete repair with multiple fractions per day

Problem

A patient with squamous cell carcinoma of the head and neck is prescribed 70 Gy in 2 Gy fractions over 7 weeks. After 50 Gy he has an intercurrent pneumonia and cannot attend radiotherapy for one week. In order to finish treatment on time, it is decided to give the last 20 Gy as 2 Gy fractions twice per day on the last five treatment days. What is the isoeffective dose in 2 Gy fractions for subcutaneous fibrosis for a 6-hour interval or an 8-hour interval?

Solution

First, we need to choose values for α/β and $T_{1/2}$. In Table 13.1 we see that skin fibrosis has a value of $\alpha/\beta = 1.7$ Gy and in Table 13.2 we find $T_{1/2} = 4.4$ hours. We now use Eqn 12.7:

$$EQD_2 = D \frac{d(1 + H_m) + (\alpha/\beta)}{2 + (\alpha/\beta)} \qquad (12.7)$$

In this case, $m = 2$ and we use Table 12.2 to look up the values of H_2. For an inter-fraction interval of 6 hours, we see that H_2 is between 0.35 ($T_{1/2} = 4.0$ hours) and 0.44 ($T_{1/2} = 5.0$ hours). Interpolation between these values yields $H_2 = 0.39$ for $T_{1/2} = 4.4$ hours and therefore

$$EQD_2 (\Delta t = 6 \, h) = 50 + 20 \cdot \frac{1.7 + 2 \cdot [1 + 0.39]}{1.7 + 2}$$

$$= 74.2 \, Gy$$

For an 8-hour interval the value of H_2 is between 0.25 ($T_{1/2} = 4.0$ hours) and 0.33 ($T_{1/2} = 5.0$ hours). Interpolation between these values yields $H_2 = 0.28$ for $T_{1/2} = 4.4$ hours and therefore

$$EQD_2 (\Delta t = 8 \, h) = 50 + 20 \cdot \frac{1.7 + 2 \cdot [1 + 0.28]}{1.7 + 2}$$

$$= 73.0 \, Gy$$

Thus, there is still some sparing from increasing inter-fraction intervals from 6 to 8 hours.

As mentioned above, this calculation assumes that the overnight interval is sufficiently long to ensure complete repair of sublethal damage. This assumption starts to break down when $T_{1/2}$ is as long as 4.4 hours. A calculation using the formula of Guttenberger *et al.* (1992) gives an EQD_2 of 25.2 Gy for the last week of b.i.d. treatment (rather than 24.2 Gy as calculated in the example) for the 6-hour interval and 24.2 Gy (rather than 23.0 Gy) for the 8-hour interval.

13.5   CONTINUOUS IRRADIATION

In brachytherapy, repair takes place not only after irradiation but also during the application (see Section 18.2). In this case, the apparent dose per fraction is modified by a function of the exposure time and the repair half-time, $T_{1/2}$ (see Equation 12.8 and the appendix to Chapter 12). The isoeffective dose depends strongly on the repair half-time as shown in Figure 18.6. As these half-times are usually not known with any useful precision from clinical data, great care should be taken when interpreting the results of isoeffect calculations for continuous irradiation.

13.6   CHANGING THE OVERALL TREATMENT TIME

Changes in overall treatment time often occur in clinical radiotherapy and there is commonly a need to correct for this. There are good reasons to believe that overall treatment time has very little, if any, influence on *late* radiation effects (Bentzen and Overgaard, 1996). However, for most tumour types and for *early* end-points, the biological effect of a given schedule will decrease if the overall treatment time is increased. In other words, an extra dose will be needed to obtain the same level of effect in a longer schedule. This is

Table 13.3 *Values for* D$_{prolif}$ *from clinical studies*

Tissue	D$_{prolif}$ (Gy d^{-1})	95% CI	T$_k$** (days)	Source
Early reactions				
Skin (erythema)	0.12	[−0.12; 0.22]	<12 days	Bentzen et al. (2001)
Mucosa (mucositis)	0.8	[0.7; 1.1]	<12 days	Bentzen et al. (2001)
Lung (pneumonitits)	0.54	[0.13; 0.95]		Bentzen et al. (2000) (R)
Tumours				
Head and neck				
—Larynx	0.74	[0.30; 1.2]		Robertson et al. (1998)
—Tonsils	0.73		30 days	Withers et al. (1995)
—Various	0.8	[0.5; 1.1]	21 days	Robers et al. (1994)
—Various	0.64*	[0.42; 0.86]		Hendry et al. (1996)
Non-small cell lung cancer	0.45			Koukourakis et al. (1996)
Medulloblastoma	0.52	[0.29; 0.75]	0 or 21 days	Hinata et al. (2001)

* Pooled estimate from a review of studies in the literature. ** T$_k$ is the assumed time for the onset of accelerated proliferation. Reference details are available from Søren Bentzen and Michael Baumann.

mainly the result of proliferation of target cells in the irradiated tissue or tumour and many attempts have been made to include this effect in the LQ model. As illustrated in Figures 12.10 and 12.11, experimental animal studies have shown that this is a non-linear effect as a function of time, in other words the dose recovered per unit time will change as a function of the time since the initial trauma. At present, there is no mathematical model describing this recovery over extended time intervals. The most cautious approach (see Section 12.9) is to use a simple linear relationship in a fairly narrow interval around the overall time of the schedule from which it has been estimated.

The magnitude of the time effect is most conveniently quantified by D$_{prolif}$, which is the dose recovered per day due to proliferation, values for which are given in Table 13.3. For minor changes in overall time, say, a 4-day protraction of a schedule, the simple estimate would then be that the EQD$_2$ has to be reduced by 4 × D$_{prolif}$. Using this method, the iso-effective doses in 2 Gy fractions delivered over two different times, T and t, will be related as

$$EQD_{2,T} = EQD_{2,t} - (T - t) \cdot D_{prolif} \quad (13.1)$$

Note that if T > t, then EQD$_{2,T}$ < EQD$_{2,t}$. There is no simple rule to indicate the maximum difference between the two times, T and t, for which this linear correction is reasonable. For a 1-week difference this approximation would probably be acceptable whereas for a 3–4-week difference this would not be a safe assumption.

Another concern is that D$_{prolif}$ may depend on the intensity of the schedule, in particular that a very short

intensive schedule may give rise to an increased value of D$_{prolif}$. It is important to stress that available values for D$_{prolif}$ in human tumours and normal tissues (Table 13.3) are not very reliable and that most of the published values apply only towards the end of a standard 6–8-week schedule. For tumours the majority of available estimates are for squamous cell carcinoma of the head and neck. As mentioned above, it appears safe to assume that D$_{prolif}$ is zero for late end-points, at least for overall treatment times up to 6–8 weeks. For early reactions, a linear correction is also applicable over a limited range of treatment times (Bentzen et al., 2001).

Example 3: correcting for overall treatment time

Problem

The Danish Head and Neck Cancer Group conducted a randomized controlled trial of 66 Gy in 33 fractions, randomizing between 5 and 6 fractions per week (Overgaard et al., 2000). This trial, DAHANCA 6, comprised patients with squamous carcinomas of the pharynx and supraglottic larynx. What is the expected difference in biological dose to the tumours between the two arms of the trial?

Solution

Starting treatment on a Monday, 33 fractions delivered with five fractions per week will take 6 full weeks + 3 additional treatment days, a total of 45 days. With six fractions per week, the overall treatment time becomes 5 full weeks + 3 additional treatment days, that is a total of 38 days. From Table 13.3 we see that D_{prolif} for HNSCC is about 0.7 Gy per day. There is no demonstrable difference in D_{prolif} among the various subsites of the head and neck region, which gives a measure of confidence to this calculation. We insert these values into Eqn 13.1 and get

$$EQD_{2,38} = EQD_{2,45} - (38 - 45) \cdot 0.7$$
$$= 66 + 4.9 = 70.9\,Gy$$

Thus, 66 Gy delivered over 38 days is biologically equivalent to 70.9 Gy in 2 Gy fractions delivered over 45 days for HNSCC.

If the two schedules in this example had employed doses per fraction that were different from 2 Gy, we would first have calculated the equivalent EQD_2 values before doing the time correction.

13.7 UNPLANNED GAPS IN TREATMENT

A frequently encountered problem in radiotherapy practice is the management of unscheduled treatment interruptions. Studies have shown that until recently about a third of all patients with HNSCC experienced one or more unplanned gaps in treatment, leading to a protraction of overall treatment time of more than 6 days. These interruptions were typically due to patient-related factors (e.g. intercurrent disease or severe radiation reactions) or logistic factors (e.g. public holidays, treatment machine downtime, transport difficulties). The management of treatment gaps has been considered in some detail by a working party of the UK Royal College of Radiologists (Hendry et al., 1996). The priority to avoid gaps or actively modify treatment after a gap is based on the strength of clinical evidence for a negative therapeutic effect of gaps in radiotherapy schedules; this evidence is strongest for squamous carcinomas of the head and neck and uterine cervix. There is also some support for the importance of overall treatment time in squamous carcinomas of the skin, lung and vagina and in medulloblastoma. Less satisfactory evidence exists for other radical treatments and there is no reason to believe that overall treatment time is a significant factor in palliative radiotherapy.

When unscheduled gaps do occur in curative radiotherapy, it is recommended that the remaining part of the treatment be modified in order to adjust for the interruption. One option is to accelerate radiotherapy after the gap. In a planned schedule delivering one fraction per day, 5 days per week, this can be accomplished by giving more than five fractions per week, either as two fractions per day, or preferably by treating on Saturday and/or Sunday. The intention is to deliver the planned total dose, with the prescribed dose per fraction, in as near the planned overall time as possible. If two fractions per day are delivered, these should be separated by the maximum possible interval, at least 6 hours and preferably more. Note that with long repair half-times, incomplete repair between the dose fractions may require a dose reduction if the risk of late complications is to be kept constant.

An alternative is to deliver the remaining part of the treatment with *hypo*fractionation, i.e. an increased dose per fraction. As a result of the differences in fractionation sensitivity between SCC and late-responding normal tissues (Table 13.1), this type of adjustment will be expected to lead to increased late sequelae or decreased tumour control or both, and should be avoided.

Equation 13.1 may be used to estimate the dose lost due to proliferation during a gap. Note that this correction does not depend on the position (i.e. time) of an eventual gap: any interruption of treatment will add a number of days beyond the planned last day of radiotherapy.

Example 4: change in fraction size, gap correction

Problem

A patient with colorectal cancer is planned to receive preoperative radiotherapy with five fractions of 5 Gy from Monday to Friday (e.g. Kapiteijn et al., 2001). Due to machine breakdown, no treatment is given on the Wednesday. It is planned to deliver the isoeffective tumour dose by increasing the size of the last two fractions in order to finish as planned on Friday. We assume that $\alpha/\beta = 10$ Gy for colorectal tumours. What is the required dose per fraction for the last two fractions? And what is the corresponding risk of rectal complications from this modified fractionation schedule?

Solution

The tumour EQD_2 from the planned three fractions (Wednesday to Friday) is

$$EQD_2 = 15 \cdot \frac{5 + 10}{2 + 10} = 18.75 \, \text{Gy}$$

We want to estimate the dose per fraction (x) so that delivering two fractions of this size gives an EQD_2 of 18.75 Gy to the tumour. We have:

$$EQD_2 = 2 \cdot x \cdot \frac{x + 10}{2 + 10}$$

We rearrange this to find a quadratic equation:

$$18.75 = 2 \cdot x \cdot \frac{x + 10}{2 + 10}$$

$$18.75 \times 12 = 2x^2 + 20x$$

$$2x^2 + 20x - 225 = 0$$

The solution to a quadratic equation of the form $ax^2 + bx + c = 0$ is

$$x = \frac{-b + \sqrt{b^2 - 4ac}}{2a}$$

and only the positive root produces a physically meaningful dose:

$$x = \frac{-20 + \sqrt{20^2 - 4 \cdot 2 \cdot (-225)}}{2 \cdot 2}$$

$$= \frac{-20 + \sqrt{400 + 1800}}{4} = \frac{-20 + 46.9}{4} = 6.7$$

Remember that the units of x are Gy. In other words, we would have to give fractions of 6.7 Gy on Thursday and Friday, a total of 13.4 Gy, in order to achieve the same tumour effect. This is of course less than the 3×5 Gy originally planned for Wednesday to Friday and the reason for this is the larger effect per Gy deriving from the increased dose per fraction in the modified schedule.

How will this affect the risk of bowel damage? From Table 13.1 we find an α/β ratio of 3.9 Gy. The EQD_2 of the modified schedule is now

$$EQD_2 = 10 \cdot \frac{5 + 3.9}{2 + 3.9} + 2 \times 6.7 \cdot \frac{6.7 + 3.9}{2 + 3.9} = 39.2 \, \text{Gy}$$

This value does not take the very short overall treatment time of 5 days into consideration and it is possible that such short schedules could involve an increased risk of consequential late reactions. Here,

we only focus on the change in biological dose arising from the change in dose fractionation and we note that the overall treatment time is unchanged in the two schedules compared here. The originally planned five doses of 5 Gy correspond to an EQD_2 for bowel of about 37.7 Gy. If we were to use a lower α/β value, for example the 1.7 Gy estimated for fibrosis, the change in EQD_2 for this end-point would be from 45.3 Gy to 48.5 Gy. Thus, according to these calculations, the risk of late bowel morbidity will be increased if this modification were implemented.

Clinically, one would be concerned about increasing the dose per fraction from 5 to 6.7 Gy; biologically, it may be questioned whether the use of the LQ model is safe anyway at these large doses per fraction. An alternative strategy would be to keep the 5 Gy per fraction, simply to accept one day of protraction and to give the fifth fraction on the Saturday.

13.8 RE-IRRADIATION

A specific problem in clinical practice is the radiotherapeutic management of patients with a new primary tumour or a loco-regional recurrence in an anatomical site that necessitates re-irradiation of a previously irradiated tissue or organ. Experimental animal data demonstrate that various end-points differ markedly in their capacity for long-term recovery of radiation tolerance (see Chapter 21). Quantitative clinical data are sparse and it may not be safe to assume any particular value of the recovery factor in a clinical setting. The most reasonable approach is probably to use the LQ model to estimate the EQD_2 values for organs and tissues at risk without any assumed recovery and then to apply a clinical assessment of the re-irradiation tolerance. Obviously, such an assessment would also include other clinical aspects such as the life expectancy of the patient in relation to the latent period for late damage, and the prospects for long-term benefit from the re-treatment.

13.9 WHAT CHANGE IN RESPONSE RATE FOLLOWS A CHANGE IN DOSE?

This is a pertinent question in a number of clinical situations and we may be concerned either with change in tumour control probability or in normal-tissue complication probability. If the response rate is n after a dose D, then the change in response rate, in percentage points, after an increment in dose ΔD is approximately

$$\Delta R \approx \frac{\Delta D}{D} \cdot 100 \cdot \gamma_n$$

where γ_n is the *local value* of the normalized dose–response gradient (see Section 10.4). The use of this formula is illustrated by the following example.

Example 5: converting from change in dose into change in response rate

Problem

For the DAHANCA 6 trial, we calculated in example 3 that acceleration in the six fractions per week arm corresponded to a 4.9 Gy dose increment. This trial comprised 791 patients with SCC of the pharynx and the supraglottic larynx. Assuming that the local tumour control probability in the five fractions per week arm is 56%, what is the expected increase in tumour control probability from the treatment acceleration?

Solution

First we need to choose the value of γ. From Figure 10.4 we find that γ_{50} is around 1.8 for pharynx and supraglottic larynx tumours. Table 10.1 shows that at the 56% level this value is still valid. We therefore calculate:

$$\Delta R = \frac{4.9}{66} \cdot 100 \times 1.8 = 13\%$$

Thus, the local tumour control probability is expected to increase by 13%. The observed local tumour control rates in the trial were 56% and 68% in the five- and six-fraction per week arms, respectively (Overgaard *et al.*, 2000). This means that the tumour control rate increased by 12%, in very good agreement with the expected increase calculated here.

13.10   DOUBLE TROUBLE

Dosimetric hotspots receive not only a higher total dose but also a higher dose per fraction and Withers (1992) called this phenomenon 'double trouble'.

A hotspot could arise due to internal and external tissue inhomogeneity or due to the radiation field arrangement. A special case is in the match zone between two abutted fields, where, depending on the geometrical matching technique used, a small tissue volume could be markedly over- or under-dosed.

Example 6: double trouble

Problem

The peak absorbed dose in the match zone between two abutted photon fields is measured by film dosimetry to be 118% of the dose on the central axis of one of the abutting fields. A total dose of 50 Gy is delivered in 25 fractions. The peak physical absorbed dose per fraction in the match zone is 2.36 Gy and the corresponding total dose is 25×2.36 Gy = 59.0 Gy. What is the peak biologically isoeffective dose in 2 Gy fractions in the match zone for a late-responding tissue with $\alpha/\beta = 2$ Gy and for a tumour with $\alpha/\beta = 10$ Gy?

Solution

This is a straightforward application of Withers' formula (Eqn 12.6). For the late-responding normal tissue we find:

$$EQD_2 = 59 \cdot \frac{2.36 + 2}{2 + 2} = 64.3 \, Gy$$

and for the tumour:

$$EQD_2 = 59 \cdot \frac{2.36 + 10}{2 + 10} = 60.8 \, Gy$$

The greater fractionation sensitivity of late-responding normal tissues relative to a tumour of this type means that the biological effect of a hotspot is relatively more important for late effects than for tumour control. There is therefore a therapeutic detriment associated with the hotspot. Clearly, volume effects should also be considered in relation to the double-trouble phenomenon.

Historically, match-zone overdosage of the brachial plexus has been associated with an unacceptable incidence of radiation plexopathies in patients receiving postoperative radiotherapy for breast cancer (Bentzen and Dische, 2000). These problems can largely be avoided by using a more optimal treatment technique.

13.11 UNCERTAINTY IN BIOLOGICAL EFFECT ESTIMATES

A simple impression of the uncertainty in biological effect estimates may be obtained simply by varying the value of α/β, D_{prolif} or γ. The idea is to insert the lower and upper 95% confidence limits of the parameter in question and use these as 95% confidence limits for the biological effect estimate. This technique is only straightforward if we are concerned with a single source of uncertainty, say, uncertainty in the α/β ratio. If we wish to evaluate the effect of uncertainty in two parameters, for example D_{prolif} and γ, it is necessary to use more advanced methods. It is *not* a good approximation simply to insert the lower and upper confidence limits for both parameters in the calculation.

Example 7: estimating uncertainty

Problem

We will repeat the calculation in example 6 but this time we will use the α/β ratio for subcutaneous fibrosis from Table 13.1. We wish to estimate the EQD$_2$ for subcutaneous fibrosis for a schedule delivering 59 Gy in 25 fractions, a dose per fraction of 2.36 Gy. What is the isoeffective dose in 2 Gy fractions for subcutaneous fibrosis and its associated 95% confidence interval?

Solution

Table 13.1 gives $\alpha/\beta = 1.7$ Gy with 95% confidence limits 0.6 and 2.6 Gy. Using the central value of α/β:

$$EQD_2 = 59 \cdot \frac{2.36 + 1.7}{2 + 1.7} = 64.7 \text{ Gy}$$

Similarly, for $\alpha/\beta = 2.6$ Gy, the lower 95% confidence limit for EQD$_2$ becomes 63.6 Gy, and using $\alpha/\beta = 0.6$ Gy, the upper 95% confidence limit becomes 67.2 Gy. Thus, our best estimate of EQD$_2$ for subcutaneous fibrosis is 64.7 Gy with 95% confidence limits 63.6 Gy and 67.2 Gy.

The confidence interval in the above example is untypically narrow. Most α/β values for human tissues and tumours are known with poorer precision than the value for subcutaneous fibrosis. Also, when the LQ formula is used to extrapolate to doses that are further away from 2 Gy than the 2.18 Gy considered in the example, uncertainty in α/β becomes more important.

An essential aspect of these calculations is to identify the main clinical concern. In examples 6 and 7, the main concern is the added risk of complications associated with the overdosage in the match zone. In example 4, the main concern is the possible increase of late effects after hypofractionation. In these cases, it is of course cautious to assume a *low value* for α/β. If on the other hand, we wish to estimate the sparing from hyperfractionation in a given patient, it would be conservative (i.e. would not be overestimating the benefit) if we assumed a relatively *high value* for α/β.

Confidence intervals for α/β derived from animal studies are generally narrower than for the corresponding human end-point. We would suggest that the full calculation, including the estimation of confidence limits, is done for the human data whenever possible, and that an independent calculation is done using the animal data.

13.12 APPLIED CLINICAL RADIOBIOLOGY: TWO CASE HISTORIES

The following clinical cases illustrate the importance of incorporating radiobiological information into clinical practice. They comprise quite complex clinical situations requiring the simultaneous application of several of the radiobiological principles presented in this book.

Example 8: clinical case I

A 48-year-old male patient presented in July 1980 with a T2 N2 M1 (single involved right cervical lymph node) squamous cell carcinoma of the left upper lobe of the lung. The patient was referred for palliative radiotherapy and treatment was delivered in five fractions of 5 Gy over 7 days using parallel-opposed anterior-posterior fields on a ^{60}Co machine. The clinical target volume included the primary tumour, the mediastinum, both supraclavicular fossae and the cervical lymph nodes on both sides. The dose was prescribed to the midplane at the level of the manubrium sterni.

Six weeks after the end of radiotherapy, the patient was reassessed. The tumour and all lymph nodes had almost completely regressed. Because of the good response of the tumour, the attending physician planned to continue the treatment to achieve a better long-term effect.

Based on the Ellis formula (see Section 12.2) the remaining tolerance of normal tissues was estimated at 28 Gy in 2 Gy fractions. This dose was applied in October 1980 to the same target volume as before, again using parallel-opposed fields and ^{60}Co. Treatment was tolerated without any remarkable early normal-tissue reactions.

In July 1981, the patient developed weakness of the right leg. Two months later there was a loss of sensory function in the left leg and the skin of the abdomen. Shortly after this, the lower extremities became completely paralysed and the patient developed bladder and bowel incontinence. After exclusion of alternative diagnoses, particularly of vertebral metastases leading to spinal cord compression, a diagnosis of radiation myelopathy of the thoracic spinal cord was established.

In 1983 the patient developed a squamous cell carcinoma of the right tonsil. Staging revealed no lymph node metastases of the tonsil tumour and no local or distant recurrence of the lung cancer. Since the patient refused surgery, the tumour was locally irradiated to 60 Gy using 2.0 Gy fractions without elective irradiation of the cervical lymph nodes. There was a small overlap with the previously treated volume, which was accepted. Because of severe mucositis, the treatment was interrupted for 6 weeks after 44 Gy in 4.5 weeks, and the overall treatment time was 12 weeks. The tumour had regressed completely at the end of radiotherapy in November 1983. In July 1984 a lymph node metastasis developed in the right upper neck, at the margins of the fields used for irradiation of the tonsil. The tonsil cancer was locally controlled. The metastasis was partially removed by surgery and a further 30.6 Gy were locally applied using 1.8 Gy fractions in August 1984 without any remarkable normal-tissue reactions. The metastatic tumour continued to progress and the patient died in May 1985 from arterial bleeding.

Clinical and radiobiological considerations

In view of the cervical lymph node metastases, a lung cancer patient today would be treated with palliative intent, most likely by chemotherapy, and possibly combined with radiotherapy. Usually a change of therapeutic aim, from a hypofractionated palliative schedule to a radical treatment, is discouraged because the high doses per fraction typically used in palliative schedules may be too toxic for late-responding normal tissues to allow the application of a high enough total dose to give a fair probability of local tumour control. However, there are the rare clinical situations where a change from a palliative to a curative schedule must be seriously taken into consideration, for example if after some high-dose fractions the histological diagnosis is proven to be incorrect or if suspected distant metastases during the course of radiotherapy turn out to be benign lesions. Similar considerations apply to situations in which high-dose fractions were accidentally applied because of overlapping fields or because of errors in monitor unit calculations (Section 13.10).

In the case presented here, 5×5 Gy were given using parallel-opposed anterior-posterior (AP) fields. Large parts of the lung were shielded and in this case spinal cord is the most critical normal tissue. As ^{60}Co was used and because the AP diameters of the lower neck are less than the AP diameter of the thorax at the level of the manubrium sterni, the maximum dose to the spinal cord was approximately 110% of the dose prescribed to the reference point for the thoracic spinal cord (i.e. 27.5 Gy in 5.5 Gy fractions) and may have been as high as 120% (30 Gy in 6 Gy fractions) for the cervical spinal cord.

Table 13.1 shows that the α/β ratio for spinal cord can be taken to be 2 Gy. Using Eqn 12.6, the isoeffective dose to the thoracic spinal cord becomes

$$EQD_2 = 27.5 \cdot \frac{5.5 + 2.0}{2.0 + 2.0} = 51.6 \text{ Gy}$$

Similarly, for the cervical spinal cord, we get $EQD_2 = 60.0$ Gy.

Following example 7, we may get an impression of the uncertainty in these estimates. The animal data in Table 12.1 suggest that α/β for the cord is somewhere in the interval 1.5–3.0 Gy and this is consistent with the human estimate in Table 13.1. Inserting these two bounds on α/β, we get a dose range of 47–55 Gy for the thoracic spinal cord and 54–64 Gy for the cervical spinal cord. Table 4.1 indicates that for a dose of 60 Gy given in 2 Gy fractions, the incidence of radiation myelopathy is 1–5%.

Thus, after the first five fractions, this patient may already have received a dose that is close to or even slightly above the acceptable dose to spinal cord. Further irradiation of the tumour and mediastinum cannot avoid increasing the spinal cord dose and would therefore be associated with a very high risk of radiation myelopathy. The fact that there was a treatment-free interval of 6 weeks will not reduce this risk because effects on late normal-tissue damage tend to be independent of overall treatment time (see Section 4.4) except for the very long intervals that may be relevant for re-irradiation (see Section 21.5). These considerations lead to the conclusion that further irradiation should not be given in this case.

This patient was further irradiated with 14 fractions of 2 Gy and 11 months later radiation myelopathy developed. Neurological examination indicated that the damage was located to the upper thoracic cord. The total EQD_2 in this area was approximately 80–85 Gy, corresponding to more than an 80% risk of radiation myelopathy. It should be noted that the clinical decision to continue radiotherapy in this patient was based on the Ellis NSD concept: this case is a good example of how the Ellis formula may overestimate late normal-tissue tolerance and therefore should not be used in clinical practice.

A final interesting aspect of this case is the long overall treatment time of almost 3 months for treatment of the lung tumour, also for the tonsil cancer. The effect of overall time on outcome is discussed in Sections 12.9 and 14.4. There is considerable heterogeneity of radiobiological parameters between individual tumours (see Section 14.8) and in the case considered here the lung tumour did not recur during follow-up of almost 5 years, indicating that either radiosensitvity was extremely high or that repopulation was very slow. Alternatively, the histological diagnosis may have been incorrect and this was not re-evaluated in this case.

Example 9: clinical case II

A 26-year-old male patient was treated in 1990 for stage IIA Hodgkin's disease with involved cervical, supraclavicular, axillary and mediastinal lymph nodes. A dose of 36 Gy was prescribed in 1.5 Gy fractions to all supra-diaphragmatic and para-aortic lymph nodes. The cervical spinal cord was shielded by ventral and dorsal blocks. Radiotherapy was associated with mild early reactions. Because of incomplete disease regression, six cycles of polychemotherapy were applied, after which all manifestations of disease were absent. At the time of treatment the patient suffered from compensated chronic nephritis.

In 1998, a squamous cell carcinoma of the left dorsal mobile tongue extending to the base of tongue was diagnosed and operated on by partial glossectomy and left supraomohyoid neck dissection. The postoperative stage was pT2 G2, pN2b (2 positive nodes) M0. The resection margins were histologically free of disease although very close. Further surgery was not compatible with maintenance of function and the patient was referred for postoperative radiotherapy. Doses to normal tissues from the previous treatment were re-evaluated to be less than 10 Gy (0.4 Gy per fraction) for the cervical spinal cord and maximally 43 Gy in 1.8 Gy fractions in soft tissues and bone.

A dose of 50.4 Gy was given to the tumour region and the cervical and supraclavicular nodes on both sides using two daily fractions of 1.2 Gy with a minimum time interval of 9 hours between the fractions. 6 MV x-rays from a linear accelerator with parallel-opposed lateral fields were used, also an anterior field for the lower neck. The spinal cord was excluded from the irradiated volume after 30 Gy and electrons were applied to the dorsal cervical nodes. After this, a boost of 15.6 Gy with the same fractionation schedule was applied to the tumour region and the left subdigastric lymph node region using a pair of wedged fields. The overall treatment time was 40 days. The patient developed grade 3 mucositis, and grade 2 xerostomia and dermatitis during treatment, and complete loss of taste. Grade 3 mucositis persisted for 3 weeks after the end of treatment and the patient lost a total of 15 kg and required tube feeding. In the following 3 weeks, he recovered rapidly. Three years after radiotherapy the tumour is loco-regionally controlled and there is no evidence of distant metastasis. Late sequelae were mild: grade 1 subcutaneous fibrosis in the left upper neck and grade 2 xerostomia, but chronic nephritis developed and the patient has now to undergo dialysis.

Clinical and radiobiological considerations

Because of the close margins and the positive lymph nodes, the patient was a candidate for postoperative radiotherapy. There is currently no unequivocal evidence that radiotherapy should be combined with chemotherapy in this situation, and it would have been associated with increased risks because of the previous chemotherapy given in 1990 and the associated damage to the kidneys.

The 36 Gy delivered in 1990 needs to be considered when evaluating the present radiotherapy. The interval of 8 years is clearly long enough to raise the possibility of long-term recovery and re-irradiation tolerance is considered in Chapter 21. Spinal cord tolerance is not a major concern in this case, as it was effectively shielded during the second treatment and because the cord received a low dose from the 1990 treatment. Data from animal experiments show that spinal cord is capable of substantial long-term recovery from radiation damage, especially if the initial biological effective dose is low (see Section 21.5). Salivary glands are also not a primary concern as the dose in 1998 was above tolerance and the degree of xerostomia depends on whether part of the parotid gland is be spared. Soft tissues and bone are therefore the most important normal tissues to consider in this case. Unfortunately, there are no good estimates of dose–response relationships after re-irradiation of these tissues. However, there are several clinical reports showing that re-irradiation in the head and neck region is possible even to total doses of more than 100 Gy (see Section 21.9).

In the present case, hyperfractionated radiotherapy was prescribed with the aim of decreasing late normal-tissue effects. Was this worthwhile? Table 13.1 shows α/β values ranging from 1.7 to 3.5 Gy for soft-tissue end-points. Note, that if we want to consider the sparing of late soft-tissue effects from hyperfractionation it is conservative to use a value in the *upper end* of this range, in this case 3.5 Gy. Using Eqn 12.6 and assuming complete repair between fractions, it can be calculated that the dose of 50.4 Gy in 1.2 Gy fractions corresponds to an EQD_2 of 43.1 Gy and the dose of 66 Gy to an EQD_2 of 56.4 Gy.

With two fractions per day, we should also consider the possible influence of incomplete repair in the 9-hour interval between fractions. As in example 2, we assume $T_{1/2} = 4.4$ hours and from Table 12.2 we find that for an 8-hour interval the value of H_2 is between 0.25 ($T_{1/2} = 4.0$ hours) and 0.33 ($T_{1/2} = 5.0$ hours). Interpolation between these values yields $H_2 = 0.28$ for $T_{1/2} = 4.4$ hours. Likewise, interpolation for a 10-hour interval gives $H_2 = 0.21$ and we therefore obtain an interpolated value for a 9-hour interval

of 0.25. Using Eqn 12.7, we have:

$$EQD_2(\Delta t = 9h) = 50.4 \cdot \frac{3.5 + 1.2 \cdot [1 + 0.25]}{3.5 + 2.0}$$
$$= 45.8 \, Gy$$

In the same way, we find that the 66 Gy in 1.2 Gy per fraction with a 9-hour interval corresponds to 60 Gy. Thus, *assuming complete repair* between fractions, hyperfractionation spares about 15% of the biologically effective dose in the high-dose region and for incomplete repair about 9% compared with conventional fractionation. A more precise calculation incorporating incomplete repair in the overnight interval yields an EQD_2 in the high-dose volume of 61.2 Gy and this corresponds to a 7% sparing compared with conventional fractionation. This appears to be a useful gain, considering the steep dose–response curve for late normal-tissue reactions (see Section 10.5).

Without long-term recovery in normal tissue, the total biologically effective dose from the first and second courses of radiotherapy in this patient would be about 85 Gy in the low-dose region and about 100 Gy in the boost area. At these doses, fibrosis would be expected to be very severe and there would be a considerable risk of severe sequelae such as ulceration and necrosis. This case is therefore in line with the conclusions of Chapter 21 that long-term recovery does occur in some (but not all!) human normal tissues and that re-irradiation, even to curative doses, may be a good option in well-selected patients.

The final consideration in deciding whether or not to hyperfractionate the re-irradiation is to calculate the EQD_2 for possible subclinical HNSCC disease. Delivering 66 Gy in 2 Gy fractions requires an overall treatment time of 6.5 weeks whereas the 66 Gy in 1.2 Gy fractions twice a day requires 5.5 weeks (the actual treatment time in this patient was 40 days; however, the prescription of a schedule has to be based on the theoretical overall time of the schedule). Assuming $\alpha/\beta = 10$ Gy for HNSCC and that repair is complete between fractions (again, this is conservative) we take the 6.5 weeks as our reference overall time. The dose recovered per day has not been estimated for subclinical disease but it is probably at least equivalent to the 0.7 Gy per day estimated for macroscopic disease (Section 13.6). Using Eqns 12.6 and 13.1 we obtain:

$$EQD_{2,HF} = 66 \cdot \frac{10 + 1.2}{10 + 2} + 7 \, days \times 0.7 \, Gy/day$$
$$= 66.5 \, Gy$$

Thus the hyperfractionation schedule is approximately isoeffective on the tumour with the alternative 66 Gy in 33 fractions over 6.5 weeks. Hyperfractionation in this case yields a *therapeutic gain* of about 7% in terms of biological dose to late-responding soft tissues.

13.13 CONCLUSIONS

Clinical studies of tumour and normal-tissue response to radiotherapy, including several randomized controlled trials of altered fractionation in head and neck cancer, have shown results that are in broad agreement with the predictions from isoeffect calculations similar to those presented here. It should be noted, however, that most estimates of radiobiological characteristics for human tumours are for squamous cell carcinoma of the head and neck. For most other tumour histologies, quantitative estimates are sparse, and isoeffective dose calculation becomes highly speculative. Quantitative estimates for early and, in particular, late normal-tissue end-points are relatively more abundant and often associated with less statistical uncertainty than the tumour parameters. As stressed in the introduction, it is important that any numerical estimates are seen in a clinical context and counterbalanced with clinical experience. The approach presented here is fundamentally a tool for extrapolating clinical experience over a relatively narrow range of dose–time–fractionation values and extrapolation to more unusual schedules cannot be assumed to be safe. If numerical isoeffect calculations are of critical importance in a given clinical case, it may be a good idea to seek advice from someone who has experience in such calculations and who is aware of the limitations of the biological data that are used in the calculations. Dose–volume models are briefly discussed in Section 10.9, but here numerical parameter estimates from analyses of clinical data are almost non-existent at the time of writing. Finally, it should be noted that decision-making *without* the support from numerical estimates can also put patients' health at risk.

BIBLIOGRAPHY

Bentzen SM, Dische S (2000). Morbidity related to axillary irradiation in the treatment of breast cancer. *Acta Oncol* 39: 337–47.

Bentzen SM, Overgaard J (1996). Clinical normal-tissue radiobiology. In: *Current Radiation Oncology* (eds Tobias JS, Thomas PR), Vol. 2. Arnold, London.

Bentzen SM, Saunders MI, Dische S (1999). Repair half-times estimated from observations of treatment-related morbidity after CHART or conventional radiotherapy in head and neck cancer. *Radiother Oncol* 53: 219–26.

Bentzen SM, Saunders MI, Dische S, Bond S (2001). Radiotherapy-related early morbidity in head and neck cancer: quantitative clinical radiobiology as deduced from the CHART trial. *Radiother Oncol* 60: 123–35.

Dische S, Saunders MI (1989). Continuous, hyperfractionated, accelerated radiotherapy (CHART): an interim report upon late morbidity. *Radiother Oncol* 16: 65–72.

Dische S, Saunders MI, Sealy R, Werner ID, Verma N, Foy C, Bentzen SM (1999). Carcinoma of the cervix and the use of hyperbaric oxygen with radiotherapy: a report of a randomized controlled trial. *Radiother Oncol* 53(2): 98–8.

Guttenberger R, Thames HD, Ang KK (1992). Is the experience with CHART compatible with experimental data? A new model of repair kinetics and computer simulations. *Radiother Oncol* 25: 280–6.

Hendry JH, Bentzen SM, Dale RG et al. (1996). A modelled comparison of the effects of using different ways to compensate for missed treatment days in radiotherapy. *Clin Oncol (R Coll Radiol)* 8: 297–307.

Kapiteijn E, Marijnen CA, Nagtegaal ID et al. (2001). Preoperative radiotherapy combined with total mesorectal excision for resectable rectal cancer. *N Engl J Med* 345: 638–46.

Lee AW, Sze WM, Fowler JF, Chappell R, Leung SF, Teo P (1999). Caution on the use of altered fractionation for nasopharyngeal carcinoma. *Radiother Oncol* 52: 207–11.

Overgaard J, Hansen HS, Grau C et al. (2000). The DAHANCA 6 & 7 trial. A randomized multicenter study of 5 versus 6 fractions per week of conventional radiotherapy of squamous cell carcinoma of the head and neck. *Radiother Oncol* 56(Suppl): S4.

Stuschke M, Thames HD (1999). Fractionation sensitivities and dose-control relations of head and neck carcinomas: analysis of the randomized hyperfractionation trials. *Radiother Oncol* 51(2): 113–21.

Thames HD, Bentzen SM, Turesson I, Overgaard M, Van den Bogaert W (1990). Time-dose factors in radiotherapy: a review of the human data. *Radiother Oncol* 19: 219–35.

Withers HR (1992). Biological basis of radiation therapy. In: *Principles and Practice of Radiation Oncology* (eds Perez CA, Brady LW), pp. 64–9. Lippincott, Philadelphia.

14

Modified fractionation

MICHAEL BAUMANN, MICHELE I SAUNDERS AND MICHAEL C JOINER

14.1 INTRODUCTION

The optimal distribution of dose over time has been a major issue throughout the history of radiotherapy and important progress has been made in this area over the past few years. The clinical evaluation and implementation of modified fractionation schedules based on biological rationales is an important focus of 'translational research' in radiation oncology. The relationships between total dose and fraction number for late-responding normal tissues, early-responding normal tissues and tumours provide the basic information required to optimize radiotherapy dose per fraction. Much work still needs to be done to determine the time of onset, the rate and the mechanisms of repopulation in tumours and normal tissues during radiotherapy, but enough is now known about the time factor to support the view that the overall duration of fractionated radiotherapy should not be prolonged above the prescribed time and that a reduction in the overall treatment time should be considered in a number of clinical situations. Evidence is emerging that inter-fraction time intervals have to be as long as possible in order to gain full benefit from fractionation schedules employing multiple fractions per day. This chapter summarizes the current status of modified fractionation in clinical radiotherapy.

14.2 CONVENTIONAL FRACTIONATION

Conventional fractionation is the application of daily doses of 1.8–2 Gy and 5 fractions per week. The dose per week is 9–10 Gy. Depending on tumour histology, tumour size and localization, total doses ranging from 40 to 70 Gy are given for macroscopic disease and lower doses when treating microscopic disease. The conventional fractionation schedule was developed on an empirical basis (Fletcher, 1988) and has been the mainstay of curative radiotherapy over the past decades in most departments in Europe and the USA.

Radiosensitive tumours such as lymphomas and seminomas can be controlled with low doses of 45 Gy or even less, and in this situation there is a low incidence of normal-tissue damage. By contrast, glioblastoma multiforme is a very resistant tumour that is not controlled even after doses as high as 70 Gy. Most tumour types, including squamous cell carcinomas and adenocarcinomas, are of intermediate sensitivity

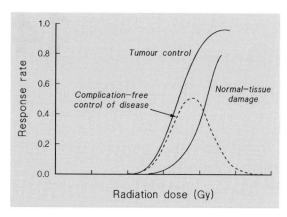

Figure 14.1 *Dose–response curves for tumour control and normal-tissue damage. The uncomplicated local tumour control rate initially increases with increasing dose after which it falls again because of a steep increase in the incidence of normal-tissue damage. Adapted from Holthusen (1936).*

(see Section 17.1). Small tumours, for example T1 or T2 carcinomas of the head and neck, are well controlled with acceptable normal-tissue damage using conventional fractionation and total doses between 60 and 70 Gy. However, local tumour control rates rapidly decline for larger tumours (see Section 17.4). As local tumour control increases with the total dose of radiotherapy, the question may be asked whether improved management of larger tumours could be gained by increasing the total dose of conventional fractionation above 70 Gy, say to doses between 80 and 100 Gy. Such a dose escalation is currently being tested for non-small-cell lung cancer and for carcinoma of the prostate. One constraint is that not only tumour control rates but also the incidence and severity of normal-tissue damage increase with increasing total doses (see Section 10.6). This was recognized as early as 1936 when Holthusen pointed out that the uncomplicated local tumour control rate initially increases with increasing dose but then falls again because of the steep increase in the incidence of normal-tissue damage. Figure 14.1 is redrawn from one of Holthusen's papers: the frequency of 'uncomplicated tumour control' follows a bell-shaped curve. Once the optimum dose is established, further improvements in uncomplicated tumour control can only be achieved by either moving the dose–effect curve for local tumour control to lower doses or the curve for normal-tissue damage to higher doses; the

latter is the objective of hyperfractionated schedules (Section 14.3). Conformal radiotherapy is another option currently used in dose escalation protocols, reducing the volume of normal tissue irradiated to high dose and therefore also the probability of late normal-tissue damage (see Section 5.5). As dose escalation using conventional fractionation is always associated with the prolongation of overall treatment time, some of the potential gain may be lost as a consequence of tumour-cell repopulation and this is considered in Section 14.4.

Radiotherapy is highly effective in dealing with a small number of cancer cells as in the treatment of microscopic disease. Thus lower doses of irradiation are used postoperatively after complete resection of breast or head and neck cancer.

14.3 MODIFICATION OF DOSE PER FRACTION

Hyperfractionation

This is the use of doses per fraction less than the 1.8–2.0 Gy given in conventional fractionation. The total number of fractions must be increased, hence the prefix *hyper*; usually two fractions are administered per day. The biological rationale of hyperfractionation is to exploit the difference between the small effect of dose per fraction on tumour control versus the larger effect of dose per fraction on the incidence and severity of late normal-tissue damage. As pointed out in Sections 12.3 and 12.6, this differential between tumours and late-responding normal tissues is thought to be caused by a different capacity of target cells in these tissues to recover from sublethal radiation damage between fractions.

In clinical practice, hyperfractionation is usually applied to escalate the total dose compared with conventional fractionation, thereby aiming at improved tumour control rates without increasing the risk of late complications (see Figure 12.7). Dose-escalated hyperfractionation has been tested in two large multicentre randomized clinical trials on head and neck squamous cell carcinoma (EORTC No. 22791 and RTOG No. 9003). The results of the EORTC trial are shown in Figure 14.2. The right-hand panel shows that hyperfractionated treatment with 70 fractions of 1.15 Gy (two fractions per day with a 4–6-hour

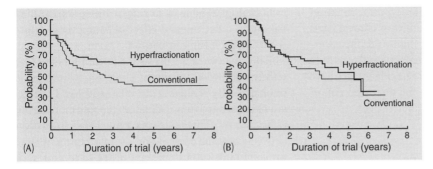

Figure 14.2 *Results of the EORTC (22791) trial of dose-escalated hyperfractionation. (A) Loco-regional tumour control (logrank, P = 0.02); (B) patients free of late radiation effects, grade 2 or worse (logrank P = 0.72). From Horiot* et al. *(1992), with permission.*

interval, total dose 80.5 Gy) produced a similar incidence of pooled grade 2 and 3 late tissue damage to a conventional schedule of 35 fractions of 2 Gy (70 Gy given in the same overall time of 7 weeks). However, the larger total dose in the hyperfractionated treatment produced an increase of about 19% in long-term local tumour control (left-hand panel). Survival appeared higher after hyperfractionation but this difference did not reach statistical significance. In the RTOG trial (Fu *et al.*, 2000), local tumour control was increased by 8% after hyperfractionation (68 fractions of 1.2 Gy, two fractions per day, 6 hours apart, total dose 81.6 Gy) compared with conventional fractionation using 2 Gy fractions to 70 Gy in the same overall time of 7 weeks. Survival was not significantly different but the prevalence of grade III late effects was significantly increased after hyperfractionation. Both these clinical trials thus confirm the radiobiological expectation that local tumour control can be increased by dose-escalated hyperfractionation, thereby supporting a high average α/β ratio for squamous cell carcinoma of the head and neck (see Table 13.1). However, while the EORTC trial supports the view that hyperfractionation allows the total dose to be increased without a simultaneous increase in late complications, the RTOG trial indicates that this is not always the case. The potential therapeutic gain from hyperfractionation is debated by Beck-Bornholdt *et al.* (1997), Baumann *et al.* (1998) and Bentzen *et al.* (1999). Factors that contribute to an increased risk of late normal-tissue damage when multiple fractions are applied per day are discussed in Section 14.5.

Hypofractionation

This is the use of doses per fraction higher than 2.0 Gy; the total number of fractions is reduced, hence the prefix *hypo*. As explained in Section 12.6, the radiobiological expectation is that hypofractionation will *lower* the therapeutic ratio between tumours and late-responding normal tissues, compared with conventional fractionation given in the same overall time. This expectation depends on the α/β ratio for the tumour being considerably higher than for late-responding normal tissues; exceptions could therefore occur for tumours that have very low α/β ratios, for example some melanomas, liposarcomas, and possibly prostate carcinomas (see Table 13.1) where hypofractionation may be as good as or even better than conventional fractionation.

Single-dose irradiation or hypofractionation with only a few large fractions are widely applied in palliative radiotherapy. These schedules use lower total doses than those applied in curative radiotherapy. For this reason, and because the patients have a limited life expectancy, late normal-tissue damage is of only minor concern. A number of randomized clinical trials have shown that symptom control after palliative hypofractionated schedules is comparable to that achieved with more fractionated schedules. These schedules have the advantage of being more convenient for the patient and they help to spare resources.

Moderate hypofractionation with dose per fraction up to approximately 3 Gy is the standard fractionation schedule for curative radiation therapy in several centres in different countries. To reduce the risk of late normal-tissue damage, slightly lower total doses are applied than for conventional fractionation. For tumours with a high α/β ratio, this decrease in total dose may well lead to a reduction in tumour control probability. However, some or all of this negative effect may be compensated by the shorter overall treatment times often used for moderate hypofractionation (Section 14.4). There is growing interest in the use of moderate hypofractionation to escalate total doses in the context of clinical trials of conformal radiation therapy: this avoids the necessity to prolong the overall treatment time and conserves treatment resources. However, these advantages have to be carefully weighed against the increased risk of late normal-tissue damage.

14.4 THE TIME FACTOR FOR FRACTIONATED RADIOTHERAPY IN TUMOURS

In the 1960s and 1970s, the prevailing view among clinicians was that prolonged overall treatment times of fractionated irradiation did not impair local tumour control. In contrast to this general view, studies on experimental tumours found that clonogenic cells proliferate rapidly after irradiation (see Sections 2.8 and 17.4) so that the ability of fractionated radiotherapy to achieve local tumour control would be expected to decrease with increasing overall treatment time. Several studies support the view that repopulation of clonogenic tumour cells accelerates at some point during fractionated radiotherapy; however, the mechanisms underlying this phenomenon are not fully understood (see Sections 12.9 and 13.6). It should also be noted that other mechanisms such as long repair half-times or increasing radiobiological hypoxia during treatment might contribute to a detrimental effect of long overall treatment times on tumour control.

The concept of a time factor in tumours became widely acknowledged among clinicians following the publication by Withers *et al.* (1988) entitled 'The hazard of accelerated tumor clonogen repopulation during radiotherapy'. This review examined the correlation between tumour control and overall treatment time for squamous cell carcinomas of the head and neck and led to the diagram shown in Figure 14.3A: this shows the dose required to achieve tumour control in 50% of cases (i.e. TCD_{50} values) plotted against the overall treatment time. Since a variety of doses per fraction were used in the various original studies summarized in this plot, the LQ model was used with an α/β ratio of 25 Gy to convert from the actual doses per fraction used into equivalent doses using 2 Gy per fraction. The various studies also achieved different tumour control rates and it was therefore necessary to interpolate or extrapolate to the 50% control level. This required an assumed value for the steepness of the dose–response relationship for the tumours; it was assumed that the dose to increase control from 40% to 60% was 2.9 Gy. As can be seen from Figure 14.3A, this retrospective review of head and neck cancer data found a clear trend: as overall time was increased, a greater total radiation dose has been required to control these tumours. The other important conclusion was that there seemed to be an initial

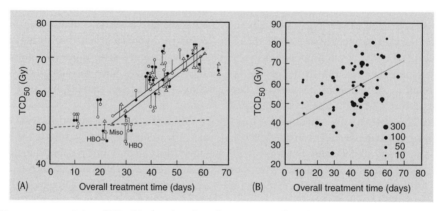

Figure 14.3 *Tumour control dose (TCD$_{50}$) in head and neck cancer as a function of overall treatment time, normalized to a dose per fraction of 2 Gy. The same large set of clinical studies has been retrospectively summarized by (A) Withers et al. (1988) and (B) Bentzen and Thames (1991). In panel B, each point indicates the result of a particular trial, the size of the symbol indicating the size of the trial. There is a trend for the curative radiation dose to increase with overall treatment time, although the details of this association differ between the two studies.*

flat portion to this relationship (the so-called 'dog-leg'). This implied that for treatment times shorter than 3–4 weeks proliferation had little effect and that, as shown for experimental tumours, it also takes time for accelerated repopulation to be switched on in human tumours. Withers *et al.* (1988) concluded that for treatment times longer than this, the effect of proliferation was equivalent to a loss of radiation dose of about 0.6 Gy per day.

This publication gave rise to considerable debate. Subsequent analyses of the same clinical data carried out by Bentzen and Thames (1991) and by Dubben (1994) are shown in Figures 14.3B and 14.4. The analysis of Bentzen and Thames made a different assumption about the steepness of dose–response curves for tumour control: the dose to increase control from 40% to 60% was taken to be 10.5 rather than 2.9 Gy, thought to be more clinically realistic. In addition, the data points in Figure 14.3B have been drawn to indicate the size of the patient sample from which the estimate of TCD_{50} had been made. Figure 14.3B suggests that the 'lag' period before commencement of repopulation may have been somewhat exaggerated by the plot shown in panel A, although this issue is still actively being discussed. The analysis by Dubben used the same radiobiological assumptions as the review by

Withers *et al.* (1988) and showed that the actual local tumour control rates could be replaced by random numbers without changing the conclusion of Figure 14.3A. As shown in Figure 14.4, the reason for this completely unexpected finding was a highly significant correlation between TCD_{50} and the prescribed total dose (normalized to 2 Gy fractions). Dubben's conclusion was that the increase of TCD_{50} with increasing treatment duration in Figure 14.3A reflects only dose–time prescriptions and that these data neither confirm nor exclude a time factor of fractionated radiotherapy. The comparison among these three analyses of the same data set is a good example of how difficult it is to draw reliable conclusions based on retrospective analyses of clinical data.

If we accept the data summarized in Figure 14.3B, the slope of the line indicates that 0.48 Gy per day is recovered during fractionated radiotherapy of head and neck squamous cell carcinoma. If we further accept that this effect is caused by repopulation and assume reasonable estimates of tumour cell radiosensitivity, we can deduce a clonogen doubling time of less than 1 week, similar to the values of pre-treatment potential doubling times measured in human tumours (see Tables 2.3 and 2.4). The potential doubling time (T_{pot}) is a cell kinetic parameter that indicates the rate at which cells are proliferating in an untreated tumour. Although there is much uncertainty about this, it has been suggested that during treatment the rate at which clonogenic cells within the tumour repopulate may also resemble the T_{pot} value. Thus accelerated fractionation, which uses a reduced overall treatment time below the conventional 6–7 weeks, should increase tumour cure rates by restricting the time available for tumour cell proliferation. From Figure 14.3B, for example, the dose in a 5-week schedule would be effectively larger than that in a 7-week schedule by a factor $0.48 \times (7 - 5) \times 7 = 6.7$ Gy, or nearly 10% of a 70-Gy treatment.

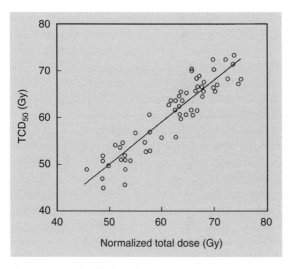

Figure 14.4 *The clinical data shown in panels A and B of Figure 14.3 as reanalysed by Dubben (1994). Tumour control dose is plotted against the prescribed total dose, normalized to a dose per fraction of 2 Gy. The positive trend in these data indicates a possible prescription bias.*

14.5 CLINICAL EVALUATION OF ACCELERATED RADIOTHERAPY

Through the joint activities of radiation biologists and clinicians, accelerated fractionation schedules have been developed that aim to counteract the rapid repopulation of clonogenic cells during therapy. *Accelerated fractionation* is defined as a shortening

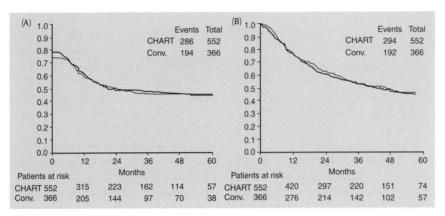

Figure 14.5 *Results of a phase III randomized trial of CHART in squamous cell carcinoma of the head and neck. (A) Probability of loco-regional tumour control; (B) probability of overall survival of patients treated by CHART (bold line) and by conventional radiotherapy (solid line). From Dische* et al. *(1997), with permission.*

of the overall treatment time or, more precisely, as an increase of the average dose per week above the 10 Gy given in conventional fractionation. *Early normal-tissue reactions are expected to increase using accelerated radiotherapy (see Section 11.2). By contrast, if recovery from sublethal radiation damage between fractions is complete (see Section 12.8), *late normal-tissue damage is expected to be constant for accelerated fractionation schedules using 1.8–2 Gy fractions and total doses comparable to conventional fractionation. If the total dose and/or the dose per fraction is reduced (sometimes termed *accelerated hyperfractionation*), late normal-tissue damage is expected to decrease.

During the past decade, a large number of randomized clinical trials of accelerated radiotherapy have been set up. At present, 10 trials have been reported, some of these so far only as abstracts. Nine of these trials (7/7 in head and neck squamous cell carcinoma, 1/2 in non-small-cell lung cancer, 1/1 in small-cell lung cancer) indicate that, for a given total dose, accelerated fractionation schedules are more effective to obtain local tumour control than conventional fractionation schedules. They therefore support the validity of the concept of a time factor for tumours.

Three randomized trials of accelerated radiotherapy have provided detailed actuarial data on tumour control and survival as well as on normal-tissue damage, and they will now be described. The strategy known as CHART (Continuous Hyperfractionated Accelerated Radiotherapy) is an example of strongly

accelerated fractionation. This protocol applies 36 fractions over 12 consecutive days (starting on a Monday and including the weekend), using three fractions per day with an interval of 6 hours between the fractions within each day. Dose per fraction is 1.5 Gy to a total of 54 Gy. Total dose is therefore reduced compared with conventional therapy, in order to remain within the tolerance of acutely responding epithelial tissues. Dische *et al.* (1997) have reported the results of a phase III clinical trial of CHART in 918 patients with head and neck cancer. Patients were randomized between CHART and conventional fractionation in 2 Gy fractions to 66 Gy. Figure 14.5A shows that loco-regional tumour control was identical in both treatment arms. CHART used 12 Gy less than conventional therapy in an overall time reduced by 33 days. If this dose reduction is thought to just offset repopulation, this would correspond to 0.36 Gy per day lost through tumour cell proliferation, which is somewhat lower than the 0.48 Gy per day from the data in Figure 14.5B. This might indicate that the lag period before onset of accelerated repopulation in head and neck carcinoma is longer than the 12-day duration of a course of CHART, but further data are necessary to confirm this. Overall patient survival was identical in both treatment arms (Figure 14.5B). As expected for accelerated radiotherapy, radiation mucositis was more severe with CHART; it occurred earlier but settled sooner and was in nearly all cases healed by 8 weeks in both arms. Unexpectedly, skin reactions were less severe and settled more quickly in the CHART-treated

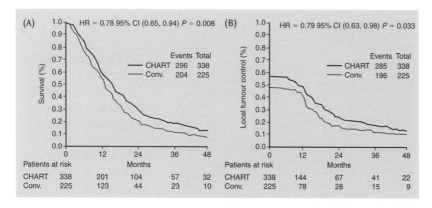

Figure 14.6 *Results of a phase III randomized trial of CHART in non-small-cell lung cancer. (A) Overall survival; (B) local tumour control of patients treated by CHART or by conventional radiotherapy (CHART results are indicated by the upper lines). From Saunders* et al. *(1999), with permission.*

patients. Life-table analysis showed evidence of reduced severity in a number of late morbidities in favour of CHART but the magnitude of these differences in late reactions would not allow a substantial increase in the total dose of CHART without increasing the risk of late damage over the rate observed for conventional fractionation. The overall conclusion is that CHART improved the therapeutic ratio in head and neck cancer by a small margin.

Saunders *et al.* (1997, 1999) reported the results of the CHART-Bronchus trial. A total of 563 patients with non-small-cell lung cancer were randomized between CHART (as described above) and conventional fractionation to 60 Gy in 2 Gy fractions. Despite the lower total dose, survival after 2 years was significantly increased by 9% from 21% to 30% in the CHART arm (Figure 14.6A). Exploratory analysis revealed that this was a consequence of improved local tumour control (Figure 14.6B) and, in squamous cell carcinoma, also a reduced incidence of distant metastases. Oesophagitis occurred earlier and reached higher scores in CHART patients, but symptoms also settled earlier and were of no major concern on longer follow-up. Pneumonitis was not decreased in the CHART arm. The overall conclusion of this study was that compared with conventional fractionation with 60 Gy, CHART offers a significant therapeutic benefit for patients with non-small cell lung cancer.

In the EORTC trial No. 22851 (Horiot *et al.*, 1997) 512 patients with head and neck cancer were randomized to receive their treatment either conventionally in a median overall time of 54 days (using 1.8–2 Gy per fraction each day, total 35–40 fractions, treatment on 5 days per week) or accelerated in a median of 33 days

(using 1.6 Gy per fraction three times per day with 4 hours minimum inter-fraction interval, total 45 fractions, treatment on 5 days per week, overall time allocated to 8 days radiotherapy, 12–14 days gap, 17 days radiotherapy). The report of the EORTC trial indicates that patients who received the accelerated treatment showed a 13% increase in loco-regional tumour control from 46% to 59% at 5 years (Figure 14.7A); there was no increase in survival compared with patients receiving conventional treatment. Early radiation effects, particularly mucositis, was much more pronounced in the accelerated arm. Thirty-eight per cent of patients had to be hospitalized for acute toxicity compared with only 7% of the patients in the conventional arm. Figure 14.7B shows that grade 3 and 4 late damage (according to the EORTC/RTOG scale) also occurred significantly more frequently after accelerated fractionation than after conventional fractionation ($P < 0.001$). The probability of being free of severe late damage at 3 years was 85% in the conventional arm but only 63% in the accelerated arm. With increasing follow-up this difference is even increasing. Most of the difference in late effects was attributable to late damage to connective tissues and mucosal sequelae.

In summary, accelerated fractionation has been shown in randomized clinical trials to counteract the time factor in head and neck and lung cancer. Some of the trials indicate an improved therapeutic ratio compared with conventional fractionation. However, one of the most intriguing biological observations from the clinical trials on accelerated fractionation is that sparing of late normal-tissue morbidity compared to conventional fractionation was much less than anticipated. In fact, late damage in the EORTC trial was even higher than after conventional fractionation.

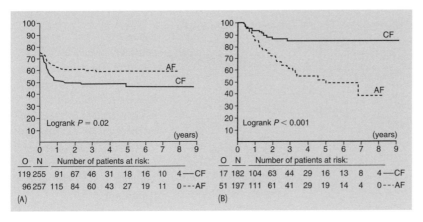

Figure 14.7 *Results of the EORTC (22851) trial of accelerated fractionation. (A) Loco-regional tumour control (logrank P = 0.02); (B) patients free of severe radiation effects, grade 3 and 4 (logrank P < 0.001). From Horiot* et al. *(1997), with permission.*

Possible reasons for these unexpected findings are discussed below.

14.6   SPLIT-COURSE RADIOTHERAPY

Intentional gaps in radiation therapy have sometimes been introduced in order to allow recovery of early-responding normal tissues. If such gaps prolong the overall treatment time, then local tumour control rates are expected to decrease. Studies on experimental tumours suggest that, for a given overall treatment time, the magnitude of the time factor is the same for continuous fractionation or for fractionation protocols including gaps (Baumann *et al.*, 2001). This supports the current clinical guidelines for the compensation of unscheduled treatment gaps that have been described in Section 13.7.

14.7   REASONS FOR INCREASED LATE NORMAL-TISSUE DAMAGE AFTER MODIFIED FRACTIONATION

Hyperfractionation and accelerated radiotherapy both require multiple radiation treatments per day. In the case of hyperfractionation, this is because in order to give an adequate number of small fractions, one per day, the overall treatment time would have to be very long; in the EORTC and RTOG trials mentioned above, the fraction number was increased to 68–70, thus requiring once-daily treatment over 14 weeks. This would be unacceptable in view of the time factor for tumour-cell repopulation. In the case

of accelerated radiotherapy, shortening the overall time but still giving one fraction per day requires an increase in dose per fraction; this would be expected to lead to an increase in late effects, although moderate hypofractionation is clinically acceptable in some situations (Section 14.3).

A radiobiological constraint in giving multiple fractions per day is that these should not be given too close together because of incomplete repair (see Section 12.8). As indicated in Section 6.7, the damage inflicted by radiation is very largely repaired in most cell types, both normal and malignant. The repair of normal-tissue stem cells is vital for their tolerance to radiation therapy and if fractions are given so close together that repair is incomplete, tolerance will be reduced. Repair half-times for many tumours and normal tissues are in the region of 0.5–2 hours (see Table 13.2). Assuming exponential decay of radiation damage, it takes six half-times for the damage to decay to 1/64, i.e. 1–2% of its initial value. The problem is that, as shown in the table, some late-responding normal tissues appear to have unusually long repair half-times. These tissues will be relatively disadvantaged by radiotherapy given with multiple fractions at a short inter-fraction interval; the therapeutic index will be impaired and the total radiation dose will have to be lowered in order to remain within tolerance. Most current schedules with multiple fractions per day employ inter-fraction times of at least 6 hours; in some situations even this gap may be too short.

New evidence on the clinical impact of incomplete repair comes from an analysis by Bentzen *et al.* (1999) of data from the CHART head and neck trial. As noted above, several late-damage end-points were significantly reduced after CHART, compared with conventional treatment. The reduction was much less than expected on the basis of LQ calculations and analysis of these data yielded repair half-times in the range of 4–5 hours for the three investigated late morbidities: laryngeal oedema, skin telangiectasia and subcutaneous fibrosis. Even the lower ends of the confidence intervals were around 3 hours. This suggests that even 6 hours between dose fractions in multiple-fractions-per-day-schedules may be too short for complete repair. Long repair half-times for late effects in human normal tissues pose a significant problem for the development of novel fractionation schedules.

Consequential late effects (see Sections 4.1 and 11.2) may also contribute to more-than-expected late morbidity after modified fractionation. Compared with conventional fractionation, the dose per week is increased, both in accelerated radiotherapy and in hyperfractionation. This is expected to produce an increase in *early* normal-tissue damage such as mucositis and more severe or more prolonged early damage may then lead to more pronounced consequential *late* effects.

14.8 IS THE SAME MODIFIED FRACTIONATION SCHEDULE OPTIMAL FOR ALL PATIENTS?

Figure 14.8 summarizes the results of experiments testing different modified fractionation schedules in two experimental squamous cell carcinoma xenografts (FaDu and GL) in mice. For a constant number of 30 fractions in FaDu tumours, the TCD_{50} increased by roughly 0.6 Gy for each day of prolongation for overall treatment times up to 40 days but more steeply for longer times (Figure 14.8, panel A); this effect was much less pronounced (0.28 Gy per day) in GL squamous cell carcinomas. By contrast, when the number of fractions was increased from 12 to 60 in a constant overall treatment time of 6 weeks (panel B), the TCD_{50} in FaDu tumours appeared to be constant while in GL tumours the TCD_{50} increased with increasing fraction number. Both dose-escalated hyperfractionation and accelerated fractionation (using constant or reduced total doses) would be advantageous in human tumours that behave like FaDu. By contrast, for tumours like GL, dose-escalated hyperfractionation would at best yield identical control rates, while after accelerated fractionation with reduced total dose such tumours would do worse than with conventional radiotherapy. These results show that the response of experimental tumours to modified fractionation may be variable and it may well be that such heterogeneity also exists between tumours in patients. There is a clear need for research on how to select patients for the newer fractionation schedules.

Results from clinical studies always reflect the average effect of a treatment modification. For example, after the accelerated CHART treatment the local control rates of head and neck cancer were identical to those obtained after conventional fractionation with a 12 Gy higher total dose (Section 14.4). Under the

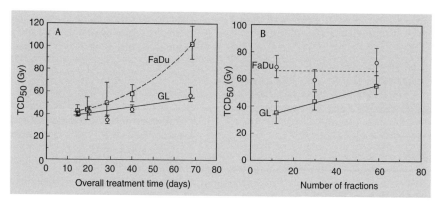

Figure 14.8 *Tumour control dose in two experimental squamous cell carcinoma xenografts (FaDu, GL) as a function of overall treatment time for irradiation with 30 fractions (panel A) or as a function of number of fractions in a constant overall treatment time of 6 weeks (panel B). There are considerable differences in the response of these tumours to modification of the fractionation schedule. See Baumann et al. (2001) for sources.*

assumption of inter-tumour heterogeneity, this would mean that some tumours with a small time factor that would have been controlled after conventional treatment to 66 Gy recurred after CHART treatment because of the reduction in total dose. This negative effect may have been compensated for by additional local control achieved in tumours that showed greater repopulation and a more pronounced time factor, i.e. tumours in which the dose recovered per day was higher than the average value of 0.36 Gy. To further improve the results of modified fractionation we need to identify subgroups of patients who are likely to benefit from a particular modification and thus to individualize treatment. As indicated in Chapter 22, considerable efforts are being made to develop predictive tests, for instance for the rate of tumour-cell repopulation; so far these investigations have not identified strong predictors that could be employed in clinical practice.

KEY POINTS

1. *Hyperfractionation* is the use of a reduced dose per fraction over a conventional overall treatment time, employing multiple fractions per day. A therapeutic advantage is thought to derive from the more rapid increase in tolerance with decreasing dose per fraction for late-responding normal tissues than for tumours.
2. *Accelerated radiotherapy* is the use of a reduced overall treatment time with a conventional dose per fraction, achieved using multiple fractions per day. The aim is to reduce the protective effect of tumour-cell repopulation during radiotherapy.
3. Multiple fractions per day should be given as far apart as possible and certainly not closer than 6 hours.

BIBLIOGRAPHY

Baumann M, Bentzen SM, Ang KK (1998). Hyperfractionated radiotherapy in head and neck cancer: a second look at the clinical data. *Radiother Oncol* **46**: 127–30.

Baumann M, Petersen C, Wolf J *et al.* (2001). No evidence for a diffferent magnitude of the time factor for continuously fractionated irradiation and protocols including gaps in two human squamous cell carcinoma in nude mice. *Radiother Oncol* **59**: 187–94.

Beck-Bornholdt HP, Dubben H-H, Liertz-Petersen C, Willers H (1997). Hyperfractionation: where do we stand? *Radiother Oncol* **43**: 1–21.

Bentzen SM, Thames HD (1991). Clinical evidence for tumor clonogen regeneration: interpretations of the data. *Radiother Oncol* **22**: 161–6.

Bentzen SM, Saunders MI, Dische S (1999). Repair halftimes estimated from observations of treatment-related morbidity after CHART or conventional radiotherapy in head and neck cancer. *Radiother Oncol* **53**: 219–26.

Dische S, Saunders M, Harvey A *et al.* (1997). A randomised mutlicentre trial of CHART versus conventional radiotherapy in head and neck cancer. *Radiother Oncol* **44**: 123–36.

Dubben HH (1994). Local control, TCD_{50} and dose-time prescription habits in radiotherapy of head and neck tumours. *Radiother Oncol* **32**: 197–200.

Fletcher GH (1988). Regaud Lecture: Perspective on the history of radiotherapy. *Radiother Oncol* **12**: 253–71.

Fu KK, Pajak TF, Trotti A *et al.* (2000). A radiation therapy oncology group (RTOG) phase III randomized study to compare hyperfractionation and two variants of accelerated fractionation to standard fractionation radiotherapy for head and neck squamous cell carcinomas: first report of RTOG 9003 [see comments]. *Int J Radiat Oncol Biol Phys* **48**: 7–16.

Holthusen H (1936). Erfahrungen über die Verträglichkeitsgrenze für Röntgenstraholen und deren Nutzanwendung zur Verhütung von Schäden. *Strahlentherapie* **57**: 254–68.

Horiot J-C, Le Fur R, N'Guyen T *et al.* (1992). Hyperfractionation versus conventional fractionation in oropharyngeal carcinoma: final analysis of a randomized trial of the EORTC cooperative group of radiotherapy. *Radiother Oncol* **25**: 231–41.

Horiot J-C, Bontemps P, van den Bogaert W *et al.* (1997). Accelerated fractionation compared to conventional fractionation improves loco-regional control in the radiotherapy of advanced head and neck cancers: results of the EORTC 22851 randomized trial. *Radiother Oncol* **44**: 111–21.

Saunders MI, Dische S, Barrett A *et al.* (1997). Continuous hyperfractionated accelerated radiotherapy (CHART) vs. Conventional radiotherapy in non-small-cell lung cancer: a randomised multicentre trial. *Lancet* **350**: 161–6.

Saunders MI, Dische S, Barrett A *et al.* (1999). Continuous, hyperfractionated, accelerated radiotherapy (CHART) versus conventional radiotherapy in non-small cell lung cancer: mature data from the randomised multicentre trial. *Radiother Oncol* **52**: 137–48.

Withers HR, Taylor JMG, Maciejewski B (1988). The hazard of accelerated tumor clonogen repopulation during radiotherapy. *Acta Oncol* **27**: 131–46.

FURTHER READING

Baumann M, Bentzen SM, Doerr W *et al.* (2001). The translational research chain: is it delivering the goods? *Int J Radiat Oncol Biol Phys* **49**: 345–51.

Thames HD, Peters LJ, Withers HR, Fletcher G (1983). Accelerated fractionation vs hyperfractionation: rationales for several treatments per day. *Int J Radiat Oncol Biol Phys* **9**: 127–38.

Thames HD, Withers HR, Peters LJ *et al.* (1982). Changes in early and late radiation responses with altered dose fractionation: implications for dose-survival relationships. *Int J Radiat Oncol Biol Phys* **8**: 219–26.

Withers HR, Maciejewski B, Taylor JMG (1989). Biology of options in dose fractionation. In: *The Scientific Basis of Modern Radiotherapy* (ed. McNally NJ), pp. 27–36. British Institute of Radiology, London.

15

The oxygen effect and tumour microenvironment

MICHAEL R HORSMAN AND JENS OVERGAARD

15.1 THE IMPORTANCE OF OXYGEN

The response of cells to ionizing radiation is strongly dependent upon oxygen (Gray et al., 1953; Wright and Howard-Flanders, 1957). This is illustrated in Figure 15.1 for mammalian cells irradiated in culture. Cell surviving fraction is shown as a function of radiation dose administered either under normal aerated conditions or under hypoxia, generally achieved by flowing nitrogen gas over the surface of the cell suspensions for a period of 30 minutes or more. The enhancement of radiation damage by oxygen is dose-modifying, i.e. the radiation dose that gives a particular level of survival is reduced by the same factor at all levels of survival. This allows us to calculate an oxygen enhancement ratio (OER):

$$\text{Oxygen enhancement ratio} = \frac{\text{Radiation dose in hypoxia}}{\text{Radiation dose in air}}$$

for the same level of biological effect. For most cells the OER for x-rays is around 3.0. However, some studies suggest that at radiation doses of 3 Gy

or less the OER is actually reduced (Palcic and Skarsgard, 1984). This is an important finding because this is the dose range for clinical fractionation treatments.

It has been demonstrated from rapid-mix studies that the oxygen effect only occurs if oxygen is present either during irradiation or within a few milliseconds thereafter (Howard-Flanders and Moore, 1958; Michael et al., 1973). The dependence of the degree of sensitization on oxygen tension is shown in Figure 15.2. By definition, the OER under anoxic conditions is 1.0. As the oxygen level increases, there is a steep increase in radiosensitivity (and thus in the OER). The greatest change occurs from 0 to about 20 mmHg; further increase in oxygen concentration, up to that seen in air (155 mmHg) or even to 100% oxygen (760 mmHg), produces a small though definite increase in radiosensitivity. Also shown in Figure 15.2 are the oxygen partial pressures typically found in arterial and venous blood. Thus, from a radiobiological standpoint most normal tissues can be considered to be well oxygenated, although it is now recognized that moderate hypoxia is a feature of some normal tissues such as cartilage and skin.

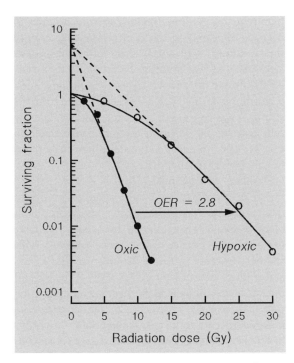

Figure 15.1 *Survival curves for cultured mammalian cells exposed to x-rays under oxic or hypoxic conditions (diagrammatic), illustrating the radiation dose-modifying effect of oxygen. Note that the broken lines extrapolate back to the same point on the survival axis (n = 5.5).*

The mechanism responsible for the enhancement of radiation damage by oxygen is generally referred to as the oxygen-fixation hypothesis and is illustrated in Figure 15.3 (see Section 8.1). When radiation is absorbed in a biological material, free radicals are produced. These radicals are highly reactive molecules and it is these that break chemical bonds, produce chemical changes, and initiate the chain of events that results in biological damage. They can be produced either directly in the target molecule (usually DNA) or indirectly in other cellular molecules and diffuse far enough to reach and damage critical targets. Most of the indirect effects occur by free radicals produced in water, since this makes up 70–80% of mammalian cells. It is the fate of the free radicals ultimately produced in the critical target, designated as R$^\cdot$ in Figure 15.3, that is important. If oxygen is present, then it can react with R$^\cdot$ to produce RO$_2^\cdot$ which then undergoes further reaction ultimately to yield ROOH in the target molecule. Thus we have a change in the chemical composition of the target and the damage is chemically fixed. Subsequently this damage can be processed enzymatically and perhaps repaired (see Section 6.7). In the absence of oxygen, or in the presence of reducing species, R$^\cdot$ can react with H$^+$, thus restoring its original form.

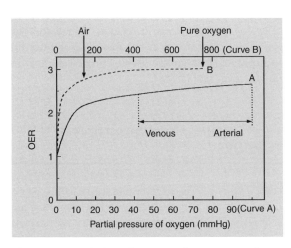

Figure 15.2 *Variation of oxygen enhancement ratio (OER) with oxygen tension. The horizontal arrows indicate the range of physiological blood oxygen tensions on the lower scale (for conversion of mmHg to kPa, multiply by 0.133). Adapted from Denekamp (1989), with permission.*

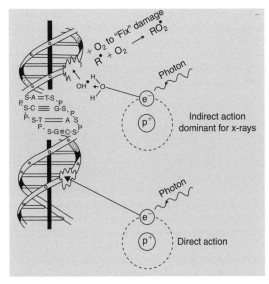

Figure 15.3 *The oxygen fixation hypothesis. Free radicals produced in DNA either by a direct or indirect action of radiation can be repaired under hypoxia but fixed in the presence of oxygen. Adapted from Hall (1988), with permission.*

15.2 THE TUMOUR MICROENVIRONMENT

Oxygen also plays an important role in the radiation response of tumours. For most solid tumours to grow they need to develop their own blood supply. This new vasculature is formed from the already established normal-tissue vessels by a process which is referred to as *angiogenesis*. However, the formation of the neovasculature usually lags behind the more rapidly increasing number of neoplastic cells; the tumours are said to 'outgrow' their blood supply. As a result, the neovasculature is unable to meet the increasing nutrient demands of the expanding tumour mass. The vasculature that is formed is also very primitive in nature and, like the cancerous tissue it supplies, is morphologically and functionally abnormal. All these factors combine to result in the development of microregional areas within tumours that are nutrient deprived, highly acidic and oxygen deficient, yet the hypoxic cells existing in these areas may still be viable, at least for a time.

The first clear indication that hypoxia could exist in tumours was made in 1955 by Thomlinson and Gray from their observations on histological sections of fresh specimens from human carcinoma of the bronchus (Figure 15.4). They observed viable tumour regions surrounded by vascular stroma from which the tumour cells obtained their nutrient and oxygen

requirements. As these regions expanded, areas of necrosis appeared at the centre. The thickness of the resulting cylindrical shell of viable tissue (100–$180\,\mu m$) was found to be similar to the calculated diffusion distance of oxygen in respiring tissues; it was thus suggested that as oxygen diffused from the stroma it was consumed by the cells and, while those cells beyond the diffusion distance were unable to survive, cells immediately bordering on to necrosis might be viable yet hypoxic.

Tannock (1968) made similar observations in mouse mammary tumours. The extent of necrosis in these tumours was much greater and each patent blood vessel was surrounded by a cord of viable tumour cells outside which was necrosis. This 'corded' structure is also seen in other solid tumours and is illustrated in Figure 15.5. Cells at the edge of the cords are thought to be hypoxic and are often called 'chronically hypoxic cells'. Tannock showed, however, that since the cell population of the cord is in a dynamic state of cell turnover, these hypoxic cells will have a short lifespan, being continually replaced as other cells are displaced away from the blood vessel, and in turn become hypoxic. More recently it has been suggested that some tumour blood vessels may periodically open and close, leading to transient or acute hypoxia (Figure 15.5). The mechanisms responsible for intermittent blood flow in tumours are not entirely clear. They might include the plugging of vessels by blood cells or by circulating tumour cells; collapse of vessels in regions of high tumour interstitial pressure; or spontaneous vasomotion in incorporated host arterioles affecting blood flow in downstream capillaries.

15.3 HYPOXIA IN EXPERIMENTAL TUMOURS

Since hypoxic cells are resistant to radiation, their presence in tumours is critical in determining the response of tumours to treatment with large doses of radiation. The presence of such cells in experimental tumours can easily be demonstrated, as shown in Figure 15.6. This shows the cell survival response of KHT mouse sarcomas, irradiated *in situ* in air-breathing mice; or in nitrogen-asphyxiated (i.e. hypoxic) mice; or as a single-cell suspension *in vitro* under fully oxic conditions. The studies in

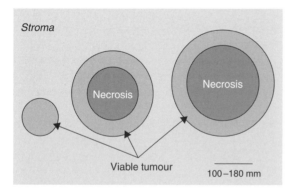

Figure 15.4 *Idealized description of the development of microscopic regions of necrosis in tumours. Conclusions by Thomlinson and Gray from studies on histological sections of human bronchial carcinoma showing the development of necrosis beyond a limiting distance from the vascular stroma. Adapted from Hall (1988), with permission.*

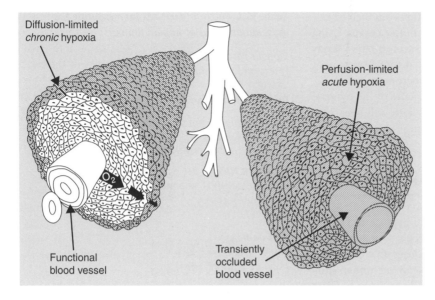

Figure 15.5 *Schematic representation of diffusion-limited* chronic *hypoxia and perfusion-limited* acute *hypoxia within tumour cords. From Horsman (1998), with permission.*

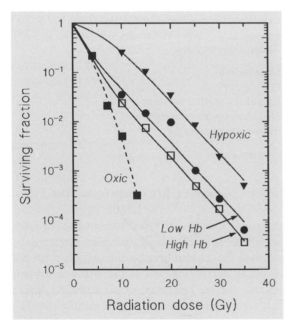

Figure 15.6 *Cell survival curves for KHT mouse sarcoma cells irradiated under aerobic or hypoxic conditions. The hypoxic data were obtained by killing the mice shortly before irradiation. Two sets of data for tumours in air-breathing mice are shown, with high and low haemoglobin levels. The dashed curve shows the* in vitro *survival of oxic cells. From Hill* et al. *(1971), with permission.*

air-breathing mice were made under both normal and anaemic conditions. Cell survival was estimated immediately after irradiation using a lung colony assay (see Section 6.4). The survival curves for tumours in air-breathing mice are biphasic. At low radiation doses, the response is dominated by the aerobic cells and the curves are close to the oxic curve; at larger radiation doses, the presence of hypoxic cells begins to influence response and the survival curve eventually parallels the hypoxic curve. The proportion of hypoxic cells (the *hypoxic fraction*) can be calculated from the vertical separation between the hypoxic and air-breathing survival curves in the region where they are parallel. In this mouse sarcoma, the hypoxic fraction was calculated to be 0.06 in mice with a high haemoglobin level ($\sim$16.5 g%) and 0.12 in anaemic mice (haemoglobin level $\sim$9.5 g%). These data thus illustrate not only the presence of hypoxic cells in these tumours but also the influence of oxygen transport.

Two other techniques are routinely used to estimate hypoxia in animal tumours. These are the so-called 'clamped tumour growth-delay assay', which involves measuring the time taken for tumours to grow to a specific size after irradiation; and the 'clamped tumour-control assay', in which the percentage of animals showing local tumour control at a certain time after treatment is recorded. For both techniques it is necessary to produce full radiation dose–response curves under normal and clamped

conditions and the hypoxic fractions can then be calculated from the displacement of these curves. Using
these assays, and the paired survival-curve assay
described above, it has been demonstrated that
most experimental solid tumours contain radiation-
resistant hypoxic cells, with estimates of the hypoxic
fractions ranging from below 1% to well over 50%
of the total viable cell population.

15.4   HYPOXIA IN HUMAN TUMOURS

Attempts to estimate the level of hypoxia in human
tumours have proven more difficult. A major reason
is that the experimental procedures that have just
been described are not applicable to the human situation. Instead it is necessary to rely on more indirect
approaches as listed in Table 15.1. The end-points
have included measurements of:

- tumour vascularization, since the oxygenation
  status of tumours is strongly dependent on vascular supply;
- haemoglobin-oxygen saturation, because this
  controls oxygen delivery to tumours;
- tumour metabolic activity, which changes under
  hypoxic conditions;
- estimating the degree of DNA damage, since
  hypoxic cells are likely to show less DNA damage
  than aerobic cells for a given radiation dose;
- hypoxic markers, which are based on the observations that certain nitroaromatic compounds are
  reduced under hypoxic conditions to reactive
  species that subsequently bind to hypoxic cells
  and then can be identified; and
- estimates of tumour oxygen partial pressure (pO_2)
  distributions.

The technique that has received by far the greatest
attention has been the use of polarographic
oxygen electrodes for measuring tumour pO_2. The
popularity of this approach came about with the
development of the Eppendorf histograph. This differs from older oxygen electrodes in employing more
robust and re-usable electrodes plus an automatic
stepping motor, thus making it possible to obtain
large numbers of oxygen measurements along several
tracks within a short time period. Using this machine,
a direct relationship between electrode estimates of
tumour oxygenation and the actual percentage of

Table 15.1 *Potential methods for measuring the
oxygenation status of human tumours*

Tumour vascularization
Intercapillary distance
Vascular density
Distance from tumour cells to nearest vessel

Haemoglobin-oxygen saturation
Cryospectroscopy
Near-infrared spectroscopy

Tumour metabolic activity
Biochemical/HPLC analysis
Bioluminescence
NMR/PET

DNA damage
Comet assay
Alkaline elution

Hypoxic markers
Immunohistochemistry (e.g. PIMO/EF5/NITP)
[18F]Fluoromisonidazole
[123I]Iodoazomycin arabinoside

Oxygen partial pressure distributions
Polarographic oxygen electrodes
19F-NMR spectroscopy

Miscellaneous
ESR spectroscopy
Tumour interstitial pressure
Phosphorescence imaging
Hypoxic stress proteins

From Horsman *et al.* (1998), with permission.

hypoxic clonogenic cells has been found. This is illustrated in Figure 15.7 in which the hypoxic fraction,
determined using a clamped tumour-control assay,
was altered in a C3H mouse mammary carcinoma by
allowing the mice to breathe different gas mixtures.
A strong correlation was found between hypoxic
fraction and the percentage of measured pO_2 values
that were equal to or less than 5 mmHg (665 Pa).
These oxygen electrodes have also been used to
measure pO_2 distributions in human tumours and
in at least two sites (cervical cancers and tumours of
the head and neck region) the pO_2 measurements
have been related to outcome after radiation therapy
(Table 15.2). In general, good correlations between
treatment outcome and pre-treatment pO_2 measurements were observed for both tumour types, with the
less well oxygenated tumours showing the poorest
results. This is clearly illustrated for head and neck

tumours in Figure 15.8, in which those patients with tumours where the percentage of low pO_2 values measured was greater than the median value for all 66 tumours had a significantly poorer local regional tumour control.

Additional, albeit more indirect, evidence that hypoxia exists in human tumours and can influence radiation response comes from those clinical trials in which some form of hypoxic modification has been

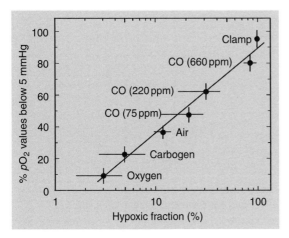

Figure 15.7 *Relationship between pO_2 electrode measurements and the hypoxic fraction in a C3H mouse mammary carcinoma. Results were obtained from normal air-breathing mice, in clamped tumours, and in mice allowed to breathe oxygen, carbogen (95% oxygen + 5% carbon dioxide), or various concentrations of carbon monoxide (CO). From Horsman et al. (1993), with permission.*

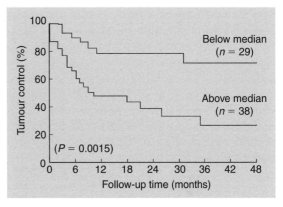

Figure 15.8 *Local control correlates with pre-treatment oxygen levels in tumours. Oxygen levels were measured with an Eppendorf electrode in 65 lymph nodes and 1 primary advanced squamous cell carcinoma of the head and neck. Tumours were stratified by whether the fraction of pO_2 values $\leqslant 2.5\,mmHg$ were above or below the median for the whole group. The lines show Kaplan–Meier estimates of actuarial tumour control probability up to 4 years after receiving conventional external radiotherapy (66–68 Gy in 33–34 fractions). Modified from Nordsmark and Overgaard (2000).*

Table 15.2 *Clinical studies in which Eppendorf estimates of pre-treatment pO_2 have been related to radiotherapy outcome*

Study	Number of patients	Influence of hypoxia
Head and neck cancer		
Adam *et al.* (*Laryngoscope* 1998)	25	No
Brizel *et al.* (*Int J Radiat Oncol Biol Phys* 1998)	43	Yes
(*Radiother Oncol* 1999)	63	Yes
Eschewege *et al.* (*Int J Radiat Oncol Biol Phys* 1997)	35	No
Nordsmark *et al.* (*Radiother Oncol* 1996)	35	Yes
(*Radiother Oncol* 2000)	66	Yes
Rudat *et al.* (*Radiother Oncol* 2001)	41	Yes
Stradler *et al.* (*Int J Radiat Oncol Biol Phys* 1997)	59	Yes
Cancer of the uterine cervix		
Fyles *et al.* (*Radiother Oncol* 1998)	74	Yes
Hoeckel *et al.* (*Cancer Res* 1996)	89*	Yes
Knocke *et al.* (*Radiother Oncol* 1999)	51	Yes
Sundfor *et al.* (*Radiother Oncol* 2000)	40	Yes

*47 patients received surgery as the primary treatment with adjuvant chemotherapy with or without radiation.
From M. Nordsmark (unpublished information).

attempted and found to improve tumour response. Using hyperbaric oxygen, chemical radiation sensitizers, or improved oxygen supply, a significant improvement in local tumour control has been seen, particularly in head and neck cancers (see Chapter 16). This is also illustrated in Figure 15.9, in which loco-regional control of tumours is expressed as a function of pre-treatment haemoglobin concentration in male or female patients treated with radiotherapy for squamous cell carcinoma of the larynx and pharynx. Local tumour control was lower in those patients with reduced haemoglobin concentrations. Such a reduction in haemoglobin would make less oxygen available to the tumour and thus increase the level of tumour hypoxia.

15.5   REOXYGENATION

The time-course of changes in the hypoxic fraction of a tumour before and after irradiation is illustrated in Figure 15.10. Tumours less than 1 mm in diameter have been found to be fully oxygenated (Stanley *et al.*, 1977). Above this size they usually become partially hypoxic. If tumours are irradiated with a large single dose of radiation, most of the radiosensitive aerobic cells in the tumour will be killed. The cells that survive will predominantly be hypoxic and therefore the hypoxic fraction immediately after irradiation will be close to 100% (note that the oxygenation status of cells in the tumour has not been changed at this point: selective abolition of colony-forming ability has led to *survivors* having a raised hypoxic fraction). Subsequently, the hypoxic fraction falls and approaches its starting value. This phenomenon is termed reoxygenation. The process of reoxygenation has been reported to occur in a variety of tumour systems, although the speed of reoxygenation varies widely, occurring within a few hours in some tumours and taking several days in others. Furthermore, the final level of hypoxia after reoxygenation can also be higher or lower than its value prior to irradiation.

The mechanisms underlying reoxygenation in tumours are not clearly understood. A number of possible processes are listed in Table 15.3. If reoxygenation occurs rapidly, then it may be due either to recirculation of blood through vessels that were temporarily closed or to a decreased cellular respiration

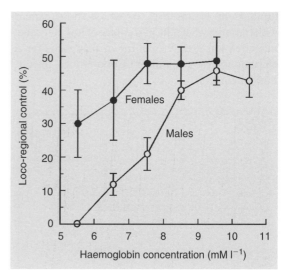

Figure 15.9 *Loco-regional tumour control as a function of sex and pre-treatment haemoglobin value in 1112 patients treated with radiotherapy for squamous cell carcinoma of the larynx and pharynx. From Overgaard (1988), with permission.*

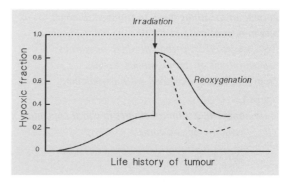

Figure 15.10 *The time-course of changes in the hypoxic fraction during the life history of a tumour. Small lesions are well oxygenated but as the tumour grows the hypoxic fraction rises perhaps in excess of 10%. A large single dose of radiation kills oxic cells and raises the hypoxic fraction. The subsequent fall is termed* reoxygenation.

(which will increase the oxygen diffusion distance). Reoxygenation occurring at longer time intervals is probably the result of cell death leading to tumour shrinkage and a reduction in intercapillary distances, thus allowing oxygen to reach hypoxic cells.

Reoxygenation has important implications in clinical radiotherapy. Figure 15.11 illustrates the

Table 15.3 *Mechanisms and time-scales of tumour reoxygenation*

Recirculation through temporarily closed vessels	Minutes
Reduced respiration rate in damaged cells	Minutes to hours
Ischaemic death of cells without replacement	Hours
Mitotic death of irradiated cells	Hours
Cord shrinkage as dead cells are resorbed	Days

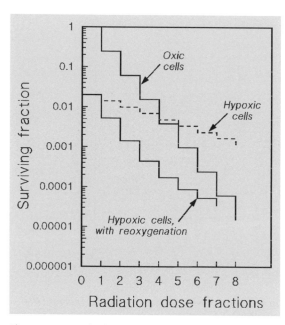

Figure 15.11 *Calculated survival curves for a tumour containing 98% well-oxygenated cells and 2% hypoxic cells when given repeated fractions of radiotherapy. The upper two lines show the progressive depletion of oxic and hypoxic cells in the absence of reoxygenation. The lower line assumes that after each dose fraction reoxygenation restores the hypoxic fraction to its pre-treatment level.*

hypothetical situation in a tumour following fractionated radiation treatments. In this example, 98% of the tumour cells are considered well oxygenated and 2% are hypoxic. The responses of oxic and hypoxic cells to repeated large dose fractions are illustrated. If no reoxygenation occurs, then each dose of radiation would be expected to kill only a small number of the hypoxic cells and the resultant curve would therefore be much shallower than that for oxic cells. At the end of treatment the tumour response will be dominated by the hypoxic cell population. However, if reoxygenation occurs between fractions, then the radiation killing of initially hypoxic cells will be greater and the hypoxic cells then have less impact on response. It has not been possible to detect reoxygenation directly in human tumours, but its existence is supported by the fact that local control can be achieved in a variety of tumours given fractionated radiotherapy with 30 fractions of 2 Gy, consistent with the measured SF_2 values for oxic tumour cells (see Section 17.5).

15.6 DRUG RESISTANCE AND MALIGNANT PROGRESSION

The presence of hypoxic cells in tumours not only has a significant impact on radiation therapy; there are also strong indications that these same cells may be responsible for tumour resistance to certain types of chemotherapy. Evidence from animal studies has shown that drugs like bleomycin, 5-fluorouracil, methotrexate and cisplatin are less effective at killing tumour cells when they are hypoxic than when they are well oxygenated (Grau and Overgaard, 1992). Whether this is a consequence of hypoxia *per se* or because hypoxic cells are normally distant from blood vessels, thus creating problems for drug delivery, or because such cells are typically non-cycling and exist in areas of low pH (both of which can influence drug activity), has never been fully established.

More recent studies are now suggesting that hypoxia may also contribute to malignant progression through its effects on signal transduction pathways and the regulation of transcription of various genes (Giaccia, 1996; Sutherland *et al.*, 1996). A number of different types of genes/proteins have been shown to be up-regulated by hypoxia and examples of these are listed in Table 15.4. These include factors involved in cellular metabolism, as well as those that help cells deal with oxidative stress (induced by

Table 15.4 *Some examples of genes/proteins that are up-regulated by hypoxia*

Glucose-regulated proteins	ORP80 (GRP78), ORP100 (GRP94)
Redox stress enzymes/molecules	ORP33 (haemoxygenase I), ORP7 (metallothionein IIA)
Metabolic enzymes	ALDA, PGK1, PKM, PFKL, LDHA
Transcription factors and signalling molecules	cJun, cFos, Jun b, AP-1, p53, NF-κB, RB, HIF-1, SP-1, PKC
Growth factors/receptors/cytokines	EPO, VEGF (VPF), ET-1, EGFR, PDGF-B, IL-1α, GADD45, GADD153

Adapted from Sutherland *et al.* (1996).

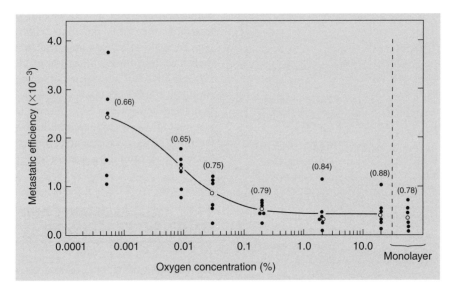

Figure 15.12 *Effect of different levels of hypoxia on metastatic potential of KHT fibrosarcoma cells. Tumour cells were grown in suspension culture and exposed to differing oxygen levels for 24 hours. They were then transferred to monolayer culture for a further 18 hours before being harvested and assayed for plating efficiency and the ability to form metastasis. Each point represents the number of metastases seen in the lungs of individual mice 20 days after intravenous injection of tumour cells. Open symbols represent median values. Numbers in parenthesis are plating efficiencies. Data for KHT cells grown continuously as monolayers are shown on the right. From Young and Hill (1990), with permission.*

radiation, hydrogen peroxide and metals) and the detoxification of drugs and chemicals. More importantly, hypoxia has been shown to induce factors that are associated with apoptosis (e.g. p53) and angiogenesis (e.g. vascular endothelial growth factor, VEGF), both of which are likely to have profound influences on the growth and development of tumours.

More direct pre-clinical evidence that hypoxia can influence malignant progression is shown in Figure 15.12. In these experiments, KHT fibrosarcoma cells were grown under hypoxic conditions before being reoxygenated and then intravenously injected into mice. Twenty days later the mice were

killed, their lungs removed and the number of lung metastases counted. Cells kept at oxygen concentrations below 0.3% clearly induced more metastases. There is also strong clinical evidence using Eppendorf oxygen electrodes to support the contention that hypoxia affects malignancy and this is illustrated in Figure 15.13 for soft-tissue sarcomas. Stratifying patients into hypoxic or well-oxygenated categories based on the pO_2 estimates made in the primary tumour prior to therapy clearly showed that those patients with the most hypoxic tumours had a statistically poorer disease-specific and overall survival at 5 years.

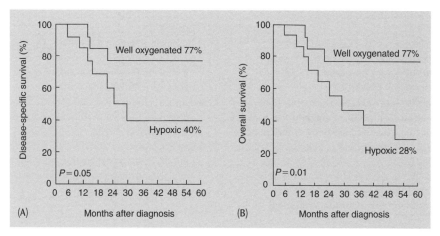

Figure 15.13 *Oxygenation status measured with an Eppendorf oxygen electrode in 28 soft tissue sarcomas: (A) disease-specific survival; (B) overall survival. Tumours with median pO_2 above 19 mmHg were classified as well oxygenated and those below or equal to 19 mmHg as hypoxic. Five-year disease-specific and overall survival rates were estimated by actuarial tumour control probability using Kaplan–Meier estimates. Patients with the most hypoxic tumours had a significantly poorer disease-specific and overall survival probability when compared with well-oxygenated tumours. From Nordsmark* et al. *(2001), with permission.*

KEY POINTS

1. Hypoxic cells are much less sensitive to radiation than well-oxygenated cells.
2. Hypoxic cells probably occur in most animal and human tumours; they are believed to be an important cause of failure by radiotherapy, especially using a small number of large dose fractions.
3. Hypoxia in tumours can be chronic or acute, for which the underlying mechanisms differ. Attempts to eliminate radioresistant tumour cells require treatments that are effective against each of these types of hypoxia.
4. Reoxygenation has been shown to occur in animal tumours; some tumours reoxygenate rapidly, others more slowly. The evidence for reoxygenation in human tumours is less direct.
5. Hypoxic cells in tumours are also known to be resistant to certain chemotherapeutic agents. They may also play an important role in malignant progression.

BIBLIOGRAPHY

Denekamp J (1989). Physiological hypoxia and its influence on radiotherapy. In: *The Biological Basis of Radiotherapy* (eds Steel GG, Adams GE, Horwich A), 2nd edn. Elsevier Science, Amsterdam.

Giaccia A (1996). Hypoxic stress proteins: survival of the fittest. *Semin Radiat Oncol* **6**: 46–58.

Grau C, Overgaard J (1992). Effect of etoposide, carmustine, vincristine, 5-fluorouracil, or methotrexate on radiobiologically oxic and hypoxic cells in a C3H mouse mammary carcinoma *in situ*. *Cancer Chemother Pharmacol* **30**: 277–80.

Gray LH, Conger AD, Ebert M *et al.* (1953). The concentration of oxygen dissolved in tissues at the time of irradiation as a factor in radiotherapy. *Br J Radiol* **26**: 638–48.

Hall EJ (1988). *Radiobiology for the Radiologist*. Lippincott, Philadelphia.

Hill RP, Bush RS, Yeung P (1971). The effect of anaemia on the fraction of hypoxic cells in an experimental tumour. *Br J Radiol* **44**: 299–304.

Horsman MR (1998). Measurement of tumour oxygenation. *Int J Radiat Oncol Biol Phys* **42**: 701–4.

Horsman MR, Khalil AA, Nordsmark M *et al.* (1993). Relationship between radiobiological hypoxia and direct estimates of tumour oxygenation in a

C3H mouse tumour model. *Radiother Oncol* **28**: 69–71.

Horsman MR, Nordsmark M, Overgaard J (1998). Techniques to assess the oxygenation of human tumors – state of the art. *Strahlenther Onkol* **174**(Suppl IV): 2–5.

Howard-Flanders P, Moore D (1958). The time interval after pulsed irradiation within which injury in bacteria can be modified by dissolved oxygen. I. A search for an effect of oxygen 0.02 seconds after pulsed irradiation. *Radiat Res* **9**: 422–37.

Michael BD, Adams GE, Hewitt HB *et al.* (1973). A post-effect of oxygen in irradiated bacteria: a submillisecond fast mixing study. *Radiat Res* **54**: 239–51.

Nordsmark M, Overgaard J (2000). A confirmatory prognostic study on oxygenation status and loco-regional control in advanced head and neck squamous cell carcinoma treated by radiation therapy. *Radiother Oncol* **57**: 39–43.

Nordsmark M, Alsner J, Keller J *et al.* (2001). Hypoxia in human soft tissue sarcomas: adverse impact on survival and no association with p53 mutations. *Br J Cancer* **84**: 1070–5.

Overgaard J (1988). The influence of haemoglobin concentration on the response to radiotherapy. *Scand J Clin Lab Invest* **48**(Suppl 189): 49–53.

Palcic B, Skarsgard LD (1984). Reduced oxygen enhancement ratio at low doses of ionizing radiation. *Radiat Res* **100**: 328–39.

Stanley JA, Shipley WU, Steel GG (1977). Influence of tumour size on hypoxic fraction and therapeutic sensitivity of Lewis lung tumour. *Br J Cancer* **36**: 105–13.

Sutherland RM, Ausserer WA, Murphy BJ, Laderoute KR (1996). Tumour hypoxia and heterogeneity: challenges and opportunities for the future. *Semin Radiat Oncol* **6**: 59–70.

Tannock IF (1968). The relation between cell proliferation and the vascular system in a transplanted mouse mammary tumour. *Br J Cancer* **22**: 258–73.

Thomlinson RH, Gray LH (1955). The histological structure of some human lung cancers and the possible implications for radiotherapy. *Br J Cancer* **9**: 539–49.

Wright EA, Howard-Flanders P (1957). The influence of oxygen on the radiosensitivity of mammalian tissues. *Acta Radiol* **48**: 26–32.

Young SD, Hill RP (1990). Effects of reoxygenation on cells from hypoxic regions of solid tumors: anticancer drug sensitivity and metastatic potential. *J Natl Cancer Inst* **82**: 371–80.

FURTHER READING

Brown JM (1979). Evidence for acutely hypoxic cells in mouse tumours and a possible mechanism of reoxygenation. *Br J Radiol* **52**: 650–6.

Chaplin DJ, Durand RE, Olive PL (1986). Acute hypoxia in tumors: implication for modifiers of radiation effects. *Int J Radiat Oncol Biol Phys* **12**: 1279–82.

Chapman JD (1984). The detection and measurement of hypoxic cells in solid tumors. *Cancer* **54**: 2441–9.

Kallman RF, Rockwell S (1977). Effects of radiation on animal tumour models. In: *Cancer* (ed. Becker FF), Vol. 6. Plenum Press, New York.

Moulder JE, Rockwell S (1984). Hypoxic fractions of solid tumors: experimental techniques, methods of analysis and a survey of existing data. *Int J Radiat Oncol Biol Phys* **10**: 695–712.

Overgaard J (1989). Sensitization of hypoxic tumour cells – clinical experience. *Int J Radiat Biol* **56**: 801–11.

Vaupel P, Kallinowski F, Okunieff P (1989). Blood flow, oxygen and nutrient supply, and metabolic micro-environment of human tumors: a review. *Cancer Res* **49**: 6449–65.

Overcoming tumour radioresistance resulting from hypoxia

MICHAEL R HORSMAN AND JENS OVERGAARD

16.1 INTRODUCTION

The radiobiological problem presented by hypoxia in tumours is set out in the previous chapter; the present chapter describes a number of therapeutic approaches that have been designed to overcome this source of resistance. These primarily include decreasing hypoxia by increasing oxygen availability; chemically or physically radiosensitizing the hypoxic cells; or preferentially killing this resistant population. Since inadequacy of the abnormal vascular supply to tumours is one reason why hypoxia develops, more recent attempts to improve tumour radiation response have involved specifically targeting the tumour blood supply.

16.2 RAISING THE OXYGEN CONTENT OF INSPIRED GAS

One of the earliest clinical attempts to eliminate hypoxia involved patients breathing high-oxygen-content gas under hyperbaric conditions (Churchill-Davidson, 1968). An increase in barometric pressure of the gas breathed by the patient during radiotherapy is termed 'hyperbaric oxygen (HBO) therapy' with pressures up to around 3 atmospheres having been used. Most trials were small in size and suffered from the use of unconventional fractionation schedules, but the results demonstrated that HBO therapy was superior to radiotherapy given in air, especially when a few large fractions were applied (Overgaard, 1989a). This was clearly seen in the largest multicentre clinical trials of HBO, by the British Medical Research Council, in which the results from both advanced head and neck cancer and uterine cervix cancer showed a significant benefit in local tumour control and subsequent survival (Figure 16.1). Benefit was not observed in bladder cancer, nor were these results confirmed by a number of smaller studies (Dische, 1985; Overgaard, 1989a). In retrospect, the use of HBO therapy was discontinued somewhat prematurely. This was partly due to the introduction of chemical radiosensitizers and because of problems with patient compliance. It has been claimed that hyperbaric treatment caused

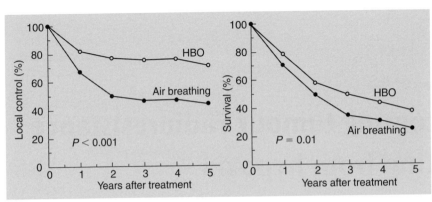

Figure 16.1 *Results from the Medical Research Council hyperbaric oxygen trial showing actuarial local tumour control and survival in patients with stage III carcinoma of the cervix randomized to receive either HBO (open symbols; 119 patients) or air breathing (closed symbols; 124 patients) in conjunction with conventional radiotherapy. Modified from Watson et al. (1978).*

significant suffering, but the discomfort associated with such a treatment must be considered minor compared with the life-threatening complications associated with chemotherapy that is used with a less restrictive indication.

High-oxygen-gas breathing, either as 100% oxygen or carbogen (95% oxygen + 5% carbon dioxide) under *normobaric* conditions has also been used clinically to radiosensitize tumours, but has failed to show significant therapeutic gain (Horsman *et al.*, 2000). One reason for this may have been the failure to achieve the optimum pre-irradiation gas breathing time (PIBT); a number of experimental studies have shown this to be critical for the enhancement of radiation damage and that results can vary from tumour to tumour. The failure of this approach may also have been related to the fact that normobaric oxygen would only be expected to deal with diffusion-limited chronic hypoxia and not with perfusion-limited acute hypoxia (see Section 15.2). Both the PIBT and the acute hypoxia phenomenon have been taken into account in the current ARCON clinical trials (Section 16.6).

16.3 HYPOXIC CELL RADIOSENSITIZERS

The concept of chemical radiosensitization of hypoxic cells was introduced by Adams and Cooke (1969) when they showed that certain compounds were able to mimic oxygen and thus enhance radiation damage. They also demonstrated that the efficiency of sensitization was directly related to the electron affinity of the compounds. It was postulated that such agents would diffuse out of the tumour blood supply and, unlike oxygen, which is rapidly metabolized by tumour cells, they would be able to diffuse further, reach the more distant hypoxic cells, and thus sensitize them. Since these drugs mimic the sensitizing effect of oxygen, they would not be expected to increase the radiation response of well-oxygenated cells in surrounding normal tissues; radiation tolerance should therefore not be compromised. The first electron-affinic compounds to show radiosensitization were the nitrobenzenes. These were followed by the nitrofurans and finally nitroimidazoles, the most potent of which was found to be the 2-nitroimidazole, *misonidazole*. Its *in vitro* activity is illustrated in Figure 16.2. Note that in these experiments misonidazole is radiation *dose-modifying*: the survival curves have the same extrapolation number (i.e. 4). The radiation response of hypoxic cells can thus be enhanced substantially by irradiating the cells in the presence of misonidazole; in fact, at a drug concentration of 10 mM, the radiosensitivity of hypoxic cells approaches that of aerated cells. The response of the aerated cells is unaffected, as expected for an oxygen-mimetic agent.

Radiosensitizers such as misonidazole also enhance radiation damage in experimental tumours *in vivo*, as shown in Figure 16.3. The magnitude of the sensitizing effect is usually expressed by the sensitizer

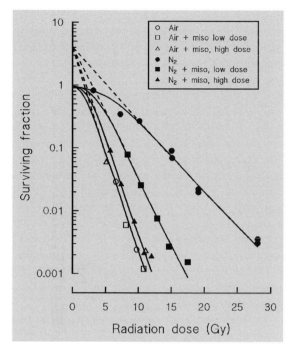

Figure 16.2 *Survival curves for aerated and hypoxic Chinese hamster cells irradiated in the presence or absence of misonidazole. Low dose: 1 mM; high dose: 10 mM. From Adams (1977), with permission.*

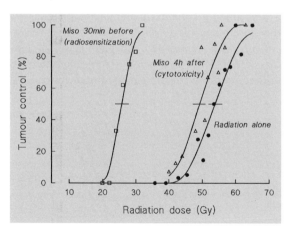

Figure 16.3 *Local tumour control in C3H mouse mammary carcinomas measured 120 days after tumour irradiation. Mice were given misonidazole (1 g kg^{-1}, i.p.) either 30 minutes before or 4 hours after irradiation. The TCD$_{50}$ dose was reduced from 54 Gy in control animals to 26 Gy in the misonidazole-pretreated mice, equivalent to an enhancement ratio (SER) of 2.1. Misonidazole given 4 hours after irradiation gave a TCD$_{50}$ of 49 Gy, an SER of 1.1.*

enhancement ratio (SER):

Sensitizer enhancement ratio = (Radiation dose without sensitizer)/(Radiation dose with sensitizer)

for the same biological effect. Large enhancement ratios (>2.0) have been found in a variety of animal tumours when the sensitizer was administered prior to single-dose irradiation. When misonidazole was combined with *fractionated* radiation, the SER values were lower. This probably results from reoxygenation between radiation fractions reducing the therapeutic impact of hypoxia. Also shown in Figure 16.3 is the effect of giving misonidazole *after* irradiation, where a small but significant enhancement was seen. This obviously cannot be due to hypoxic cell radiosensitization; it is probably due to the well-demonstrated observation that mizonidazole is directly toxic to hypoxic cells, the level of cell killing increasing considerably with the duration of exposure to the sensitizer.

The first clinical studies of radiosensitizers were with metronidazole in brain tumours and together with encouraging laboratory studies of misonidazole they were followed by a boom in the late 1970s of trials exploring the potential of this latter agent as a radiosensitizer (Dische, 1985; Overgaard, 1989a). Most of the trials with misonidazole were unable to demonstrate a significant improvement in radiation response, although benefit was seen in some trials in certain subgroups of treated patients. This was certainly true for the Danish head and neck cancer trial (DAHANCA 2), which found a highly significant improvement in pharynx tumours but not in the prognostically better glottic carcinomas (Overgaard *et al.*, 1989). The generally disappointing clinical results with misonidazole may be partly because it was evaluated in unpromising tumour sites and with too few patients. However, the most likely explanation is the fact that the misonidazole doses were too low, limited by the risk of neurotoxicity. Figure 16.4 summarizes data in mice for the dependence of sensitization on misonidazole concentration, in comparison with *in vitro* results. Although the SER for misonidazole increases with drug dose, the maximum tolerated misonidazole dose that can be given with standard clinical fractionated radiotherapy is around 0.5 g m^{-2}, which results in a tumour concentration of about 15 μg g^{-1}, and it is clear from the laboratory animal data that such a dose could only be expected to yield a small sensitizer enhancement ratio. The difficulty of achieving sufficiently large clinical doses of misonidazole has led to a search for better radio-sensitizing drugs (Coleman, 1988; Overgaard, 1994). Of the many compounds synthesized and tested, two of the most promising were *etanidazole* and *pimonidazole* (Overgaard, 1994). Etanidazole was selected as being superior to misonidazole for two reasons. First, although it has a sensitizing efficiency equivalent to that of misonidazole, it does have a shorter half-life *in vivo*, which should lead to reduced toxicity. Second, it also has a reduced lipophilicity (a lower octanol/water partition coefficient) and is therefore less readily taken up in neural tissue, leading to less neurotoxicity. Pimonidazole contained a side chain with a weakly basic piperidine group. This compound is more electron-affinic than misonidazole and thus is more effective as a radiosensitizer; it is also uncharged at acid pH, thus promoting its accumulation in ischaemic regions of tumours. A pimonidazole trial was started in uterine cervix, but was stopped when it became evident that those patients who received pimonidazole showed a poorer response. Etanidazole was tested in two large head and neck cancer trials, one in the USA and the other in Europe. In neither case was there a significant therapeutic benefit, although in a later subgroup analysis a positive benefit was reported (Overgaard, 1998).

In Denmark, an alternative strategy was taken that involved searching for a less toxic drug and thus *nimorazole* was chosen. Although its sensitizing ability was less than could theoretically be achieved by misonidazole, nimorazole was far less toxic and thus could be given in much higher doses. At a clinically relevant, dose the SER was approximately 1.3. Furthermore, the drug could be given in association with a conventional radiation therapy schedule and was therefore amenable to clinical use. When given to patients with supraglottic and pharyngeal carcinomas (DAHANCA 5) a highly significant benefit in terms of improved loco-regional tumour control and

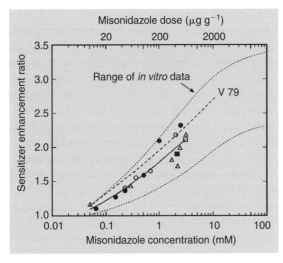

Figure 16.4 *Sensitizer enhancement ratios determined in* vivo *using large single radiation doses as a function of misonidazole dose (upper scale). The symbols indicate different tumour types. The solid line shows the best fit to the* in vivo *results. The dotted lines enclose the range of* in vitro *data (lower scale); data on V79 cells indicated by the dashed line. From Brown (1989), with permission.*

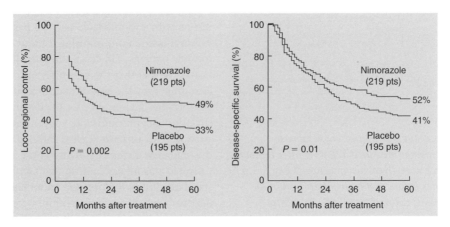

Figure 16.5 *Results from the DAHANCA 5 study showing actuarial estimated loco-regional tumour control and disease-specific survival rate in patients randomized to receive nimorazole or placebo in conjunction with conventional radiotherapy for carcinoma of the pharynx and supraglottic larynx. From Overgaard* et al. *(1998), with permission.*

disease-free survival were obtained (Overgaard *et al.*, 1998). These results are shown in Figure 16.5 and are consistent with the earlier DAHANCA 2 study for misonidazole. As a consequence, nimorazole has now become part of the standard treatment schedule for head and neck tumours in Denmark.

16.4 META-ANALYSIS OF CONTROLLED CLINICAL TRIALS OF MODIFIED TUMOUR HYPOXIA

The clinical role of hypoxia is one of the most thoroughly addressed issues in radiotherapy and has been under investigation for many years. Of the numerous clinical trials that have been conducted during the past three decades, most have been inconclusive and this has raised serious concerns about the real importance of hypoxia. This was addressed in a meta-analysis of all randomized clinical trials in which some form of hypoxic modification was performed in solid tumours undergoing radiotherapy with curative intent. The

survey of published and unpublished data identified more than 11 000 patients treated in 91 randomized clinical trials. The median number of patients per trial was 76 (range 14–626) and the trials involved hyperbaric oxygen (HBO, 31 trials), hypoxic cell radiosensitizers (53 trials), HBO and radiosensitizer (1 trial), oxygen or carbogen breathing (5 trials) and blood transfusion (1 trial). Tumour sites were bladder (16 trials), uterine cervix (20 trials), CNS (13 trials), head and neck (29 trials), lung (10 trials), oesophagus (2 trials) and mixed (1 trial). These trials were analysed with regard to local tumour control (65 trials), survival (77 trials), distant metastases (21 trials) and complications resulting from radiotherapy (26 trials). The overall results are given in Table 16.1. The most relevant end-point was considered to be local tumour control in view of the local nature of the radiation treatment, and this showed a significant improvement. This improvement persisted when the trials were evaluated separately for radiosensitizer or HBO treatment. When analysed according to site, significant improvements were found only for uterine cervix and head and neck cancers. Overall survival

Table 16.1 *Meta-analysis of randomized clinical trials of radiotherapy with a hypoxic-cell modifier*

(A) Summary of randomized trials

End-point	No. of trials	No. of patients	RT + modifier (%)	RT alone (%)	Odds ratio (95% CL)
Loco-regional control	65	8652	52	45	1.29 (1.19–1.41)
Survival	77	10 037	35	31	1.19 (1.09–1.29)
Distant metastases	21	4138	20	21	0.93 (0.80–1.07)
RT complications	26	3916	18	17	1.09 (0.93–1.29)

(B) Loco-regional tumour control as a function of type of hypoxic modification

Hypoxic modifier	No. of trials	No. of patients	RT + modifier (%)	RT alone (%)	Odds ratio (95% CL)
HBO/oxygen*	24	2667	59	49	1.47 (1.26–1.71)
Hypoxic sensitizer*	41	5974	48	42	1.24 (1.12–1.38)
Transfusion	1	135	84	69	2.27 (1.00–5.20)

(C) Loco-regional tumour control as a function of tumour type and location

Tumour site	No. of trials	No. of patients	RT + modifier (%)	RT alone (%)	Odds ratio (95% CL)
Head and neck	27	4250	46	39	1.35 (1.20–1.53)
Bladder	12	707	50	45	1.24 (0.93–1.67)
Uterine cervix	16	2877	65	58	1.31 (1.13–1.52)
Lung (NSCLC)	8	624	37	33	1.19 (0.85–1.65)
Oesophagus	2	192	30	26	1.25 (0.66–2.34)
All (group C) trials	65	8652	52	45	1.29 (1.19–1.41)

*Including 1 trial with hyperbaric oxygen (HBO) + misonidazole (124 patients).

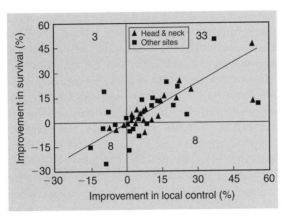

Figure 16.6 *Results from 52 randomized trials of radiotherapy with/without hypoxic modification in which both local tumour control and survival data were obtained. A positive improvement either in survival or local control indicates that the hypoxic-modified arms were better than those of the controls. A strong correlation between both end-points is indicated (r = 0.69; slope = 0.81). The figure shows that patients with head and neck carcinoma seem to have the most impressive benefit.*

was also significantly improved, again dominated by the head and neck patients, but no difference was found for distant metastases or radiation complications. The trials did use different fractionation schedules, including some large doses per fraction, but even for head and neck trials using conventional fractionation, the effect of hypoxic modification was still maintained with an odds ratio of 1.25 (1.08–1.45). Figure 16.6 shows the relationship between improvement in local control and subsequent improvement in survival. The trials shown in this figure are all of epithelial carcinomas, but patients with head and neck tumours generally achieved the highest improvement in both local control and subsequent survival.

From this meta-analysis it appears that the hypoxic problem in radiotherapy may be marginal in most adenocarcinomas. Future efforts should therefore be focused on squamous cell carcinoma, especially of the head and neck, at least when radiotherapy is given in conventional treatment schedules. The variation in the results among the trials certainly points towards a considerable heterogeneity among tumours with the same localization and histology. Thus the need to *predict* the presence of hypoxia and especially the capacity for reoxygenation appears to be a key issue

in order to optimize future clinical applications. The observations that polarographic oxygen electrode measurements were highly predictive for the outcome of radiotherapy in head and neck and cervix (see Section 15.4) indicates that a better selection of patients may be possible. The significant improvement obtained by manipulation of the hypoxic status of squamous tumours of the head and neck, and to a lesser extent cervix, indicates that the underlying biological rationale is probably sound, at least in these tumour sites. It would be logical, therefore, to direct future clinical studies of the hypoxic problem at these tumour types and sites.

16.5 MODIFICATION BASED ON HAEMOGLOBIN

It is well established that haemoglobin concentration is an important prognostic factor for the response to radiotherapy in certain tumour types, especially squamous cell carcinomas (Overgaard, 1989a; Grau and Overgaard, 1997; Horsman *et al.*, 2000). Generally, patients with low haemoglobin levels have a reduced loco-regional tumour control and survival probability (see Figure 15.9). While several mechanisms can be proposed to explain this relationship, tumour hypoxia is clearly one of the major factors.

Although there is no clear relationship between the 'steady-state' haemoglobin concentration and the extent of tumour hypoxia, experimental and clinical studies have both indicated that a rapid, albeit transient, *increase* of the haemoglobin concentration by transfusion can result in an increase in tumour oxygenation (Hirst, 1986). Furthermore, studies have shown that the amount of oxygen delivered to tumours by the blood is especially important for a curative result. This is clearly illustrated in Figure 16.7, in which head and neck cancer patients who smoke were found to have a significantly lower loco-regional control than those who did not. Smoking can lead to a loss of more than 30% of the oxygen-unloading capacity of the blood and this would be expected to significantly reduce tumour oxygenation and subsequently decrease tumour control (Grau and Overgaard, 1997).

The importance of haemoglobin has led to two randomized trials of the effect of transfusion in patients with low haemoglobin values (Overgaard *et al.*, 1998; Fyles *et al.*, 2000). Despite an initial positive report

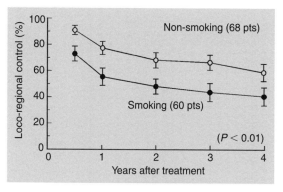

Figure 16.7 *Influence of smoking during treatment on the outcome of radiotherapy in patients with advanced head and neck carcinoma. The local control probability was significantly poorer in patients who continued to smoke during radiotherapy, probably due to reduced oxygen delivery to the tumour. Results from a prospective study in patients treated with curative radiotherapy alone; modified from Grau and Overgaard (1997).*

from the Canadian trial in uterine cervix carcinoma, both studies concluded that the use of such transfusions did not significantly improve treatment outcome. In the DAHANCA 5 study, transfusion was given several days prior to radiotherapy and adaptation may have occurred. Using pre-clinical data, Hirst (1986) hypothesized that any increase in tumour hypoxic fraction induced by anaemia will be only transient, with tumours adapting to the lowered oxygen delivery. Transfusing anaemic animals decreased tumour hypoxia, but this effect also was only transient and the tumours were able to adapt to the increased oxygen level. This suggests that when correcting for anaemia it may not necessarily be the final haemoglobin concentration by itself that is important. Rather, an increasing haemoglobin concentration occurring at the time when the tumours are regressing during radiotherapy may be more likely to result in an increased oxygen supply to tumours and a subsequent improvement in response to radiotherapy.

Although a well-documented causal relationship between haemoglobin concentration, tumour oxygenation and response to radiotherapy has not been shown, it is likely that such a relationship does exist and there is thus a rationale for investigating the possibility of improving the outcome of radiotherapy in relevant tumour sites in patients with low haemoglobin concentration given curative radiotherapy. The use of erythropoietin (EPO) is another approach for

increasing haemoglobin levels and, unlike transfusion, such an increase would result in a gradual increase of oxygen supply over time. Several studies have now shown that EPO is capable of producing such a gradual increase in haemoglobin concentration in patients with head and neck cancer (Henke *et al.*, 1999) and currently several multicentre phase III studies are underway to evaluate the importance of EPO in radiotherapy. The prognostic significance of haemoglobin levels may be more complex than stated above. That it may involve issues other than tumour oxygenation is indicated by the fact that haemoglobin levels also have been found to predict for the response of patients treated with surgery. This of course does not eliminate the importance of tumour oxygenation nor the relevance of a high haemoglobin concentration.

16.6 OVERCOMING ACUTE HYPOXIA IN TUMOURS

Another possible explanation for the disappointing results with hypoxic modification in radiotherapy may be the fact that most of the procedures so far used clinically operate against diffusion-limited *chronic* hypoxia, and they have little or no influence on perfusion-limited *acute* hypoxia (see Section 15.2). Experimental studies have demonstrated that *nicotinamide*, a vitamin-B3 analogue, can enhance radiation damage in a variety of murine tumours using both single-dose and fractionated schedules (Horsman, 1995). Typical results are illustrated in Figure 16.8. This enhancement of radiation damage depends on tumour type, drug dose and the time of irradiation after drug administration, although it does appear to be independent of route of administration. Nicotinamide can enhance radiation damage in normal tissues but generally these effects are less than are seen in tumours.

The mechanism of action of nicotinamide seems primarily that it prevents the transient fluctuations in tumour blood flow that lead to the development of acute hypoxia (Horsman *et al.*, 1990). This finding led to the suggestion that the optimal approach would be to combine nicotinamide with treatments that specifically target chronic hypoxia. Benefit has been seen when nicotinamide was combined with hyperthermia, perfluorochemical emulsions, pentoxifylline and high-oxygen-content gas breathing (Horsman, 1995).

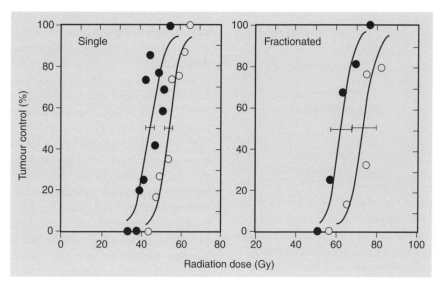

Figure 16.8 *Effect of an intraperitoneal injection of nicotinamide (500–1000 mg kg⁻¹) prior to local tumour irradiation on the level of tumour control measured as a function of the total radiation dose given either as a single treatment to C3H mammary carcinomas or in a fractionated schedule to the carcinoma NT. Results are for radiation alone (○) or nicotinamide and radiation (●). Redrawn from Horsman* et al. *(2000).*

The combination of nicotinamide with carbogen breathing is now under investigation in a number of European clinical studies in the so-called ARCON (Accelerated Radiation, CarbOgen and Nicotinamide) trials, and preliminary results in patients with head and neck cancer are encouraging (Kaanders *et al.*, 1998).

16.7 HYPERTHERMIA

The use of hyperthermia to treat cancer has a history that is more than 5000 years old. However, there has always been the problem of achieving adequate heating of deep-seated tumours. This is not the case with superficial lesions and as technology has improved, the application of hyperthermia alone or in combination with chemotherapy or radiation to such tumours has been more widespread (Nielsen *et al.*, 2001). The aim of hyperthermia is not solely to overcome hypoxic radioresistance but this is included here because of the key role of tumour ischaemia in the efficacy of hyperthermia.

Thermal damage to cells *in vitro* and *in vivo* depends both on temperature and heating time. This is illustrated in Figure 16.9, which shows that the growth delay seen in mouse tumours increased

linearly with heating time and that the slope of the relationship was critically dependent upon temperature in the range 41–45°C. The slope values at each temperature can be summarized in an Arrhenius plot which shows a breakpoint around 42.5°C, indicating a change in the mechanism of damage by heat (see insert in Figure 16.9). Sensitivity to hyperthermia varies greatly among different cell lines but in general there is no differentially enhanced sensitivity in malignant cells as compared with normal-tissue cells. However, the compromised blood flow in tumours can lead to a differential response to heat for two important reasons. First, with a reduced blood flow there is less cooling and temperature rises will be greater. Second, hypoxic cells that are present in tumours as a result of the poor blood supply exist in areas of high acidity, and cells at low pH are far more sensitive to heat damage. This preferential sensitivity of hypoxic cells to heat makes hyperthermia an excellent modality for use in combination with radiation.

When radiation and heat are combined, two distinct phenomena occur and these are illustrated in Figure 16.10. If heat and radiation are given *simultaneously*, there is sensitization. Here the thermal enhancement ratio (TER; ratio of the radiation dose without heating to that with heating to produce the same effect) simply gets larger as the heating time or

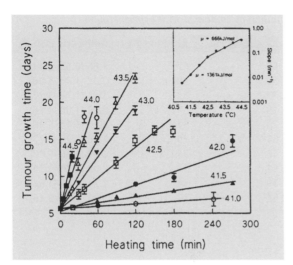

Figure 16.9 *Tumour growth time as a function of heating time for a solid mouse mammary carcinoma heated* in vivo *in the range 41.0–44.5°C. Tumour growth time was the time taken for tumours to regrow to five times their treatment volume.* Inset: *Time–temperature plot showing the slope of the dose–response curves as a function of heating temperature. From Lindegaard and Overgaard (1987), with permission.*

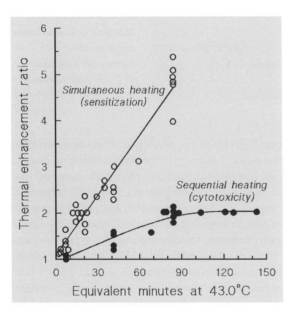

Figure 16.10 *Thermal enhancement ratio as a function of heat treatment in a mouse mammary carcinoma exposed either to simultaneous* (radiosensitization) *or sequential* (cytotoxicity) *radiation and hyperthermia (heat 4 hours after radiation). From Overgaard (1989b), with permission.*

temperature increases, an effect that occurs to the same degree in tumours and normal tissues. However, if heat treatment is given *after* irradiation in a sequential schedule, then the TER is reduced as the time interval is increased: the sensitization dissappears. If the time interval is sufficient (i.e. 4 hours as shown in Figure 16.10) no sensitization is seen and the smaller TER obtained eventually reaches a plateau. This reflects the fact that now the increase in radiation response due to heating is simply the result of direct heat killing of radiation-resistant hypoxic cells. The combination of hyperthermia with radiation has also been investigated in a number of clinical trials and in Table 16.2 shows a meta-analysis of the results from all the published multicentre randomized clinical trials (a total of 1919 patients in 23 trials). Hyperthermia significantly improved loco-regional tumour control in a number of sites, including chest wall, cervix, rectum, bladder, melanoma and head and neck. Taking all these results together, a highly significant improvement was obtained ($P < 0.0001$), clearly demonstrating the potential of hyperthermia to improve radiation therapy.

16.8 BIOREDUCTIVE DRUGS

Selective killing of hypoxic cells can also be achieved with bioreductive drugs. These are compounds that undergo intracellular reduction to form active cytotoxic species, primarily under low oxygen tensions. The development of such agents arose following the discovery that electron-affinic radiosensitizers not only sensitize hypoxic cells to radiation but also are preferentially toxic to them (Section 16.3). These drugs can be divided into three major groups, as illustrated in Figure 16.11: quinones (e.g. mitomycin C), nitroimidazoles (e.g. RSU-1069) and N-oxides (e.g. tirapazamine).

Mitomycin C (MMC) is probably the prototype *bioreductive drug*. It has been used clinically for many years as a chemo-radiosensitizer, long before it was realized it had preferential effects against hypoxic cells. It is activated by bioreduction to form products that crosslink DNA and therefore produce cell killing. Several randomized clinical trials in patients with squamous cell carcinoma of the head and neck have now been undertaken, specifically using MMC to counteract the effects of hypoxia. Initial studies

Table 16.2 *Meta-analysis of randomized clinical trials of radiotherapy combined with hyperthermia**

Tumour site	No. of trials	No. of patients	RT + heat (%)	RT alone (%)	Odds ratio (95% CL)
Advanced breast	2	143	68	67	1.06 (0.52–2.14)
Chest wall	4	276	59	38	2.37 (1.46–3.86)
Cervix	4	248	77	52	3.05 (1.77–5.27)
Rectum	2	258	19	9	2.27 (1.08–4.76)
Bladder	1	101	73	51	2.61 (1.14–5.98)
Prostate	1	49	81	79	1.16 (0.28–4.77)
Melanoma	1	128	56	31	2.81 (1.36–5.80)
Head and neck	5	274	51	33	2.08 (1.28–3.39)
Mixed	3	442	39	34	1.24 (0.84–1.82)
All trials	23	1919	52	38	1.80 (1.50–2.16)

*All results are for loco-regional control.

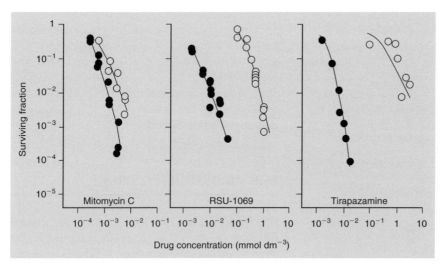

Figure 16.11 *Survival of mammalian cells exposed to either mitomycin C, RSU-1069 or tirapazamine under aerobic (○) or hypoxic (●) conditions. Redrawn from Horsman et al. (2000).*

reported an improvement in local tumour control and/or survival, without any enhancement of radiation reactions in normal tissues. However, this has not been confirmed by more recent studies, perhaps not surprising when one considers that MMC actually has a very small differential killing effect between aerobic and hypoxic cells (Figure 16.11). Also, in the clinical trials MMC was only administered once or twice during the entire course of radiotherapy, so its ability to preferentially kill hypoxic cells and thus enhance radiation therapy must have been limited. Attempts to find more efficient quinones have been undertaken and to that end porfiromycin and EO9 have been developed.

The finding that misonidazole was preferentially toxic towards hypoxic cells led to numerous efforts to find other *nitroimidazoles* that were better. To that

end RSU-1069 was developed. This compound has the classic 2-nitroimidazole radiosensitizing properties, but also an aziridine ring at the terminal end of the chain, which gave the molecule substantial potency as a hypoxic cell cytotoxin, both *in vitro* and *in vivo*. In large-animal studies it was found to cause gastrointestinal toxicity and a less toxic pro-drug was therefore developed (RB-6145), which is reduced *in vivo* to RSU-1069. Although this drug was found to have potent anti-tumour activity in experimental systems, further animal studies revealed that this drug induced blindness; this is perhaps not surprising when one realizes that the retina is hypoxic. Further development of this drug has been halted.

Perhaps the most promising group of bioreductives are the *organic nitroxides*, of which the benzotriazene di-N-oxide, tirapazamine, is the lead compound. The

Table 16.3 *Strategies targeting the tumour vasculature*

Target	Agents/approaches
Activators of angiogenesis	Antibodies/antisense to angiogenic growth factors
Matrix/cell–matrix interactions	Metalloproteinase inhibitors, Marismastat, alpha (v)-integrin antagonists
Receptors	Antibodies to vascular endothelial growth factor (VEGF) receptor, Suramin, alpha (v)-integrin binding motifs
Signal transduction pathways	Inhibitors of tyrosine kinase activity of flk-1/KDR, SU5416, SU6668, ZD4190, PD 0173073
Endothelial cell function	Angiostatin, endostatin, TNP-470, Tie2 antagonists
Existing tumour vasculature	Colchicine, flavone acetic acid (FAA), 5,6-dimethylxanthenone-4-acetic acid (DMXAA), combretastatin A-4 disodium phosphate (CA4DP), ZD6126

Adapted from Siemann *et al.* (2000).

parent moiety shows limited toxicity toward aerobic cells, but after reduction under hypoxic conditions a product is formed that has been shown to be highly toxic and can substantially enhance radiation damage to tumours *in vivo*. More recent studies have shown this bioreductive drug to be effective in enhancing the anti-tumour activity of cisplatin and it is in this context that preliminary clinical testing has been performed, with encouraging results. Other N-oxides are currently under development, including AQ4N and chlorambucil N-oxide.

16.9 VASCULAR TARGETING THERAPIES

The vascular supply to tumours is one of the major factors responsible for the development of hypoxia. The tumour vasculature develops from normal-tissue vessels by the process of 'angiogenesis'. This is an essential aspect of tumour growth, but this tumour neovasculature is primitive and chaotic in nature and is often unable to meet the oxygen demands of rapidly expanding tumour regions, thus allowing hypoxia to develop (see Section 15.2). The importance of the tumour neovasculature in determining growth and the environmental conditions within a tumour makes it an attractive target for therapy and two approaches are currently in vogue. The first and most popular is the use of drugs to prevent angiogenesis from occurring. The second involves the use of therapies that can specifically damage the already established vasculature. Examples of both anti-angiogenesis and vascular damaging agents are shown in Table 16.3.

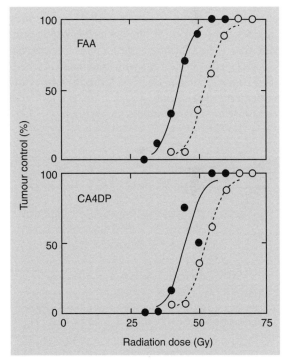

Figure 16.12 *Local tumour control in C3H mammary carcinomas measured 90 days after local tumour irradiation with single radiation doses either given alone (open symbols) or followed by a single intraperitoneal injection with FAA (150 mg kg^{-1}) or CA4DP (250 mg kg^{-1}) within 1 hour after irradiation (closed symbols).*

Damage to tumour blood vessels leads to a reduced blood flow to the affected tumour region. This may give rise to local hypoxia and ischaemia, and ultimately cell death. Since hypoxic cells are already under stress as a result of oxygen and nutrient deprivation, it is likely that these cells will be the first to die after this additional insult from vascular shutdown. It is thus to be expected that such vascular targeting drugs may enhance radiation response. A number of pre-clinical studies have investigated this interaction and shown that, indeed, the radiation response of murine tumours can be improved by administration of a vascular-targeting drug (Figure 16.12). In these experiments tumour-bearing mice were injected either with FAA or CA4DP. Both drugs can induce sustained reduction in tumour blood flow and significantly increase tumour necrosis, but on their own they have no effect on tumour control and they delay tumour growth by only a few days. However, if these drugs are administered as a single injection at the same time or shortly after local tumour irradiation, they significantly improve tumour control. Limited further studies suggest that these effects are tumour-specific and an enhancement can be seen with fractionated schedules. Several vascular-targeting drugs are currently undergoing phase-I clinical evaluation, and testing in combination with radiation is anticipated.

KEY POINTS

1. Hypoxic cell radioresistance is a significant cause of failure in the local control of tumours, especially squamous cell carcinomas of the head and neck and cervix.
2. Clinical attempts to overcome hypoxic cell radioresistance using either high-oxygen-content gas breathing, chemical radiosensitizers or blood transfusions have shown mixed results. Meta-analysis of randomized trials does, however, demonstrate a significant benefit.
3. Since these treatments are designed to negate the effects of *chronic* hypoxia, additional benefit may be obtained by including a modifier of *acute* hypoxia such as nicotinamide in the treatment protocol.
4. Hypoxic cell cytotoxins (e.g. bioreductive drugs) also show promise as clinically relevant methods for eliminating radioresistance.
5. Hyperthermia also preferentially kills hypoxic cells, but in addition it can produce significant radiosensitization and a recent meta-analysis

of results from published multicentre clinical trials clearly demonstrates the benefit of combining hyperthermia with radiation.
6. Since one of the major factors responsible for hypoxia is the inadequate vascular supply of tumours, pre-clinical studies are now suggesting that drugs that specifically target tumour blood vessels may provide a new approach to overcoming the hypoxia problem.

BIBLIOGRAPHY

Adams GE (1977). Hypoxic cell sensitizers for radiotherapy. In: *Cancer* (ed. Becker FF), Vol. 6. Plenum Press, New York.

Adams GE, Cooke MS (1969). Electron-affinic sensitization: I. A structural basis for chemical radiosensitizers in bacteria. *Int J Radiat Biol* **15**: 457–71.

Brown JM (1989). Hypoxic cell radiosensitizers: where next? *Int J Radiat Oncol Biol Phys* **16**: 987–93.

Churchill-Davidson I (1968). The oxygen effect in radiotherapy – historical review. *Front Radiat Ther Oncol* **1**: 1–15.

Coleman CN (1988). Hypoxia in tumours: a paradigm for the approach to biochemical and physiological heterogeneity. *J Natl Cancer Inst* **80**: 310–17.

Dische S (1985). Chemical sensitizers for hypoxic cells: a decade of experience in clinical radiotherapy. *Radiother Oncol* **3**: 97–115.

Fyles AW, Milosevic M, Pintilie M, Syed A, Hill RP (2000). Anemia, hypoxia and transfusion in patients with cervix cancer: a review. *Radiother Oncol* **57**: 13–19.

Grau C, Overgaard J (1997). Significance of hemoglobin concentration for treatment outcome. In: *Medical Radiology: Blood Perfusion and Microenvironment of Human Tumors* (eds Molls M, Vaupel P), pp. 101–12. Springer-Verlag, Heidelberg.

Henke M, Guttenberger A, Barke F, Pajonk F, Pötter R, Fromhold H (1999). Erythropoietin for patients undergoing radiotherapy: a pilot study. *Radiother Oncol* **50**: 185–200.

Hirst DG (1986). Anemia: a problem or an opportunity in radiotherapy? *Int J Radiat Oncol Biol Phys* **12**: 2009–17.

Horsman MR (1995). Nicotinamide and other benzamide analogs as agents for overcoming hypoxic cell radiation resistance in tumours. *Acta Oncol* **34**: 571–87.

Horsman MR, Chaplin DJ, Overgaard J (1990). Combination of nicotinamide and hyperthermia to eliminate radioresistant chronically and acutely hypoxic tumor cells. *Cancer Res* **50**: 7430–6.

Horsman MR, Lindegaard JC, Grau C, Nordsmark M, Overgaard J (2000). Dose response modifiers in radiation therapy. In: *Clinical Radiation Oncology* (eds Gunderson LL, Tepper JE), pp. 155–68. Churchill Livingstone, New York.

Kaanders JHAM, Pop LAM, Marres HAM *et al.* (1998). Accelerated radiotherapy with carbogen and nicotinamide (ARCON) for laryngeal cancer. *Radiother Oncol* **48**: 115–22.

Lindegaard JC, Overgaard J (1987). Factors of importance for the development of the step-down heating effect in a C3H mammary carcinoma *in vivo*. *Int J Hyperthermia* **3**: 79–81.

Nielsen OS, Horsman M, Overgaard J (2001). A future for hyperthermia in cancer treatment: editorial comment. *Eur J Cancer* **37**: 1587–9.

Overgaard J (1989a). Sensitization of hypoxic tumour cells – clinical experience. *Int J Radiat Biol* **56**: 801–11.

Overgaard J (1989b). The current and potential role of hyperthermia in radiotherapy. *Int J Radiat Oncol Biol Phys* **16**: 535–49.

Overgaard J (1994). Clinical evaluation of nitroimidazoles as modifiers of hypoxia in solid tumors. *Oncol Res* **6**: 507–16.

Overgaard J (1998). Letter to the editor. *Radiother Oncol* **48**: 345–6.

Overgaard J, Sand Hansen H, Andersen AP *et al.* (1989). Misonidazole combined with split-course radiotherapy in the treatment of invasive carcinoma of larynx and pharynx. Final report from the DAHANCA 2 study. *Int J Radiat Oncol Biol Phys* **16**: 1065–8.

Overgaard J, Sand Hansen H, Overgaard M *et al.* (1998). A randomised double-blind phase III study of

nimorazole as a hypoxic radiosensitizer of primary radiotherapy in supraglottic larynx and pharynx carcinoma: results of the Danish Head and Neck Cancer Study (DAHANCA) protocol 5-85. *Radiother Oncol* **46**: 135–46.

Siemann DW, Warrington KH, Horsman MR (2000). Targeting tumor blood vessels: an adjuvant strategy for radiation therapy. *Radiother Oncol* **57**: 5–12.

Watson ER, Halnan KE, Dische S (1978). Hyperbaric oxygen and radiotherapy: a Medical Research Council trial in carcinoma of the cervix. *Br J Radiol* **51**: 879–87.

FURTHER READING

Brown JM, Giacchia AJ (1998). The unique physiology of solid tumors: opportunities (and problems) for cancer therapy. *Cancer Res* **58**: 1408–16.

Dahl O, Overgaard J (2002). Hyperthermia. In: *Oxford Textbook of Oncology* (eds Souhami RL, Tannock I, Hohenberger H, Horiot J-C), 2nd edn, pp. 511–25. Oxford University Press, Oxford.

EORTC Cooperative Group for Radiotherapy (1991). Consensus Meeting on Tumour Hypoxia. *Radiother Oncol* **20**(Suppl 1): 1–159.

Field SB, Morris CC (1983). The relationship between heating time and temperature: its relevance to clinical hyperthermia. *Radiother Oncol* **1**: 179–86.

Horsman MR (1993). Hypoxia in tumours: its relevance, identification and modification. In: *Current Topics in Clinical Radiobiology of Tumours* (ed. Beck-Bornholdt HP), pp. 11–26. Springer-Verlag, Berlin.

Raleigh JA (ed.) (1996). Hypoxia and its clinical relevance. *Semin Radiat Oncol* **6**: issue 1.

17

The radiobiology of tumours

G GORDON STEEL

17.1 THE CLINICAL PICTURE: TUMOUR CONTROL PROBABILITY

The level of success of radiotherapy for cancer varies considerably from one disease and tumour stage to another. It is common clinical experience that some tumours are curable with high probability; in other tumour types it is only a proportion of patients who achieve long-term survival; and there are yet others in which local control by radiotherapy is seldom achieved. Lymphomas, including Hodgkin's disease, are among the most radioresponsive; glioblastoma and osteosarcoma are examples of very radioresistant diseases; and between these two extremes lie the other non-lymphoid cancers that form most of the daily work of radiotherapy departments.

The task of giving a quantitative description of this clinical picture is fraught with problems. Rubin *et al.* (1974) summarized data then available on the 'prescribed tumour lethal doses for 95% tumour control probability' for various tumour types. The values ranged from 35 Gy for seminoma, Wilms' tumour and neuroblastoma to greater than 80 Gy for glioblastoma, melanoma, osteosarcoma and some other tumour types. Deacon *et al.* (1984) looked again at this classification, concluded that the data were generally inadequate to calculate TCD_{95} values,

and preferred instead to place tumour types into five categories of radioresponsiveness. They admitted that 'even this crude tabulation is open to dispute'. This table, which appeared in previous editions of this book, is not reproduced here because the doubts about its reliability continue. A summary of clinical tumour control (TCP) curves was made by Okunieff *et al.* (1995). They analysed data from 50 single-institution studies on macroscopic disease. The resulting TCD_{50} values ranged widely: breast cancer, 21.4–90.3 Gy; supraglottic cancer, 50.4–83.4 Gy; cervix cancer, 24.3–64.4 Gy. Values for the steepness of the tumour control curves (γ_{50}, see Section 10.4) were also calculated but as a result of the low quality of the data these also vary so widely as to be difficult to summarize. At this stage it must be concluded that although (as noted in the previous paragraph) differences in clinical responsiveness among tumour types are apparent, it is impossible to quantify these differences with a useful level of precision.

17.2 EXPERIMENTAL TUMOUR SYSTEMS

Research into the radiation response of tumours has been performed on a wide variety of tumour cell systems. *In vivo* studies have mainly been carried out on tumours in experimental animals, usually in mice and rats. In addition to studies carried out on permanent *in vitro* tumour cell lines, *in vitro* techniques have often been used to investigate the radiosensitivity of cells from experimental tumours (so-called *in vivo–in vitro* experiments) or on cells taken directly from human tumours. The range of cell systems that have been used may be described under the following headings, arranged roughly in order of increasing closeness to cancer in man.

In vitro cell lines

Although it is possible to grow cells from normal tissues in cell culture systems, the cultures usually fail after perhaps 20–30 passages. This is known as the Hayflick limit. It is clearly a disadvantage for most laboratory research that cultures should die out and it has been overcome in three main ways. First, some normal-cell cultures have been grown through the Hayflick limit and have become immortal. They retain some characteristic features of normal-tissue cells (contact-inhibition of growth in crowded cultures or failure to grow in immune-deficient mice, etc.) and they are usually not known to be virally transformed. Widely used examples are CHO (Chinese hamster ovary) cells and V79 fibroblasts (also from hamster). Second, there are normal-tissue cells that have been virally transformed (for instance by Simian virus SV40). These usually lose contact inhibition and retain viral sequences in their genome. The third approach is to use human or animal *tumour* cells. Tumour cells appear not to be subject to the Hayflick limit and can often be grown continuously without deterioration. A wide variety of cell lines have been used, including HeLa (derived from a human cervix carcinoma), L5178Y mouse lymphoma cells and the human tumour cell lines referred to in Section 17.5. All types of 'permanent' cell lines are subject to genetic drift and the various sublines in different laboratories may not be identical. See Freshney (1987) for a general text on tissue culture.

Multicellular spheroids

Some cell lines readily form aggregates in tissue culture that can grow up to a diameter of a fraction of a millimetre. They have been widely studied as *in vitro*

models of tumours; they of course have no vascular system but depend on diffusion of oxygen and other nutrients through the surface of the 'spheroid'. Small spheroids are fully oxygenated but as they grow they develop a hypoxic core. In larger spheroids, three or more concentric zones can sometimes be distinguished, among which cell proliferation, oxygenation and drug and radiation sensitivity may vary (Durand and Sutherland, 1973).

Transplanted tumours in experimental animals

A wide variety of tumours have been conditioned to repeated transplantation in laboratory animals. Some of these arose spontaneously; some were induced by chemicals, radiation or viruses. During repeated passage, usually subcutaneously, they grow faster and more uniformly and often lose differentiated characteristics. They are attractive as reproducible and convenient *in vivo* tumour systems but may in some respects have deviated away from the original primary tumour. Well-known examples are L1210 leukaemia, Lewis lung tumour, B16 melanoma and R1 rhabdomyosarcoma (Kallman, 1987).

A matter of some importance is the immune status of the grafts. Tumours grown in non-inbred strains of animals or in an inbred colony that differs from that in which they arose will inevitably be subject to variable host rejection (Scott, 1991). If the tumours grow fast, they may beat the developing rejection processes and the investigator may imagine that rejection is unimportant. But if the tumour is treated with radiation or cytotoxic drugs, the influence of the immune response on residual tumour may become significant; more importantly, if the anti-tumour effects of two agents are compared and one is more immune-suppressive than the other, misleading results can be obtained. This is especially the case if tumour cure is used as the end-point, for immune responses are particularly effective against a small amount of tumour remaining after therapy.

Primary animal tumours

The word *autochthonous* is sometimes used for tumours that are studied in the host within which they arose. They may be spontaneous, or they may have been induced by radiation, carcinogenic chemicals, viruses or other means. A primary tumour would be expected to bear greater resemblance to human tumours than one that has been transplanted many times: its immune status should be more realistic and it will not have undergone the growth acceleration and other changes that occur on repeated transplantation. The main drawbacks are that to generate a sufficient supply of spontaneous tumours requires large numbers of animals to be kept for a long period of time; they are therefore expensive. Second, if potent carcinogens are used to increase the induction frequency, the resulting tumours tend to be immunogenic. Mammary tumours arising spontaneously in C3H mice and their isotransplants have been used for some important radiobiological studies (Suit et al., 1965, 1992; Suit and Maeda, 1967).

Human tumour xenografts

A *xenograft* is a transplant from one species to another. In the cancer field this usually refers to a human tumour grown in a laboratory animal. If the recipient animal has a normal immune system, then a xenograft should not grow, but there are two main ways in which growth has been achieved. First, animal strains have been developed that are congenitally immune-deficient. Best known are nude mice, which, in addition to being hairless, also lack a thymus. Many human tumours will grow under the skin of nude mice (Sparrow, 1980). More recently there have been nude rats, also SCID mice which suffer from the severe combined immunodeficiency syndrome and which are deficient in both B-cell and T-cell immunity. Second, it is possible to severely immune-suppress mice to the point where they will accept human tumour grafts. It is important to recognize that neither type of host completely fails to reject the human tumour cells: rejection processes between man and mouse are still present and these complicate the interpretation of *in situ* tumour therapeutic studies. Nevertheless, xenografts do maintain many of the biological and therapeutic properties of their source tumours, and they comprise a valuable type of experimental system (Steel et al., 1983).

Clinical radiobiology

The ultimate experimental system is the cancer patient, and randomized clinical trials have an essential role in the development of new therapies. In addition, although the scope for experimenting on patients is limited, there are some radiobiological experiments, which, while not of direct benefit to the individual patient, have been carried out with appropriate informed consent. Examples are measurements of the distribution of oxygen concentration in tumours, or studies of the proliferation rate of tumour cells using flow cytometry of biopsies. Results of studies in clinical radiobiology are described in a number of parts of this book, especially Chapters 10, 11 and 16.

17.3 END-POINTS FOR MEASURING RADIATION EFFECTS ON TUMOURS

Three principal methods have been used to document and compare the effects of radiation or cytotoxic drugs on experimental tumours.

Tumour growth delay

This is especially useful for tumours growing subcutaneously, the size of which can be measured accurately with callipers. A group of tumours are selected to have closely similar size. They are divided into similar groups and given different treatments, one group being left untreated. Tumour volume is then followed at regular intervals. The usual pattern is that shown in Figure 17.1A: a period of regression followed by regrowth. In order to measure growth delay, we select an end-point (such as twice or four times the treatment size), determine the average time that treated and control tumours take to reach this size, and by subtraction find the delay.

Results obtained with different radiation doses can then be plotted as a dose–response curve (Figure 17.1B). If we wish to evaluate the effect on the tumour of some modification of treatment (adding a radiosensitizer, changing inspired oxygen level, etc.), we would perform a larger experiment in which both modified and unmodified tumours are studied together. Thus we would obtain two dose–response curves and a good way of indicating the extent of modification is to calculate a dose-modifying factor (DMF). This can be read off as the ratio of radiation doses that give the same effect: (without modification)/ (with modification). If the modification is truly

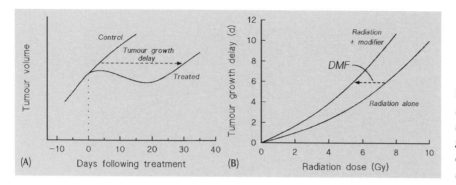

Figure 17.1 *(A) Illustrating the measurement of tumour growth delay, and (B) the calculation of a dose modifying factor (DMF).*

dose-modifying, then the DMF value should be the same at all levels of effect. It is then better to calculate the DMF (by computer) by asking what value would allow the two curves to be most nearly superimposed. A variety of terms similar to DMF have also been used and calculated in the same way, such as oxygen enhancement ratio (OER), sensitizer enhancement ratio (SER), or thermal enhancement ratio (TER).

Comparison of growth delay among tumours of different growth rate leads to uncertainties in interpretation. One approach (Kopper and Steel, 1975) is to calculate a *specific growth delay*:

Specific growth delay = $(TD_{treated} - TD_{control})/TD_{control}$

where TD indicates the time within which treated or control tumours double in volume after the time of treatment. Specific growth delay corresponds to the number of volume doubling times saved by treatment. Since the doubling time for repopulation by clonogenic cells may not bear a constant relation to volume doubling time, this approach should be regarded as only roughly satisfactory. There is no *ideal* solution to the problem of comparing growth delay among tumours of different growth rate.

Tumour control

As radiation dose is increased there will come a point where some tumours fail to regrow. We can then evaluate a modifying agent by determining its effect on this 'curative' radiation dose. The radiation dose that controls 50% of tumours is usually called the TCD_{50} and a DMF can be calculated by determining the ratio of TCD_{50} values without/with the modifier (if DMF values thus obtained are greater than 1.0, then this indicates radiosensitization). It is important

when using this assay to observe the tumour-bearing mice for a long enough time to detect almost all possible recurrences. Death of animals from metastases may frustrate this and the assay is therefore not appropriate for tumours that frequently metastasize. A further drawback is that the assay is greatly affected by any host immune reaction against the tumours (see previous section). The TCD_{50} assay has been widely and successfully used by Suit *et al.* (1965).

The use of this assay in evaluating the radiosensitization by misonidazole of first-generation transplants of C3H mouse mammary tumours is illustrated in Figure 17.2 (Fowler *et al.*, 1976). The objective was to ask: 'What duration of fractionated radiotherapy gives the best therapeutic response, in the presence or absence of the sensitizer?' Figure 17.2A shows examples of the dose–response curves for tumour control with and without the administration of the sensitizer 30 minutes before irradiation. Dose–response curves for the early skin reactions in the feet of mice were documented in parallel experiments. These allowed the radiation dose (with or without sensitizer and for any duration of treatment) that gave a fixed level of skin damage to be identified. The level of tumour control that corresponded to each of these doses (for instance, *D*) could then be read off from the corresponding tumour control curve. Figure 17.2B shows (in outline) the results: tumour control probability for a fixed level of skin damage as a function of the duration of fractionated treatment. Without misonidazole, short treatments were bad; there was an optimum treatment duration of around 8 days. Adding misonidazole thus greatly improved the results of short schedules but had little effect on the longer ones. The explanation may be one that is important for clinical radiotherapy: reoxygenation is incomplete for short treatment times and a radiosensitizer

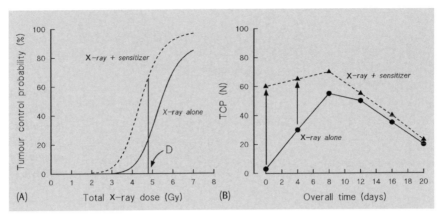

Figure 17.2 *Tumour control in the evaluation of optimum fractionation with a radiosensitizer. (A) examples of tumour control curves for a selected duration of treatment; (B) tumour control probability, TCP(N), for a fixed level of early skin damage. The effect of the sensitizer (arrows) was greatest for short overall treatment times. A diagrammatic representation of the results of Fowler* et al. *(1976), with permission.*

may counteract this deficiency; long treatment times may allow reoxygenation to occur but they may be suboptimal because of tumour cell repopulation.

Cell survival

Cell survival studies have for many years under-pinned the cellular basis of tumour response to treatment. In comparison with the other two end-points described above, clonogenic assays have the advantage of removing the cells into a growth environment that is uniform and unaffected by treatment; there is therefore less opportunity for artefacts due to the effects of treatment on the host animal. Clonogenic cell survival is dealt with in Section 6.2.

17.4 SOME CONCLUSIONS FROM THE *IN VIVO* RADIOBIOLOGY OF EXPERIMENTAL TUMOURS

The large number of radiobiological studies done on animal tumours during the 1970s and 1980s provided the basis for many important concepts, including the following.

The tumour size effect

Large tumours are more difficult to cure than small tumours but this is mainly due to the number of clonogenic cells that have to be killed. A course of

radiotherapy that can achieve a surviving fraction of, say, 10^{-9} could be curative in a tumour that has less than 10^9 clonogenic cells, but probably not in one that has 10^{12} (see Figure 2.1 and Section 6.6). The more intricate question is whether, in addition to this obvious effect, the clonogenic cells in large tumours are also *less sensitive* to therapy.

There is good evidence that this is the case. Stanley *et al.* (1977) treated Lewis lung tumours with γ-radiation, BCNU or cyclophosphamide at a wide range of tumour sizes and produced the results shown in Figure 17.3. As tumour size increased, there was in each case a steep decline in cellular sensitivity (a rise in cell survival) over the size range from 1 to 100 mm^3. This could have been due to the internal vascular supply becoming progressively poorer in the growing tumours, thus decreasing the access of chemotherapeutic agents and increasing the proportion of cells that were hypoxic and therefore resistant to radiation treatment.

Accelerated repopulation

The notion that clonogenic cells that survive radiation treatment may quickly repopulate the tumour was suggested by the classic study of Hermens and Barendsen (1969). They irradiated rat R1 rhabdomyosarcoma transplants with a single 20 Gy dose of x-rays and measured both tumour volume and the fraction of surviving clonogenic cells over the following few weeks (Figure 17.4). Tumour volume showed a

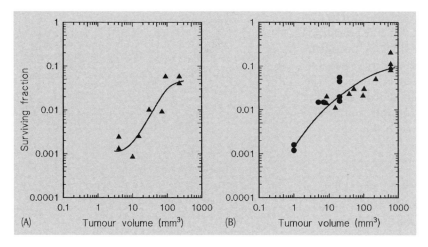

Figure 17.3 *Variation with tumour size of cell survival in the Lewis lung tumour treated with (A) 75 mg/kg cyclophosphamide or (B) 10 Gy γ-rays. ▲, subcutaneous tumours; ●, lung tumours. From Stanley* et al. *(1977), with permission.*

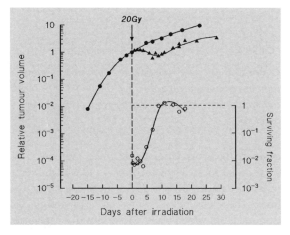

Figure 17.4 *Response of the R1 tumour to 20 Gy x-rays showing the volume response and the surviving fraction of clonogenic cells. From Hermens and Barendsen (1969), with permission.*

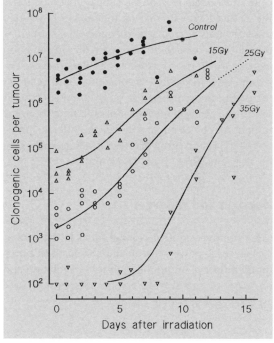

Figure 17.5 *Estimated number of clonogenic cells per tumour in the Lewis lung tumour following various doses of γ-radiation: △, 15 Gy; ○, 25 Gy; ▽, 35 Gy. From Stephens* et al. *(1978), with permission.*

slight regression, followed by regrowth. Surviving fraction immediately after irradiation was around 10^{-2} and it remained at that level for 4 days. It then increased rapidly to reach unity at post-irradiation days 10–12. Although this appears to demonstrate rapid tumour repopulation, it should be noted that surviving fraction does not take into account the loss of countable but doomed cells from the tumour which presumably was increasing during this 12-day period: a rapid rise in surviving fraction could be due to the loss of non-clonogenic doomed cells.

More reliable, therefore, are the results of Stephens *et al.* (1978), who in the Lewis lung tumour carefully measured not only the surviving fraction but also the number of viable cells per tumour and were thus able to make an estimate of the *total clonogenic cells per tumour* (Figure 17.5). Following single radiation doses in the range 15–35 Gy, there was clear evidence for accelerated repopulation and the speed of repopulation was greater following the larger doses.

An important notion that is well illustrated by the data in Figure 17.4 is that tumour volume provides a poor reflection of clonogenic cell kill. A treatment that produces only slight and temporary regression may depress surviving fraction by as much as two decades (99% clonogenic cell kill). It is the slow rate of tumour regression that prevents this from being revealed in the volume change (see Section 2.5).

The tumour bed effect

Careful measurement of the growth rate of experimental tumours that recur following radiation treatment has often shown that it is slower than the growth rate of untreated tumours of the same size. This is called the *tumour bed effect*. A similar phenomenon is the reduced growth rate of tumours transplanted into previously irradiated subcutaneous sites. It is thought that both these effects are due to radiation damage to stromal (including vascular) tissues. The reason why accelerated repopulation and retarded regrowth can occur together is because the former is seen in surviving clonogenic cells at a time when the tumour may be shrinking, whereas the latter is a property of the volume growth rate of irradiated tumours; see Begg and Terry (1985) and Kallman (1987).

Hypoxia and reoxygenation

Most tumours contain clonogenic cells that are at various levels of oxygenation and this fact has a profound influence on tumour control by radiation and on ways of quantifying tumour response. These aspects are dealt with in Chapter 15.

17.5 THE RADIOSENSITIVITY OF HUMAN TUMOUR CELLS

Initial slope of the cell survival curve

A key question in radiation biology applied to radiotherapy is: 'How radiosensitive are human tumour cells, and how does this relate to clinical radiocurability?' Prior to 1980 there was little information on this but interest was aroused by Fertil and Malaise (1981), who surveyed the published literature on *in vitro* human tumour cell survival curves and found

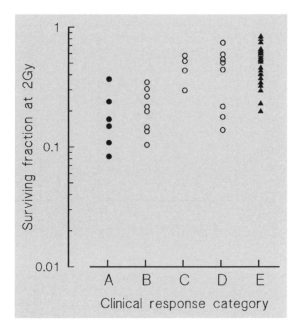

Figure 17.6 *Surviving fraction at 2 Gy for 51 human tumour cell lines, arranged in five categories of clinical radioresponsiveness. From Deacon* et al. *(1984), with permission.*

evidence for a correlation with clinical response. This survey was repeated by Deacon *et al.* (1984), who summarized data on 51 non-HeLa human tumour cell lines. These covered 17 different histopathological tumour types which were placed into five categories of local tumour radiocurability:

- Group A: lymphoma, myeloma, neuroblastoma;
- Group B: medulloblastoma, small-cell lung cancer;
- Group C: breast, bladder, cervical carcinoma;
- Group D: pancreatic, colorectal, squamous lung cancer;
- Group E: melanoma, osteosarcoma, glioblastoma, renal carcinoma.

The placing of tumour types in this list is somewhat uncertain and the underlying clinical data do not allow this to be done unequivocally. However, the ranking A–E broadly reflects clinical experience. The *in vitro* cell survival data for each cell line were analysed to determine the surviving fraction at 2 Gy (which was termed SF_2), chosen as a measure of the initial slope of the cell survival curves. The results are shown in Figure 17.6. Within each category of clinical radioresponsiveness there was considerable scatter (not surprising in view of the many different sources, cell lines and techniques used), but in confirmation of Fertil and Malaise's conclusions there was a significant trend in the data towards group A having lower and group E having higher SF_2 values. This important conclusion underlies the belief that the *steepness of the initial slope* is a significant factor in the clinical response of tumours to radiotherapy. A more recent analysis including additional data reached the conclusion that there was no significant difference between the survival data for groups C, D and E. The tumours in these groups, which include many of the solid tumours treated with radiation therapy, have an average SF_2 value of roughly 0.5: we would expect that half the oxic clonogenic cells would be killed with each 2 Gy radiation dose. The extended analysis showed that the radiosensitivity of groups A and B was significantly greater than for the three more resistant groups.

Initial slope and tumour cure

Cell lines in group A of Figure 17.6 have SF_2 values that average around 0.2 or less, while those in group E cluster around 0.5. Is this difference large enough to be of clinical significance? It may be, for the reasons shown in Figure 17.7. Imagine treating a tumour whose SF_2 is 0.5 with a succession of 2 Gy radiation doses. If the surviving fraction per dose remains constant, then the survival from 30 doses (i.e. 60 Gy) will be $(0.5)^{30} \approx 10^{-9}$. For an SF_2 of 0.2, the overall survival would be below 10^{-20}. Looking horizontally in the figure, an SF_2 of 0.5 requires a total dose of 60 Gy to reduce an initial number of 10^9 clonogenic cells down to one cell, whereas for an SF_2 of 0.2 this would be 25 Gy. The difference of a factor of two in these total doses is comparable with the difference in isoeffective total doses for the clinical response of most human tumours. This is a very simplistic argument, which assumes constant effect per fraction and ignores the effects of tumour hypoxia; what it indicates is that the steepness of the initial slope could be an important determinant of the success of multifraction irradiation.

Cell survival curves for human tumour cells

The survival curves shown in Figure 17.8A illustrate the range of radiosensitivity commonly found among

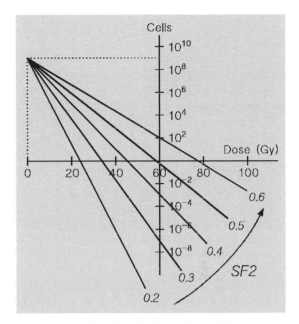

Figure 17.7 *Effect of multiple fractions of 2 Gy given to tumours whose SF_2 values range from 0.2 to 0.6. The full lines show the survival of an original 10^9 clonogenic cells during exposure to a sequence of 2 Gy doses.*

human tumour cell lines. The doses that correspond to a survival of 10^{-2} differ by approximately a factor of three. At low dose rate (panel B) the curves fan out and become straighter (see Section 18.3); these curves tend to extrapolate the initial slopes of the high-dose-rate survival curves. The full lines in Figure 17.8A are linear-quadratic (LQ) curves fitted to the data. With these and other data sets, the fit is good: there is a clear initial slope and the data are consistent with a continuously bending curve.

Since there may be a subcellular basis for regarding the separate terms of the LQ equation as mechanistically different (see Sections 7.5 and 7.6) it is interesting to examine their relative contributions to cell killing. We may separate them thus:

Linear or alpha component = $\exp(-\alpha d)$

Quadratic or beta component = $\exp(-\beta d^2)$

Having fitted the data with the LQ equation, as shown in Figure 17.8A, we know the values for α and β, and for any chosen dose we can calculate these components. This has been done in Figure 17.9 for 17 human tumour cell lines (Steel and Peacock, 1989). The chosen dose is 2 Gy, a typical dose per fraction in

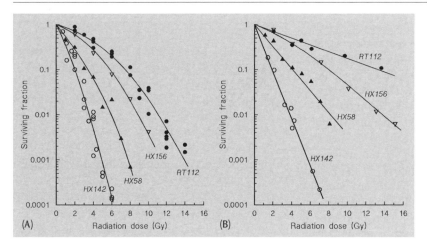

Figure 17.8 *Cell survival curves for four representative human tumour cell lines irradiated (A) at high dose rate, 150 cGy min^{-1}; or (B) at low dose rate, 1.6 cGy min^{-1}. HX142, neuroblastoma; HX58, pancreas; HX156, cervix; RT112, bladder carcinoma. From Steel (1991), with permission.*

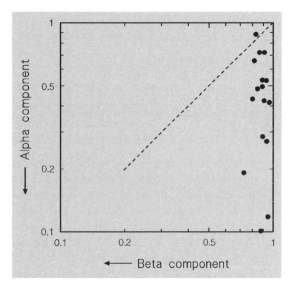

Figure 17.9 *Contributions to the surviving fraction at 2 Gy from the linear and quadratic components of radiation cell killing, for 17 human tumour cell lines. From Steel and Peacock (1989), with permission.*

realistic doses is dominated by the steepness of the linear component. The nature of this linear component is therefore a matter of considerable interest. One view is that it may be the result of DNA damage due to clusters of ionization events at the end of electron tracks, as illustrated in Figure 8.1.

How can we obtain an accurate measurement of the linear component of cell killing? By fitting the LQ model to a survival curve, it is possible to derive estimates of α and β but these are often not very accurate: 'trade-off' between α and β allows a range of combinations of the two parameters to fit the data almost equally well. A useful alternative is to use low-dose-rate irradiation. As indicated in Section 18.3, the cell survival curve at low dose rate seems to extrapolate the initial slope of the high-dose-rate curve. Furthermore, fitting data obtained at a variety of dose rates using the LPL model allows an estimate of the limiting slope at infinitely low dose rate (e.g. line B in Figure 18.2). This is the survival curve under conditions of full repair and is a useful indication of the linear component of cell killing (Steel, 1991).

clinical radiotherapy. It can be seen that the calculated points lie down the right-hand border of this diagram: the dispersion in radiosensitivity among these cell lines at 2 Gy is entirely due to differences in the steepness of the *linear component* of cell killing. The small amounts of cell kill due to the beta component (distance of the points from the right-hand boundary) do not seem to correlate with sensitivity.

The conclusion is one that derives from most of the models of radiation cell killing: cell killing at clinically

KEY POINTS

1. Growth delay, tumour control, and clonogenic cell survival are the principal experimental end-points for tumour response.
2. Human tumours differ in radiocurability and the initial slope of the cell survival curve for oxic tumour cells is one of the underlying factors.

3. In addition to the reduction in survival of clonogenic cells, tumour response is also influenced by stromal damage and factors that determine repopulation rate.
4. Cell survival curves for human tumour cells are well fitted by the linear-quadratic equation. Survival at radiation doses up to around 2 Gy is dominated by the linear term in this equation.

BIBLIOGRAPHY

Begg AC, Terry NHA (1985). Stromal radiosensitivity: influence of tumour type on the tumour bed effect assay. *Br J Radiol* **58**: 93–6.

Deacon J, Peckham MJ, Steel GG (1984). The radioresponsiveness of human tumours and the initial slope of the cell survival curve. *Radiother Oncol* **2**: 317–23.

Durand RE, Sutherland RM (1973). Dependence of the radiation response of an *in vitro* tumor model on cell cycle effects. *Cancer Res* **33**: 213–19.

Fertil B, Malaise EP (1981). Inherent radiosensitivity as a basic concept for human tumor radiotherapy. *Int J Radiat Oncol Biol Phys* **7**: 621–9.

Fowler JF, Sheldon PW, Denekamp J, Field SB (1976). Optimum fractionation of the C3H mouse mammary carcinoma using X-rays, misonidazole or neutrons. *Int J Radiat Oncol Biol Phys* **1**: 579–92.

Freshney RI (1987). *Culture of Animal Cells*. Liss, New York.

Hermens AF, Barendsen GW (1969). Changes of cell proliferation characteristics in a rat rhabdomyosarcoma before and after X-irradiation. *Eur J Cancer* **5**: 173–89.

Kallman RF (1987). *Rodent Tumor Models*. Pergamon, New York.

Kopper L, Steel GG (1975). The therapeutic response of three human tumour lines maintained in immune-suppressed mice. *Cancer Res* **35**: 2704–13.

Okunieff P, Morgan D, Niemierko A, Suit HD (1995). Radiation dose–response of human tumours. *Int J Radiat Oncol Biol Phys* **32**: 1227–37.

Rubin P, Keller B, Quick R (1974). The range of prescribed tumour lethal doses in the treatment of different human tumors. In: *The Biological and Clinical Basis of Radiosensitivity* (ed. Friedman M), pp. 435–84. Charles C Thomas, Springfield, IL.

Scott OCA (1991). Tumour transplantation and tumor immunity: a personal view. *Cancer Res* **51**: 757–63.

Sparrow S (1980). *Immunodeficient Animals for Cancer Research*. Macmillan, London.

Stanley JA, Shipley WU, Steel GG (1977). Influence of tumour size on a hypoxic fraction and therapeutic sensitivity of Lewis lung tumour. *Br J Cancer* **36**: 105–13.

Steel GG (1991). Cellular sensitivity to low dose-rate irradiation focuses the problem of tumour radioresistance. *Radiother Oncol* **20**: 71–83.

Steel GG, Peacock JH (1989). Why are some human tumours more radiosensitive than others? *Radiother Oncol* **15**: 63–72.

Steel GG, Courtenay VD, Peckham MJ (1983). The response to chemotherapy of a variety of human tumour xenografts. *Br J Cancer* **47**: 1–13.

Stephens TC, Currie GA, Peacock JM (1978). Repopulation of gamma-irradiated Lewis lung carcinoma by malignant cells and host macrophage 1 precursors. *Br J Cancer* **38**: 573–82.

Suit HD, Maeda M (1967). Hyperbaric oxygen and radiobiology of a C3H mouse mammary carcinoma. *J Natl Cancer Inst* **39**: 639–52.

Suit HD, Shalek RJ, Wette R (1965). Radiation response of C3H mouse mammary carcinoma evaluated in terms of radiation sensitivity. In: *Cellular Radiation Biology*. Williams & Wilkins, Baltimore.

Suit HD, Skates S, Taghian A *et al.* (1992). Clinical implications of heterogeneity of tumor response to radiotherapy. *Radiother Oncol* **25**: 251–60.

18

The dose rate effect: brachytherapy and targeted radiotherapy[1]

G GORDON STEEL

18.1 INTRODUCTION

There are two principal situations where low-dose-rate radiotherapy is used in cancer treatment. Irradiation using implanted solid radioactive sources (i.e. brachytherapy) is widely performed, either by implantation into tumour tissues or by intracavitary insertions. Irradiation of tumours using blood-borne radioactive materials (i.e. targeted radiotherapy) has been extensively researched and, although at the present time its efficacy is not remarkable, it still offers hope for the future.

18.2 MECHANISMS UNDERLYING THE DOSE RATE EFFECT

The dose rates used for most radiobiological studies on cells and tissues tend to be in the range 1–5 Gy min^{-1},

---

[1]Part of the text of this chapter incorporates material from Chapter 24 of the second edition of this book, written by the late Dr Tom Wheldon.

as are dose rates used clinically for external-beam radiotherapy. Exposure times for a dose of, say, 2 Gy are therefore no more than a couple of minutes. Within this time, the initial *chemical* (i.e. free radical) processes that are generated by radiation can take place but such times are not long enough for the repair of DNA damage or for any other *biological* processes to occur (see Section 1.3). As dose rate is lowered, the time taken to deliver a particular radiation dose increases; it then becomes possible for a number of biological processes to take place during irradiation and to modify the observed radiation response. These processes are best described by the *4 Rs of Radiobiology:* recovery (or repair), reassortment, repopulation, and reoxygenation (see Section 6.9).

Figure 18.1 illustrates the operation of these processes in producing the dose rate effect. The range of dose rates over which each has an effect depends upon its speed. Repair is the fastest of these processes (half-time $\sim$1 hour) and when the exposure duration is of the order of 1 hour considerable repair will take place. Calculations show that repair at this speed will modify radiation effects over the dose rate range from around 1 Gy min^{-1} down to $\sim$0.1 cGy min^{-1}

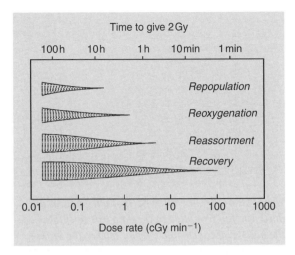

Figure 18.1 *The range of dose rates over which repair, reassortment, reoxygenation and repopulation modify radiosensitivity depends upon the speed of these processes. From Steel* et al. *(1986), with permission.*

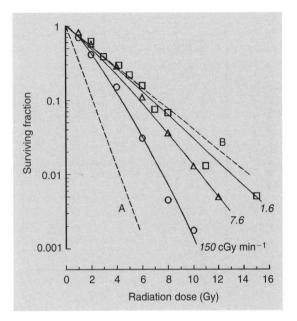

Figure 18.2 *Cell survival curves for a human melanoma cell line irradiated at dose rates of 150, 7.6 or 1.6 cGy min^{-1}. The data are fitted by the LPL model, from which the lines A and B are derived (see text). From Steel* et al. *(1987), with permission.*

(see Figures 18.4, 18.6). Even in the range of clinical external-beam dose rates, small effects on tolerance may arise from changes in dose rate. By contrast, repopulation is a much slower process. Doubling times for repopulation in human tumours or normal tissues cannot be less than 1 day; the range is probably very wide, from a few days to weeks (see Sections 2.7 and 22.4). Only when the exposure duration becomes a significant fraction of a day will significant repopulation occur during a single radiation exposure. Repopulation, either in tumours or normal tissues, will therefore influence cellular response over a much lower range of dose rates, below, say, 2 cGy min^{-1}, depending upon the cell proliferation rate. Reassortment (i.e. cell-cycle progression) will modify response over an intermediate range of dose rates, as will reoxygenation in tumours. The kinetics of reoxygenation are variable among tumour types and poorly understood; this could, nevertheless, be a significant factor reducing the effectiveness of brachytherapy given over a short overall time.

18.3 DOSE RATE EFFECT ON CELL SURVIVAL

As radiation dose rate is lowered in the range 1 Gy min^{-1} down to 1 cGy min^{-1}, the radiosensitivity of cells decreases and the shouldered cell survival curves observed at high dose rate gradually become straighter. This is illustrated in Figure 18.2. At 150 cGy min^{-1} the survival curve has a marked curvature; at 1.6 cGy min^{-1} it is almost straight (on the semi-log plot) and seems to extrapolate the initial slope of the high-dose-rate curve. The amount of sparing associated with the dose rate reduction can be expressed by reading off the radiation doses that give a surviving fraction of, say, 0.01: these values are 7.7 Gy at 150 cGy min^{-1} and 12.8 Gy at 1.6 cGy min^{-1}. The ratio of these doses (12.8/7.7 = 1.6) has been called the dose recovery factor (DRF). The data at all three dose rates in Figure 18.2 have been simultaneously fitted by the LPL model (see Section 7.6), a model that is particularly useful for simulating the dose rate effect. This allows an estimate to be made of the half-time for cellular recovery (0.16 hour) and it also predicts survival under conditions of no repair (line A) or full repair (line B). Three further examples of low-dose-rate survival curves in human tumour cell lines are shown in Figure 18.3: they well illustrate the linearity of low-dose-rate survival curves.

For four selected human tumour cell lines, Figure 17.8 shows the survival curves at these two dose rates

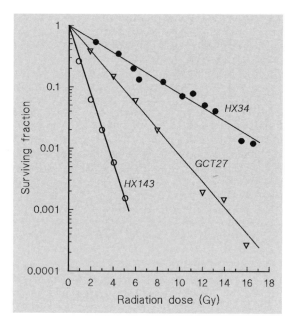

Figure 18.3 *Cell survival curves for three human tumour cell lines irradiated at the low dose rate of 1.6 cGy min⁻¹. HX143, neuroblastoma; GCT27, germ-cell tumour of the testis; HX34, melanoma. From Steel (1991), with permission.*

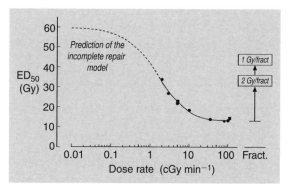

Figure 18.4 *The dose rate effect for pneumonitis in mice. The full line fitted to the data was calculated on the basis of the incomplete repair model; the broken line shows its extrapolation to very low dose rates. The boxes on the right show the ED_{50} values for fractionated irradiation. From Down et al. (1986), with permission.*

(150 and 1.6 cGy min⁻¹). These four sets of data have been chosen to illustrate the dose rate effect and the range of radiosensitivities seen among human tumour cells (Steel *et al.*, 1987). At high dose rate, there is a range of approximately 3 in the radiation dose that gives a survival of 0.01. At low dose rate, the curves fan out and become straight or nearly so: the range of $D_{0.01}$ values is now roughly 7. This illustrates an important characteristic of low-dose-rate irradiation: it discriminates better than high dose rate between cell lines of differing radiosensitivity.

18.4 DOSE RATE EFFECT IN NORMAL TISSUES

Most normal tissues show considerable sparing as dose rate is reduced. An example is shown in Figure 18.4. The thorax of conscious mice was irradiated with ⁶⁰Co γ-rays and damage to the lung was measured using a breathing-rate assay (Down *et al.*, 1986). The radiation dose that produced acute pneumonitis in 50% of the mice (i.e. the ED_{50}) was 13.3 Gy at 100 cGy min⁻¹ but it increased to 34.2 Gy at the lowest

dose rate of 2 cGy min⁻¹ (DRF = 2.6). Note that a similar degree of sparing could be achieved (in studies of other investigators) by fractionated high-dose-rate irradiation using 2 Gy per fraction, and even more sparing at 1 Gy per fraction. Note also that at 2 cGy min⁻¹ the curve is still rising rapidly. It was not possible in these experiments to go down to dose rates below 2 cGy min⁻¹ because of the difficulty of immobilizing the mice for long periods of time.

The data in Figure 18.4 have been fitted by the incomplete repair model (Thames, 1985; see Section 12.8). This model simulates the effect of recovery on tissue sensitivity; it does not take account of cell proliferation during irradiation. The model fits the data well and it also allows extrapolation down to low dose rates. It predicts, in this example, that dose sparing due to recovery will continue to increase down to about 0.01 cGy min⁻¹ at which the ED_{50} is 59 Gy and the recovery factor (i.e. DRF value) is 4.4. Proliferation of stem cells in the lung will lead to even greater sparing at very low dose rates.

The comparison between a single low-dose-rate exposure (2 cGy min⁻¹) and fractionated high-dose-rate irradiation (2 Gy per fraction) allows an important conclusion to be drawn. If the fractions are delivered once per day, then the overall time to deliver an ED_{50} dose of 34 Gy is 17 days. The same effect is produced by a single low-dose-rate treatment in 28 hours. *Continuous low-dose-rate exposure is thus the most efficient way of allowing maximum tissue recovery in the shortest overall time.* It minimizes the effects of

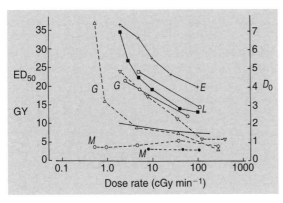

Figure 18.5 *The dose rate effect in normal tissues of the mouse: L, lung; G, gut; E, epilation; M, bone marrow. Full lines refer to left-hand scale, dashed lines to right-hand scale. See Steel* et al. *(1986) for sources.*

proliferation, which is an advantage in terms of damage to tumour cells but a disadvantage for the tolerance of early-responding normal tissues.

Figure 18.5 shows similar data from a number of other studies of the dose rate effect on normal tissues in mice. Considerable sparing of the intestine is observed, especially below 1 cGy min^{-1}, where proliferation has a marked effect. By contrast, there is little or no sparing of haemopoietic tissues. The dose rate effect on mouse lethality (LD$_{50}$, indicated in Figure 18.5 by the full line without points) is comparatively slight, probably because this is predominantly due to damage to bone marrow, no doubt also with a component of damage to the intestine.

18.5 ISOEFFECT RELATIONSHIPS BETWEEN FRACTIONATED AND CONTINUOUS LOW-DOSE-RATE IRRADIATION

A variety of theoretical descriptions of the dose rate effect have been made but for clinical application the most widely used is the incomplete repair model of Thames (1985). The calculations of Dale (1985, 1989) make the same basic assumptions, although the formulation is slightly different. The basic equation of the incomplete repair model for continuous irradiation is:

$$E = \alpha D + \beta D^2 g \qquad (18.1)$$

where E is the level of effect, α and β are parameters of the linear-quadratic (LQ) equation, D is the total

dose, and g is a function of time (both of the time between fractions and the duration of continuous exposure). Note that the time-dependent recovery factor modifies only the quadratic term in the LQ equation, a feature that is supported by experimental data (Wells and Bedford, 1983; Steel *et al.*, 1987; Figure 18.2). Note also that repopulation is ignored in these calculations.

The value of g depends upon the half-time for recovery ($T_{1/2}$) and the duration of exposure (t) according to the relation:

$$g = 2\,[\mu t - 1 + \exp(-\mu t)]/(\mu t)^2 \qquad (18.2)$$

where $\mu = 0.693/T_{1/2}$ (Thames, 1985; see Table 12.3). This model allows isoeffect relationships to be calculated and, as shown in Figure 18.4, it is successful in fitting experimental data over a range of dose rates. Further examples of calculated curves are shown in Figure 18.6. Panel A shows the fractionated case (see Section 12.8). The line in this chart corresponds to Equation 12.5, as shown in Figure 12.7. The interfraction intervals have here been assumed to be long enough to allow complete recovery between fractions, although the model can handle shorter intervals. Panel B in Figure 18.6 shows isoeffect curves for a single continuous exposure at any dose rate, on the assumption that the half-time for recovery is 1.0, 1.5 or 2.0 hours. The three curves are slightly different and this illustrates the dependence of the isoeffect curve for continuous exposure on the speed of recovery: the curve shifts laterally to lower dose rates as the half-time is prolonged. Unfortunately, recovery half-time is seldom known in clinical situations, which limits the value of calculations of this sort.

The curves in the panels of Figure 18.6 are *mutually isoeffective*. They are calculated for the same effect level and for the same values of α and β (the α/β ratio is 10 Gy), chosen to give an extrapolated dose of 72 Gy at infinitely small dose per fraction or infinitely low dose rate. This example illustrates the equivalence that is predicted by the mathematical models between a particular continuous dose rate and a corresponding dose per fraction. For the parameters assumed here (as shown by the vertical arrows), a dose rate of around 1–2 cGy min^{-1} (roughly 1 Gy h^{-1}) is equivalent to fractionated treatment with approximately 2 Gy per fraction, for both of which the isoeffective dose is 60 Gy.

A further important conclusion can be drawn from calculations of the type shown in Figure 18.6.

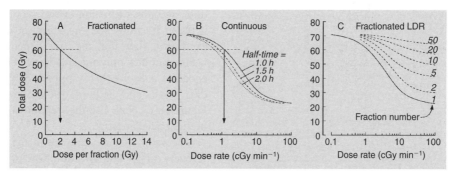

Figure 18.6 *Isoeffect curves calculated on the incomplete repair model (Thames, 1985) for fractionated, continuous, or fractionated low-dose-rate radiation exposure (the three panels are mutually isoeffective). Repopulation is ignored. The α/β ratio is 10 Gy and the extrapolated response dose (BED) is 72 Gy. Adapted from Steel (1991) and Steel et al. (1989), with permission.*

In Sections 12.6 and 14.3 (see Figure 12.7) we have seen how the use of large fraction sizes leads to a therapeutic disadvantage. The same is true for high continuous dose-rate treatments. By drawing further horizontal lines between panels A and B in Figure 18.6 it can be seen that a dose rate of $5\,\text{cGy}\,\text{min}^{-1}$ is equivalent to around 6–8 Gy per fraction and $10\,\text{cGy}\,\text{min}^{-1}$ to over 10 Gy per fraction.

Figure 18.6C shows the results of model calculations for *fractionated low-dose-rate irradiation*. Once again, using the incomplete repair model, we have calculated isoeffect curves for treatment with 2–50 fractions, each given at the dose rate shown on the abscissa and with full recovery between fractions. Again, repopulation is ignored. This diagram indicates the basic feature of fractionated low-dose-rate exposure: as the number of fractions is increased, the dose rate effect is reduced (i.e. the curves become flatter), and as the dose rate is lowered, the effect of fractionation is reduced (as seen by the vertical spread between the curves). This results from a simple principle. As irradiation is protracted, it is cellular recovery that produces all these effects and there is a limit to how much recovery the cells can accomplish. If recovery between fractions is allowed, then there is less to be recovered *during* each fraction, and *vice versa*.

An alternative approach to the description of the dose rate effect is the lethal, potentially lethal (LPL) model of Curtis (1986). This is a mechanistic model that is described in Section 7.6. It has theoretical advantages for studies that seek to describe the cellular mechanisms of radiation cell killing but is less appropriate for clinical calculations than the empirical equations of Thames and Dale referred to above.

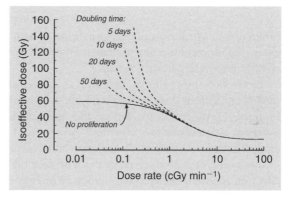

Figure 18.7 *Illustrating the effect of cell proliferation as a function of dose rate. Isoeffect curves are shown for no proliferation or with the doubling times indicated. The calculations are based on a simple model of exponential growth, ignoring radiation effects on the rate of cell proliferation.*

Effect of cell proliferation

The effect of proliferation at very low dose rates is graphically illustrated in Figure 18.7. These calculations are made for a hypothetical cell population with an α/β ratio of 3.7 Gy and a repair half-time of 0.85 hour. Cell proliferation is assumed to occur with the doubling times shown in the figure and no account has been taken of radiation effects on the rate of proliferation (if this occurred it would reduce the effect of proliferation at the higher dose rates). For these parameter values there is no effect of proliferation at dose rates above $1\,\text{cGy}\,\text{min}^{-1}$ but as the dose rate is lowered to $0.1\,\text{cGy}\,\text{min}^{-1}$ the isoeffective dose rises very steeply. The implication for brachy-therapy is that above 1 cGy min^{-1} repopulation effects can be ignored, but below this dose rate they will be substantial, both in tumours and in early-responding normal tissues.

The inverse dose rate effect

Although in situations affecting clinical practice it is a general rule that cellular sensitivity decreases with decreasing dose rate, exceptions to this rule have been noted. Mitchell and Bedford in early studies of cell killing in mammalian cell lines occasionally found a slight inversion which they attributed to a lower dose rate allowing cells to progress though the cell cycle into more sensitive phases, thus suffering greater damage. In studies of oncogenic transform-ation by high-LET radiations, the existence of an inverse dose rate effect is well recognized.

18.6   RADIOBIOLOGICAL ASPECTS OF BRACHYTHERAPY

The principal reasons for choosing interstitial or intracavitary radiotherapy in preference to external-beam treatment relate to dose delivery and dose distribution rather than to radiobiology. Irradiation from an implanted source within a tumour carries a distinct geometrical advantage for sparing the sur-rounding normal tissues that will inevitably tend to receive a lower radiation dose. Brachytherapy thus exploits the volume effect in normal tissues (see Chapter 5). Normal tissues will also often be exposed to a lower dose rate, which gives the additional advan-tage of 'negative double trouble' (see Section 13.10).

Variation in cell killing around an implanted radioactive source

The non-uniformity of the radiation field around an implanted source has important radiobiological con-sequences. Close to the source the dose rate is high and the amount of cell killing will be close to that indicated by the acute-radiation survival curve. As we move away from the source, two changes take place: cells will be less sensitive at the lower dose rates, and within a given period of implantation the accumulated

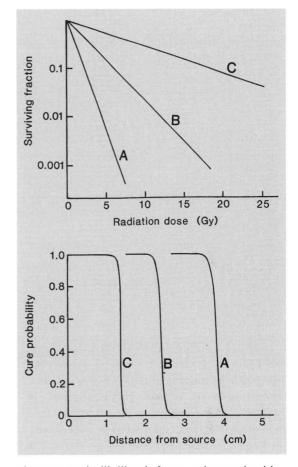

Figure 18.8 *The likelihood of cure varies steeply with distance from a point radiation source. The radius at which failure occurs depends upon the steepness of the survival curve at low dose rate (upper panel). From Steel* et al. *(1989), with permission.*

dose will also be less. These two factors lead to a very rapid change in cell killing with distance from the source. Within tissues (tumour or normal) that are close to the source the level of cell killing will be so high that cells of any radiosensitivity will be killed. Further out, the effects will be so low that even the most radiosensitive cells will survive. Between these extremes there is a critical zone in which differential cell killing will occur. As shown by Steel *et al.* (1989), for cells of any given level of radiosensitivity, model calculations imply that there will be cliff-like change from high to low local cure probability, taking place over a radial distance of a few millimetres (Figure 18.8). The distance of the cliff from the source is deter-mined by the radiosensitivity of the cells at low dose

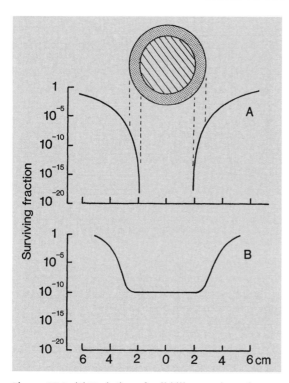

Figure 18.9 *(A) Variation of cell kill around a point source of radiation. The source gives 0.87 Gy min⁻¹ at 2 cm (i.e. 75 Gy in 6 days); there are 10⁹ cells per cm³, for which $\alpha = 0.35\,Gy^{-1}$, $\beta = 0.035\,Gy^{-2}$, half-time for recovery is 1 hour (Steel et al., 1989). The hatched area indicates the volume within which the surviving fraction is below 10^{-20}. The stippled area indicates the volume where survival is between 10^{-20} and 10^{-6}, which is the critical region for tumour control. For comparison, panel B shows the type of profile that would be aimed for with external-beam radiotherapy.*

rate, nearer for radioresistant cells and further away for radiosensitive cells (Steel, 1991). There would appear to be a strong case for introducing a predictive test of tumour cell radiosensitivity (see Section 22.2) into brachytherapy practice. If the dose distribution or the total dose administered could be adjusted on this basis a therapeutic gain might be achieved.

Figure 18.9 contrasts this situation with external-beam radiotherapy where the aim is usually to deliver uniform radiation dose across the tumour. Only in a narrow zone around an implanted source (where the surviving fraction changes from, say, 10^{-20} to 10^{-6}) will radiobiological considerations be of interest or importance in relation to tumour control. The same principle will apply to normal-tissue damage: serious

damage to normal structures depends on making sure that they are outside the corresponding 'cliff'.

Is there a radiobiological advantage in low-dose-rate radiotherapy?

The question of whether low-dose-rate irradiation itself carries a therapeutic advantage is an interesting one. There is a considerable volume of literature on the dose rate effect, both in tumours and in normal tissues, on the basis of which it would be difficult to claim that under all circumstances low-dose-rate treatment would have the best therapeutic index. As shown in Figure 17.8, cells that are the least sensitive to radiation and have the largest shoulder on the cell survival curve will show the greatest degree of dose sparing. These are not necessarily cell lines of low α/β ratio, for Peacock et al. (1992) have shown that a range of human tumour cell lines, including those shown in Figure 17.8, have similar α/β ratios: radioresistant tumour cells tend to have both a lower α *and* a lower β than more sensitive cells. In a particular therapeutic situation we could make a calculation comparing the relative DRFs between tumour and critical normal tissues. This would tell us whether the normal tissues might be spared more or less than the tumour cells if we were to lower the dose rate. But this does not answer the therapeutic question because to treat with one large high-dose-rate fraction is not normally a clinical option. In fact, we know from clinical experience in the early history of radiotherapy that large high-dose-rate treatments are bad and that changing to a single low-dose-rate exposure would be better. This is similar to comparing hypofractionation with the use of conventional or reduced dose per fraction (see Figure 14.2). The appropriate clinical question is whether a single continuous low-dose-rate treatment is better than using a conventional fractionation schedule.

As is illustrated in Figure 18.6, there is, on the basis of the incomplete repair model, an equivalence between dose per fraction in fractionated radiotherapy and dose rate for a single continuous exposure. Roughly speaking, for a given level of cell killing, the total dose required at a continuous dose rate of $1\,Gy\,h^{-1}$ is the same as that required by fractionated treatment with 2 Gy per fraction. This equivalence depends upon the half-time for recovery but it is relatively independent of the α/β ratio (Fowler, 1989). In radiobiological terms, these two treatments should be equally effective. Lowering the (fractionated) dose per fraction will spare late-responding normal tissues whose α/β ratio is low, as also will lowering the dose rate (continuous) below $1\,\mathrm{Gy\,h^{-1}}$.

The success of intracavitary therapy may result from two factors:

1. the lower volume of normal tissue irradiated to a dose that discriminates between tissue sensitivities (i.e. the annular region in Figure 18.9); and
2. the practical and radiobiological benefits of short treatment times. The clearest advantage for low-dose-rate irradiation is that for a given level of cell killing, and without hazarding late-responding normal tissues, this treatment will be complete within the *shortest overall time* (Section 18.4). Tumour cell repopulation will therefore be minimized. This could confer a therapeutic advantage for the treatment of rapidly repopulating tumours.

A potential *disadvantage* of low-dose-rate irradiation is that because of the short overall treatment time there may be inadequate time available for the reoxygenation of hypoxic tumour cells and therefore greater radioresistance due to hypoxia.

Pulsed brachytherapy

The availability of computer-controlled high-dose-rate afterloading systems provides the opportunity to deliver interstitial or intracavitary radiotherapy in a series of pulses. The gaps between pulses allow greater freedom for the patient, increased safety for nursing staff, as well as technical advantages, for instance in allowing corrections for the decay of the radioactive source that minimize effects on the quality of treatment. During the past few years there has been a surge of interest in pulsed brachytherapy, not only in radiotherapy for cancer but also in the treatment of non-neoplastic lesions in large blood vessels: vascular brachytherapy (Waksman, 2000).

In principle, any move away from continuous exposure towards treatment with gaps carries a radiobiological *disadvantage*. This is because the dose rate *within* each pulse is higher and this allows less opportunity for repair of radiation damage. Slowly repairing tissues will therefore be disadvantaged and, as argued in Section 14.7, there will be a loss of therapeutic index between tumour tissues that repair fast and those late-responding normal tissues that repair

more slowly. The magnitude of this effect was considered by Brenner and Hall (1991), who concluded that for gaps between pulses of up to 60 minutes the radiobiological deficit may be acceptable. During the ensuing years there has been much theoretical discussion of the guidelines for safe treatment with pulsed brachytherapy. There have been some attempts to obtain laboratory data that bear on this debate, and whilst this has been taking place the clinical use of pulsed treatment has continued apace. Theoretical studies have examined the effect of half-times for repair in normal and tumour tissues, including the evidence for multiple half-time components within each tissue (Fowler and Van Limbergen, 1997; Sminia *et al.*, 1998). Experimental studies in tissue culture have thrown light on the dangers of pulse times longer than 1 hour (Chen *et al.*, 1997). Brachytherapy studies on laboratory animals are technically difficult, not least because of the differences in scale between rats and humans, but detailed studies of effects in the rat spinal cord have been carried out (Pop *et al.*, 2000).

Clinical experience in the use of pulsed brachytherapy is increasing, and the availability of equipment that allows a single high-intensity source to be 'stepped' through the treatment field provides an important new degree of control. The method does, however, need to be applied with care, for there are penalties in terms of the quality of treatment when pulse sizes are allowed to be too large or when time between pulses is increased much above 1 hour. High-dose-rate afterloading systems create the temptation to shorten the overall time and, as indicated above, this could lead to increased early reactions to radiotherapy and greater tumour radioresistance due to inadequate reoxygenation. However, especially in situations where brachytherapy is used as a boost, it may well be that the very non-uniform dose distributions provide greater latitude in choice of treatment parameters than is the case with external-beam radiotherapy.

18.7 TARGETED RADIOTHERAPY

Targeted radiotherapy means the treatment of cancer by radioactive materials injected into the blood circulation and carried selectively into tumour cells by means of a suitable 'vehicle'. This has widely been perceived to be an exciting prospect, and much research effort has been (and still is) devoted to making it work. It has the potential to sterilize metastases anywhere in the body; but as with cancer chemotherapy, the key problem is *selectivity* of delivery of the toxic agent to tumour cells, coupled with the difficulty of delivering adequate amounts of radioactivity. The first clinical example of the targeted radiotherapy principle in oncology was the use of iodine-131 in the treatment of well-differentiated thyroid carcinomas; unfortunately, there are no other tumour types for which so simple a targeting agent can be used. Recent research has focused mainly on monoclonal antibodies and MIBG as targeting agents.

Monoclonal antibodies

Monoclonal antibodies target quite small molecular groups (i.e. epitopes) on the surface of cancer cells which, it is hoped, will be sufficiently different from corresponding epitopes on normal cells. Disappointingly, no really dramatic differences between normal and cancer cell surfaces have yet been found. Differences do exist, but these are usually quantitative rather than qualitative. Antibodies are large molecules that penetrate rather poorly into some tumours and there are serious problems in adequately hitting all tumour cells. Lymphoma and neuroblastoma are among the few tumour types that can be treated successfully using radiolabelled antibodies. A high-dose strategy, pioneered in Seattle, involves the administration of large activities of an ^{131}I-labelled monoclonal antibody which has moderate selectivity for B-lineage lymphocytes or lymphoma cells. The doses given are ablative and bone marrow rescue is required. This approach has given encouraging results in treating B-cell lymphoma patients in terms of long-duration remissions and possible cures (Press *et al.*, 1993). However, the high activities of ^{131}I present logistical difficulties in relation to radiation protection. Recent reviews of radioimmunotherapy for lymphomas and other diseases reflect considerable technical ingenuity but slow progress in achieving improved clinical results (Buchsbaum *et al.*, 1999; Press, 1999; Mendelsohn, 2000).

Molecular precursors of tumour-associated proteins

The catecholamine precursor analogue meta-iodobenzylguanidine (MIBG) is preferentially taken up by certain tumour types such as neuroblastoma and phaeochromocytoma. MIBG uptake requires active transport and occurs only in metabolically competent cells. Clinical studies using single-agent [^{131}I] MIBG have achieved promising responses (Lashford *et al.*, 1992), especially when this treatment is given at first presentation (de Kraker *et al.*, 1995), and this is currently one of the most successful forms of targeted radiotherapy. Heterogeneity of isotope uptake among tumour cells is a key problem and microdosimetric rationales described below suggest that [^{131}I] MIBG should be given as part of a combined modality regimen (Gaze and Wheldon, 1996) or, more speculatively, together with gene therapy (Mairs *et al.*, 2000).

18.8 RADIONUCLIDES FOR TARGETED THERAPY

The important considerations in choosing a radionuclide include the radiobiological characteristics of the particle emission (e.g. its RBE), its energy and mean range, its physical half-life and the ease and feasibility of conjugating it to appropriate targeting agents. Table 18.1 summarizes some properties of radionuclides of current interest. They may be divided into long-range β-emitters, short-range β-emitters and emitters of α-particles and Auger electrons of still shorter range. Clinical experience so far has been confined to the long-range β-emitters (^{131}I and ^{90}Y). Ultra-short-range Auger electrons are capable of direct cell kill only when incorporated into DNA itself. Physical half-lives of a few days, comparable with the biological half-lives of most vehicles, are thought to be ideal. Very short half-lives (as with the α-emitters ^{211}At and ^{212}Bi) may present considerable logistical difficulties. Chemical conjugation to carrier molecules is relatively easy for the halogens (F, Br, I, At) and becomes progressively more difficult with radiometals, which tend to detach from the carrier molecule. Work is now in progress to find new ways to bind radiometals more firmly and it is possible that these compounds will further extend the list of usable radionuclides.

Long-range β-emitters have the property of irradiating untargeted cells by cross-fire from adjacent targeted cells. This may be advantageous when tumour heterogeneity leads to non-uniformity of dose delivery, but it has the disadvantage that adjacent normal tissues may also be irradiated. A review of radionuclides and carrier molecules for therapy was published by Zweit (1996).

18.9   RADIATION DOSIMETRY

In contrast to external-beam irradiation, for which dosimetry is a precise science, the dosimetry of radiation delivered by radionuclides involves considerable uncertainties. At present, doses both to tumour and normal tissues can only be estimated approximately. Uncertainties arise from the non-uniformity of radionuclide distribution, its changing pattern with time, and its dependence on individual patient pharmacokinetics. The usual approach to dose estimation is to employ the MIRD Schema, a set of data published by the US Nuclear Medicine Society which provides tables of estimated absorbed doses in various tissues as a function of the radionuclide distribution and its variation with time.

Vaughan *et al.* (1987) collated published data on the uptake of radiolabelled antibodies into human tumours and on the kinetics of antibody clearance. They observed for systemically injected radioactivity that a tumour uptake of 0.0005% per gram of tumour was typical, and that the concentration of bound antibody usually declined exponentially with a half-life of 2–3 days. These authors then used these parameters in a dosimetric model to calculate the doses that could be delivered to tumours by monoclonal antibody-targeted ^{131}I or ^{90}Y. They concluded that if the total whole-body radiation dose had to be limited to around 2 Gy (in the absence of bone marrow rescue), then it would not be possible to deliver a curative dose (say of 60 Gy) to macroscopic solid tumours. To achieve such a dose, better targeting agents would be needed, or targeted therapy would have to be given by some strategy that was more effective in terms of therapeutic differential than simply injecting radiolabelled antibodies into the bloodstream.

Microdosimetry and radiocurability

A major difference between external-beam and radionuclide-targeted irradiation relates to microdosimetry, especially the absorption of radiation dose in small tumours where dimensions are less than the mean path length of the particles emitted by the

radionuclide (Table 18.1). In the case of ^{131}I, microdosimetric problems arise in tumours whose diameter is less than 1–2 mm. If such microtumours have radionuclide atoms uniformly distributed throughout their volume, the absorption of the emitted energy will be relatively inefficient, for a substantial proportion of nuclear particles will escape into the surrounding tissues (Figure 18.10). Microdosimetric calculations by Humm (1986) have provided estimates of the fraction of emitted energy that would be absorbed by a spherical microtumour as a function of its diameter, for several different radionuclides. Although the smaller microtumours absorb less dose, they also contain fewer clonogenic cells and therefore less dose is needed to sterilize them. These factors result in a relationship between tumour curability and tumour size that is more complex for targeted radiotherapy than for

Table 18.1 *Properties of radionuclides of current interest in targeted therapy*

Radionuclide	Half-life	Emission	Mean particle range
^{90}Y	2.7 days	β	5 mm
^{131}I	8 days	β	0.8 mm
^{67}Cu	2.5 days	β	0.6 mm
^{199}Au	3.1 days	β	0.3 mm
^{211}At	7 hours	α	0.05 mm
^{212}Bi	1 hour	α	0.05 mm
^{125}I	60 days	Auger	~1 μm
^{77}Br	2.4 days	Auger	~1 μm

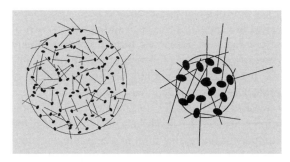

Figure 18.10 *The proportion of energy deposited outside a radiolabelled metastasis becomes considerable when its diameter is comparable with the mean range of the emitted radiation. On the left is a large lesion, on the right a small one. The particle range is considered constant. Reproduced with permission of Dr J.A. O'Donoghue.*

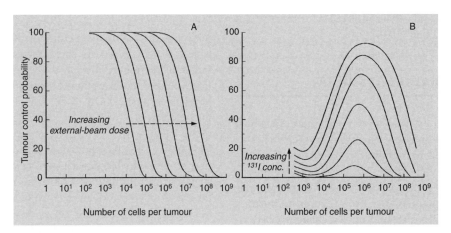

Figure 18.11 *Relationship between tumour cure probability and tumour size: for external-beam irradiation at six different dose levels (left panel) and for spherical tumours labelled uniformly with various ^{131}I concentrations (right panel). The tumour size for maximum cure rate is a property of the isotope (Table 18.2) but is independent of dose.*

Table 18.2 *Tumour size for optimal radiocurability by uniformly targeted radionuclides*

Radionuclide	Optimal tumour diameter	Equivalent cell number
^{90}Y	~2 cm	~10^{10}
^{131}I	~2 mm	~10^6
^{211}At	~60 μm	~10
^{125}I (Auger component)	~1 μm	~1

external-beam irradiation. With conventional radiotherapy, it is well known that the larger a tumour, the lower will be the chance of its being sterilized by any given dose of radiation (see Section 17.4). This is illustrated in Figure 18.11A which shows how at each of several radiation dose levels, tumour cure probability decreases steadily as a function of increasing tumour size. In contrast, Figure 18.11B shows how tumour cure probability is expected to change with tumour size for several activity levels of ^{131}I. Unlike the external irradiation situation, the family of curves shows a rising component (increasing tumour size leading to more efficient absorption of emitted energy), a peak value, and a falling component where the increasing number of cells to be sterilized dominates the response. As a result, for each radionuclide there is an optimal tumour diameter for radiocurability (Table 18.2): both smaller and larger tumours will be less radiocurable than those at the optimal size. The lower radiocurability of very small micrometastases is a

unique feature of radionuclide therapy and is one of the reasons why the combination of targeted radiotherapy with external-beam irradiation may be an effective strategy (Wheldon and O'Donoghue, 1990).

18.10 RADIOBIOLOGICAL FACTORS IN TARGETED RADIOTHERAPY

Targeted radiotherapy is given at a low and exponentially declining dose rate (Dale, 1996). As indicated in Sections 18.2 and 18.3, this means that most radiation damage will be repaired during targeted irradiation, and cell survival curves will be virtually straight. Tumours with a low α/β ratio will have shallow survival curves at these dose rates (see the data for HX34 in Figure 18.3) and will be poorly responsive. It is unlikely that *repopulation* will be a major factor for a treatment scheme that delivers most of the radiation dose over a few days, but as the dose rate falls, tumour cell proliferation will counteract the modest cell kill achieved by irradiation. Fowler (1990) has estimated that when the dose rate falls below 2–3 cGy h^{-1} the treatment is likely to be ineffective. Hypoxia and lack of complete reoxygenation could be a further cause of resistance, since most of the radiation dose delivered by targeted radiotherapy is usually given within a week, as a result of the biological clearance of the agent and radioactive decay. There is a need for hypoxic cell radiosensitizers or bioreductive drugs to be explored in conjunction with targeted radiotherapy in laboratory systems.

18.11 BORON NEUTRON CAPTURE THERAPY (BNCT)

This is a specialized approach to targeted therapy that has been under development for many years (Barth *et al.*, 1990). Its title is somewhat misleading in that this is not a form of neutron therapy but a way of generating α-particles within the tumour site; it is this secondary radiation that is responsible for any tumoricidal effect. The approach relies on the physical properties of the non-radioactive boron isotope ^{10}B. When exposed to 'slow' neutrons (i.e. with thermal or epithermal energies), this isotope has a large cross-section for neutron capture. A fission reaction ensues in which the boron nucleus splits into ^{7}Li plus ^{4}He, also emitting a pulse of γ-rays. The ^{4}He nucleus is an α-particle that produces a densely ionizing track over a range of a few cell diameters. In the absence of boron, fission neutrons at the intensities required for this process produce little biological damage.

BNCT is a two-step strategy: targeting of ^{10}B to tumour cells, followed by fission of the isotope by neutron irradiation (Figure 18.12). The use of an external neutron beam and the fact that ^{10}B itself is a 'cold' isotope gives the therapist more control over the process than is usual in targeted therapy. Boron may accumulate in organs other than in the tumour sites (e.g. the liver), but if these sites are known it may be possible to avoid irradiating them with neutrons. The effectiveness of this treatment requires sufficient difference in uptake between the tumour and local normal tissues. α-particle radiation is very damaging to targeted cells and even the most resistant cell types will be efficiently sterilized. Research effort is being directed at the production of filtered beams of epithermal neutrons, which have superior penetration properties compared with thermal neutrons. In Europe, this effort is concentrated at the nuclear reactor facility at Petten in The Netherlands, with the initial objective of treating intracranial disease (Hideghety *et al.*, 1999).

As with any form of targeted therapy, success depends critically on the availability of a suitable targeting agent, in this case one that will carry boron into tumour cells to a higher concentration than in local normal tissues (Barth *et al.*, 1990). Monoclonal

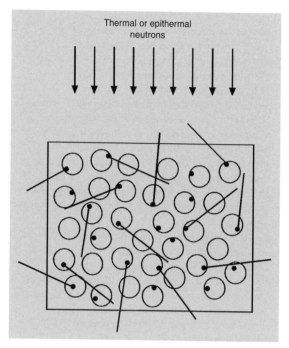

Figure 18.12 *Illustrating the local production within a small volume of tissue of isotropic α-particle radiation by neutron-induced fission of boron atoms (○, cells; ●, ^{10}B atoms; —, α-tracks).*

antibodies are an obvious candidate, but whether these are capable of carrying sufficient boron is yet to be ascertained. The use of boron-conjugated epidermal growth factor to target tumours that overexpress the EGF receptor is also being investigated. Oligonucleotides conjugated to boron are further potential candidates for exploiting specific abnormal DNA sequences in malignant tumours and these may have the advantage of requiring less boron incorporation for cell killing by BNCT. Although unique in some respects, BNCT may well be limited by factors that are common to all radioactive targeting methods. Its therapeutic effectiveness will depend on the selectivity of uptake of boron into the tumour. The α-particles generated by BNCT have a short range and the level of cell killing will depend on the homogeneity of boron uptake among tumour cells (Coderre and Morris, 1999).

BIBLIOGRAPHY

Barth RF, Soloway AH, Fairchild RG (1990). Boron neutron therapy of cancer. *Cancer Res* **50**: 1061–70.

Brenner DJ, Hall EJ (1991). Fractionated high dose rate versus low dose rate regimens for intracavitary brachytherapy of the cervix. *Br J Radiol* **64**: 133–41.

Buchsbaum DJ, Rogers BE, Khazaeli MB *et al.* (1999). Targeting strategies for cancer radiotherapy. *Clin Cancer Res* **5**: 3048s–55s.

Chen CZ, Huang Y, Hall EJ, Brenner DJ (1997). Pulsed brachytherapy as a substitute for continuous low dose rate: an *in vitro* study with human carcinoma cells. *Int J Radiat Oncol Biol Phys* **37**: 137–43.

Coderre JA, Morris GM (1999). The radiation biology of boron neutron capture therapy. *Radiat Res* **151**: 1–18.

Curtis SB (1986). Lethal and potentially lethal lesions induced by radiation – a unified repair model. *Radiat Res* **106**: 252–70.

Dale RG (1985). The application of the linear-quadratic dose-effect equation to fractionated and protracted radiotherapy. *Br J Radiol* **58**: 515–28.

Dale RG (1989). Time-dependent tumour repopulation factors in linear-quadratic equations – implications for treatment. *Radiother Oncol* **15**: 371–82.

Dale RG (1996). Dose-rate effects in targeted radiotherapy. *Phys Med Biol* **41**: 1871–84.

de Kraker J, Hoefnagel, CA, Caron H *et al.* (1995). First line targeted radiotherapy, a new concept in the treatment of advanced stage neuroblastoma. *Eur J Cancer* **31A**: 600–2.

Down JD, Easton DF, Steel GG (1986). Repair in the mouse lung during low dose-rate irradiation. *Radiother Oncol* **6**: 29–42.

Fowler JF (1989). Dose rate effects in normal tissues. In: *Brachytherapy 2* (ed. Mould RF), pp. 26–40. Proceedings of the 5th International Selectron Users' Meeting 1988. Nucletron International BV, Leersum, The Netherlands.

Fowler JF (1990). Radiobiological aspects of low dose rates in radioimmunotherapy. *Int J Radiat Oncol Biol Phys* **18**: 1261–9.

Fowler JF, Van Limbergen EF (1997). Biological effect of pulsed dose rate brachytherapy with stepping sources if short half-times of repair are present in tissues. *Int J Radiat Oncol Biol Phys* **37**: 877–83.

Gaze MN, Wheldon TE (1996). Radiolabelled MIBG in the treatment of neuroblastoma. *Eur J Cancer* **32A**: 93–6.

Hideghety K, Sauerwein W, Grochulla F *et al.* (1999). Postoperative treatment of glioblastoma with BNCT at the Petten irradiation facility. *Strahlenther Onkol* **175**(Suppl 2): 111–14.

Humm JL (1986). Dosimetric aspects of radiolabelled antibodies for tumour therapy. *J Nucl Med* **27**: 1490–7.

Lashford LS, Lewis, IJ, Fielding SL *et al.* (1992). Phase I/II study of 131-iodine metaiodobenzylguanidine in chemoresistant neuroblastoma: a United Kingdom Children's Cancer Study Group investigation. *J Clin Oncol* **10**: 1889–96.

Mairs RJ, Cunningham SH, Boyd M, Carlin S (2000). Applications of gene transfer to targeted radiotherapy. *Curr Pharm Des* **6**: 1419–32.

Mendelsohn J (2000). Jeremiah Metzger Lecture. Targeted cancer therapy. *Trans Am Clin Climatol Assoc* **111**: 95–110.

Peacock JH, Eady JJ, Edwards SM *et al.* (1992). The intrinsic α/β ratio for human tumour cells: is it a constant? *Int J Radiat Biol* **61**: 479–87.

Pop LA, Millar WT, van der Plas M, van der Kogel (2000). Radiation tolerance of rat spinal cord to pulsed dose rate brachytherapy: the impact of differences in temporal dose distribution. *Radiother Oncol* **55**: 301–15.

Press OW (1999). Radiolabelled antibody therapy of B-cell lymphomas. *Semin Oncol* **26**(Suppl 14): 58–65.

Press OW, Eary JF, Appelbaum FR *et al.* (1993). Radiolabeled-antibody therapy of B-cell lymphoma with autologous bone marrow support. *N Engl J Med* **329**(17): 1219–24.

Sminia P, Schneider CJ, Koedooder K *et al.* (1998). Pulse frequency in pulsed brachytherapy based on tissue repair kinetics. *Int J Radiat Oncol Biol Phys* **41**: 139–50.

Steel GG (1991). Cellular sensitivity to low dose rate irradiation focuses the problem of tumour radioresistance (The ESTRO Breur Lecture). *Radiother Oncol* **20**: 71–83.

Steel GG, Down JD, Peacock JH, Stephens TC (1986). Dose-rate effects and the repair of radiation damage. *Radiother Oncol* **5**: 321–31.

Steel GG, Deacon JM Duchesne GM *et al.* (1987). The dose–rate effect in human tumour cells. *Radiother Oncol* **9**: 299–310.

Steel GG, Kelland LR, Peacock JH (1989). The radiobiological basis for low dose-rate radiotherapy. In: *Brachytherapy 2* (ed. Mould RF), pp. 15–25. Proceedings of the 5th International Selectron Users' Meeting 1988. Nucletron International BV, Leersum, The Netherlands.

Thames HD (1985). An 'incomplete-repair' model for survival after fractionated and continuous irradiation. *Int J Radiat Biol* **47**: 319–39.

Vaughan ATM, Anderson P, Dykes P, Bradwell AR (1987). Limitations to killing of tumours using radiolabelled antibodies. *Br J Radiol* **60**: 567–78.

Waksman R (2000). Vascular brachytherapy: update on clinical trials. *J Invas Cardiol* **12**(Suppl A): 18A–28A.

Wells RL, Bedford JS (1983). Dose rate effects in mammalian cells. IV: Repairable and nonrepairable damage in noncycling C3H 10T1/2 cells. *Radiat Res* **94**: 105–34.

Wheldon TE, O'Donoghue JA (1990). The radiobiology of targeted radiotherapy. *Int J Radiat Biol* **58**: 1–21.

Zweit J (1996). Radionuclides and carrier molecules for therapy. *Phys Med Biol* **41**: 1905–14.

Particle beams in radiotherapy

MICHAEL C JOINER

19.1 INTRODUCTION

Modern radiotherapy is usually given by linear accelerators producing high-energy x-rays of 4–25 MV which have generally superseded therapy with lower energy ^{60}Co or ^{137}Cs γ-rays. These are all uncharged electromagnetic radiations, physically similar in nature to radio waves or visible light except that the photons ('packets' of energy) are energetic enough to ionize molecules in tissues that they penetrate. It is this ionization that results in the biological effects seen in radiotherapy. Although there is some energy dependence, these radiations have roughly the same biological effect per unit dose. Electron beams are quantum-mechanically similar to x-rays and produce similar biological effects. Two other classes of radiations for use in radiotherapy are often referred to as:

- *light particles* – e.g. protons, neutrons and α-particles;
- *heavy particles* – e.g. fully stripped carbon, neon, silicon or argon ions.

These light and heavy particles may have a greater effect per unit dose compared with conventional radiations. The charged particles have, in addition, very different depth–dose absorption profiles compared with uncharged particles (i.e. neutrons) or conventional electromagnetic radiations (x- and γ-rays) and this enables more precise dose distributions to be achieved in radiotherapy. This chapter focuses on these different types of radiation for use in cancer therapy.

19.2 MICRODOSIMETRY

It is possible to build up a picture of the submicroscopic pattern of ionizations within a cell nucleus using special techniques for measuring ionization in very small volumes, together with computer simulations: this is the field of microdosimetry. Figure 19.1 shows examples of microdosimetric calculations of ionization tracks from γ-rays or α-particles passing through a cell nucleus (Goodhead, 1988, 1989). At the scale of the cell nucleus, the γ-rays deposit much of their energy as single isolated ionizations or excitations and much of the resulting DNA damage is efficiently repaired by enzymes within the nucleus (see Section 8.5). About 1000 of these sparse tracks are produced per Gy of absorbed radiation dose. The α-particles produce fewer tracks but the intense

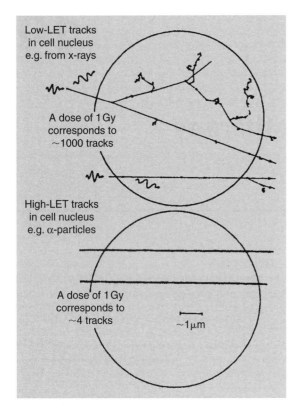

Low-LET tracks
in cell nucleus
e.g. from x-rays

A dose of 1 Gy
corresponds to
~1000 tracks

High-LET tracks
in cell nucleus
e.g. α-particles

A dose of 1 Gy
corresponds to
~4 tracks

~1 μm

Figure 19.1 *The structure of particle tracks for low-LET radiation (above) and α-particles (below). The circles indicate the typical size of mammalian cell nuclei. Note the tortuous tracks of low-energy secondary electrons, greatly magnified in this illustration. From Goodhead (1988), with permission.*

ionization within each track leads to more severe damage where the track intersects vital structures such as DNA. The resulting DNA damage may involve several adjacent base pairs and will be much more difficult or even impossible to repair; this is probably the reason why these radiations produce steeper cell survival curves and allow less cellular recovery than x-rays. At the low doses of α-particle irradiation that are encountered in environmental exposure, only some cells will be traversed by a particle and many cells will be unexposed.

Linear energy transfer (LET) is the term used to describe the density of ionization in particle tracks. LET is the average energy (in keV) given up by a charged particle traversing a distance of 1 μm. In Figure 19.1, the γ-rays have an LET of about $0.3 \, \mathrm{keV} \, \mu\mathrm{m}^{-1}$ and are described as low-LET radiation.

The α-particles have an LET of about $100 \, \mathrm{keV} \, \mu\mathrm{m}^{-1}$ and are an example of high-LET radiation.

Why are neutrons described as high-LET radiation when they are uncharged? Neutrons do not interact with the orbital electrons in the tissues through which they pass and they do not directly produce ionization. They do, however, interact with atomic nuclei from which they eject slow, densely ionizing protons. It is this secondary production of knock-on protons that confers high LET.

19.3 BIOLOGICAL EFFECTS DEPEND UPON LET

As LET increases, radiation produces more cell killing per Gy. Figure 19.2 shows the survival of human T1g cells plotted against dose for eight different radiations, with LET varying from $2 \, \mathrm{keV} \, \mu\mathrm{m}^{-1}$ (250 kVp x-rays) to $165 \, \mathrm{keV} \, \mu\mathrm{m}^{-1}$ (2.5 MeV α-particles). As LET increases, the survival curves become steeper, they also become straighter with less shoulder, which indicates either a higher ratio of lethal to potentially lethal lesions (in lesion-interaction models) or that high-LET radiation damage is less likely to be repaired correctly (in repair saturation models; see Section 7.7). For particles of identical atomic composition, LET generally increases with decreasing particle energy. However, notice that 2.5 MeV α-particles are less efficient compared with 4.0 MeV α-particles even though they have a higher LET; this is due to the phenomenon of *overkill* indicated in Figure 19.3.

The *relative biological effectiveness* (RBE) of a radiation under test (e.g. a high-LET radiation) is defined as:

$$\mathrm{RBE} = \frac{\text{dose of reference radiation}}{\text{dose of test radiation}}$$

to give the same biological effect. The reference low-LET radiation is usually 250 kVp x-rays. Figure 19.3 shows RBE values for the T1g cells featured in Figure 19.2. Curves have been calculated at cell survival levels of 0.8, 0.1 and 0.01, illustrating the fact that RBE is not constant but depends on the level of biological damage and hence on the dose level. RBE rises to a maximum at an LET of about $100 \, \mathrm{keV} \, \mu\mathrm{m}^{-1}$, then falls for higher values of LET due to overkill. For cells to be killed, energy must be deposited in a

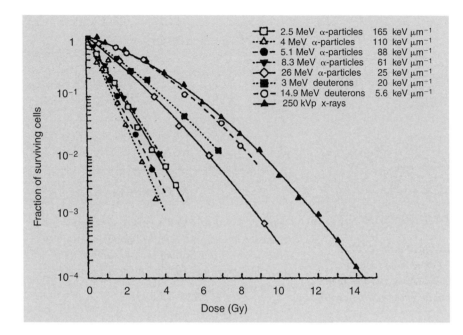

Figure 19.2 *Survival of human kidney cells exposed* in vitro *to radiations of different LET. From Barendsen (1968), with permission.*

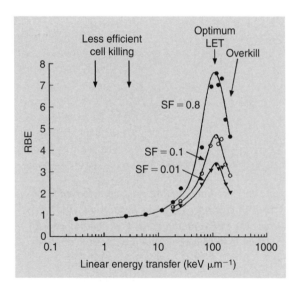

Figure 19.3 *Dependence of RBE on LET and the phenomenon of overkill by very high-LET radiations. From Barendsen (1968), with permission.*

number of critical sites in the cell (see Section 7.3). Sparsely ionizing low-LET radiation is inefficient because more than one particle may have to pass through the cell to kill it. Densely ionizing very high-LET radiation is also inefficient because it deposits more energy than necessary in critical sites. These

cells are overkilled and per Gy there is then less likelihood that other cells will be killed, leading to a reduced biological effect. Radiation of optimal LET deposits just enough energy per cell to inactivate the critical targets. This optimum LET is usually around $100\,keV\,\mu m^{-1}$ but it does vary between different cell types and depends on the spectrum of LET values in the radiation beam as well as the mean LET.

As LET increases, the oxygen enhancement ratio (OER, see Section 15.1) decreases. The measurements shown as an example in Figure 19.4 were also made with cultured T1g cells of human origin (Barendsen, 1968). The sharp reduction in OER occurs over the same range of LET as the sharp increase in RBE (Figure 19.3).

19.4 RELATIVE BIOLOGICAL EFFECTIVENESS (RBE) DEPENDS ON DOSE

As indicated in Figure 19.3, the RBE is higher if measured at lower radiation doses, corresponding to higher levels of cell survival. Figure 19.5 shows in more detail the RBE for 4.0 MeV α-particles plotted against dose of 250 kVp x-rays, for the T1g human cells irradiated *in vitro*. The data points were derived

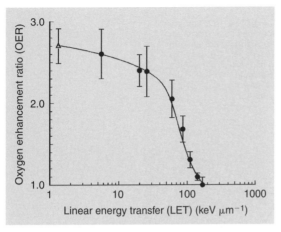

Figure 19.4 *The oxygen enhancement ratio (OER) decreases with increasing LET. Closed circles refer to monoenergetic α-particles and deuterons and the open triangle to 250 kVp x-rays. From Barendsen (1968), with permission.*

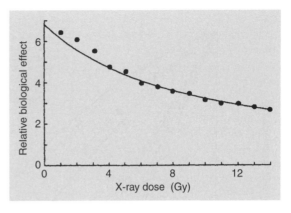

Figure 19.5 *RBE of 4 MeV α-particles increases with decreasing dose for cell lines irradiated in vitro. RBE values were calculated from the cell survival data shown in Figure 19.2. The full line is calculated as described in the text.*

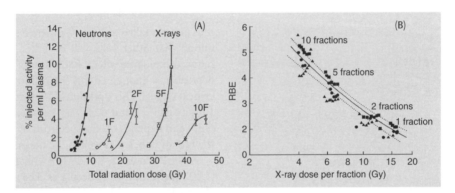

Figure 19.6 *The RBE for kidney damage increases with decreasing dose per fraction. RBE values are derived from graphs similar to panel A, which shows dose-effect curves for ^{51}Cr-EDTA clearance following irradiation with 1, 2, 3, 5 and 10 fractions of neutrons or 1, 2, 5 and 10 fractions of x-rays. The RBE values in panel B were obtained with various renal-damage end-points: isotope clearance (circles), reduction in haematocrit (squares); increase in urine output (triangles). From Joiner and Johns (1987), with permission.*

from Figure 19.2 by reading off from the α-particle survival curve the dose required to achieve the same cell survival as obtained for each x-ray dose tested. The RBE for the 4.0 MeV α-particles increases with decreasing dose because the low-LET x-ray survival response is more curved and has a bigger shoulder compared with the high-LET survival response. If linear-quadratic (LQ) equations are used to model both the low- and the high-LET responses, RBE can also be predicted mathematically from the α/β ratios

and the ratio $\alpha_{\text{high-LET}}/\alpha_{\text{low-LET}}$. This prediction is shown by the solid line.

RBE can also be measured *in vivo*. In normal tissues this may be done by comparing the relationships between damage and dose both for high- and low-LET radiations. This may be done for any end-point of damage, including tissue breakdown or loss of tissue function. Figure 19.6A shows the results of an experiment to study the loss of renal function in mice after external-beam radiotherapy. This was done by measuring the increased retention of ^{51}Cr-radiolabelled EDTA in the plasma 1 hour after injection; normally functioning kidneys completely clear this substance from the body within this time. For neutrons (produced by bombarding beryllium with 4 MeV deuterons, designated d(4)-Be), fractionation makes almost no difference to the tolerance dose but for x-rays a much higher total dose is required to produce renal damage when the treatment is split into two, five or ten fractions. This difference in the fractionation response for high- and low-LET radiations *in vivo* reflects the shape of the survival curves for the putative target cells in the tissue: almost straight for neutrons, and downwards-bending for x-rays (Figure 19.2). In this situation, RBE is calculated from the ratio of x-ray to neutron total doses required to produce the same biological effect *in the same number of fractions*. This is plotted against x-ray dose per fraction in Figure 19.6B. It can be seen that *in vivo*, RBE increases with decreasing dose per fraction in exactly the same way as RBE increases with decreasing single dose for the cells *in vitro* shown in Figure 19.5.

19.5 RESPONSE OF DIFFERENT TISSUES TO HIGH-LET RADIATION

The response to neutrons shown in Figure 19.6A suggests that for a fixed level of biological effect there should be much less change in total dose with fractionation for high-LET radiation compared with low-LET radiation. Figure 19.7 summarizes isoeffect curves relating total dose to dose per fraction for early-responding (dashed lines) and late-responding (full lines) tissues exposed to fractionated neutron irradiation (Withers *et al.*, 1982). This figure should be compared with Figure 12.1, which shows these relationships for a similar range of tissues exposed to fractionated x- or γ-rays. The following conclusions can be drawn from this comparison:

1. There is much less change in isoeffective total dose with fractionation for neutrons, either in early- or late-responding tissues. This reflects the straighter survival curves for the putative target cells for high-LET radiation.
2. For photons, the total dose increases more steeply with decreasing dose per fraction for late-responding than for early-responding tissues, reflecting the smaller α/β ratios for late-responding

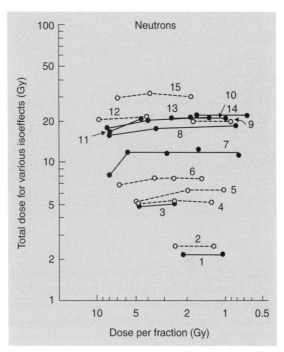

Figure 19.7 *Summary of published data on isoeffect curves for neutrons as a function of dose per fraction in various tissues of mice and rats. Broken lines indicate data on early-responding tissues; full lines are for late-responding tissues. Compare with Figure 12.1. Key: 1, thyroid function; 2, haemopoietic colonies; 3, vertebral growth; 4, spermatogenic colonies; 5, fibrosarcomas; 6, jejunum colonies; 7, lung LD$_{50}$; 8, lumbar nerve root function; 9, 12, skin desquamation; 10, skin contraction; 11, skin late changes; 13, spinal cord; 14, oral mucosa necrosis; 15, skin necrosis. From Withers* et al. *(1982), with permission.*

tissues (see Sections 12.5 and 13.2). RBE therefore rises rapidly with decreasing dose per fraction for late-responding tissues and more gradually for early-responding tissues.

3. Comparing the same tissues exposed to both photons and neutrons, RBE values for late tissue responses are *not* intrinsically higher than for early responses, but because of their faster increase as dose is reduced, the RBE values for late tissue response *tend* to be higher than for early tissue response at low doses per fraction, especially at or below 2 Gy per (x-ray) fraction.

To emphasize this last point, Figure 19.8 demonstrates the rise in neutron RBE (compared with

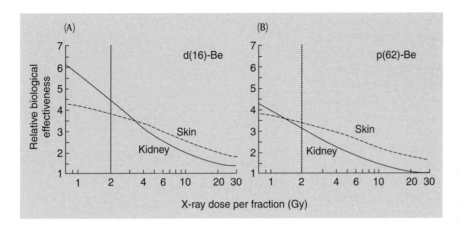

Figure 19.8 *Comparison of RBE values for mouse skin and kidney exposed to two different neutron beams. From Joiner (1988), with permission.*

x-rays) with decreasing dose per fraction in skin (an early-responding tissue) and kidney (a late-responding tissue). In this example, the RBE for d(16)-Be neutrons in kidney was greater than in skin at an x-ray dose per fraction of 2 Gy, but lower for a more highly penetrating, p(62)-Be neutron therapy beam. Therefore, compared with conventional photon therapy, late renal damage would be increased relative to acute reactions (and perhaps relative to tumour response) by treating with a low-energy neutron beam, but late renal injury would actually be spared on the high-energy machine. It is very important to understand that these relationships are specific to these tissues and these neutron beams. Similar relationships between other early-responding and late-responding tissues may not follow the same pattern and so must be evaluated individually in each case and for each treatment site to determine whether neutrons would deliver a therapeutic gain. It is not true that late reactions are always worse after neutron therapy for the same level of acute injury, but they may be in some cases. (Note: a d(16)-Be neutron beam has similar depth-dose characteristics to orthovoltage x-rays whereas a p(62)-Be neutron therapy beam can produce treatment plans comparable with a 4 MV linac.)

19.6 THE BIOLOGICAL BASIS FOR HIGH-LET RADIOTHERAPY

We have seen (Figure 19.4) that the differential radiosensitivity between poorly oxygenated (more

resistant) and well-oxygenated (more sensitive) cells is reduced with high-LET radiations. Therefore, tumour sites in which hypoxia is a problem in radiotherapy (some head and neck tumours, for example) might benefit from high-LET radiotherapy in the same way as from chemical hypoxic-cell sensitizers (see Section 16.3).

The effect of low-LET radiation on cells is strongly influenced by their position in the cell cycle, with cells in S-phase being more radioresistant than cells in G2 or mitosis (see Section 6.8). Cells in stationary (i.e. plateau) phase also tend to be more radioresistant than cells in active proliferation. Both these factors act to increase the effect of fractionated radiotherapy on more rapidly cycling cells compared with those cycling slowly or not at all, because the rapidly cycling cells that survive the first few fractions are statistically more likely to be caught later in a sensitive phase and so be killed by a subsequent dose, a process termed 'cell-cycle resensitization'. This differential radiosensitivity due to cell cycle position is considerably reduced with high-LET radiation (Chapman, 1980) and is a reason why we might expect high-LET radiotherapy to be beneficial in some slowly growing, x-ray-resistant tumours.

A third biological rationale for high-LET therapy is based on the observation that the range of radiation response of different cell types is reduced with high-LET radiation compared with x-rays. This is shown in Figure 19.9, which summarizes the *in vitro* response of 20 human cell lines to photon and neutron irradiation (Britten *et al.*, 1992). This reduced range of response affects the benefit expected, which is the balance between tumour and

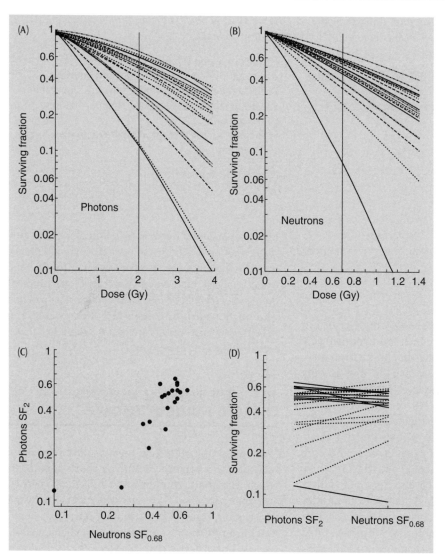

Figure 19.9 *Response of 20 human tumour cell lines to (A) 4 MVp photons, or (B) p(62.5)-Be neutrons. The vertical lines show the photon (2 Gy) and neutron (0.68 Gy) doses that give the same median cell survival; the average RBE is therefore 2/0.68 = 2.94. Panel C shows that the range of cell survival at the reference neutron dose of 0.68 Gy is less than the range of photon SF_2 values. In 9/20 of the cell lines neutrons gave lower cell survival than photons at these doses (panel D).*

normal-tissue responses. Thus, if tumour cells are already more radiosensitive to x-rays than the critical normal-cell population, high-LET radiation should not be used since this would reduce an already favourable differential. Possible examples are seminomas, lymphomas and Hodgkin's disease. However, if the tumour cells are more resistant to x-rays than the critical normal cells, high-LET radiation might reduce this difference in radiosensitivity and thus would effectively 'sensitize' the tumour cell population relative to a fixed level of normal-tissue damage. High-LET radiation would be advantageous in this case.

Clinical results with high-LET radiations

These three radiobiological arguments lead us to expect that high-LET radiotherapy might be of benefit to some cancer patients but not to others. Clinical trials of neutrons that have so far been performed have generally failed to detect such an advantage in the whole cancer patient populations that have been studied. If high-LET therapy is going to be of clinical use, it should therefore be given only to patients who are likely to respond poorly to conventional x-ray therapy, on the basis of the results of assays for tumour oxygenation, cell kinetics or radiosensitivity. The

Table 19.1 *Hypothetical clinical trials which show the importance of patient selection in determining the value of high-LET radiotherapy*

	Total number	Successful response to		*p*-value
		Neutrons	Photons	
(A)				
Subgroup	40	14	6	0.03
Remainder	160	40	40	–
Total	200	54	46	0.3
(B)				
Subgroup	40	14	6	0.03
Remainder	160	36	44	0.3
Total	200	50	50	–

From Bewley (1989).

Table 19.2 *Summary of clinical indications for fast neutron therapy*

1. Salivary gland tumours (locally extended)
2. Prostatic adenocarcinoma (locally extended)
3. Soft-tissue sarcoma (slowly growing, inoperable)
4. Paranasal sinuses (adenocarcinoma, adenoid cystic ca.)
5. Melanoma and rectal carcinoma (palliative treatment)

From Wambersie *et al.* (1994).

principles of these predictive assays are described in Chapter 22. Table 19.1 demonstrates hypothetically the importance of patient selection for neutron therapy, or indeed for any new therapy that is only expected to benefit a subgroup of patients. Suppose that 200 patients enter a trial of high-LET versus photon therapy with 100 patients in each arm. Of these, 80% respond equally well to the two treatments (and we suppose that they have a 50% cure rate), but the other 20% do better with the high-LET therapy, and this small subgroup responds with a 70% cure rate after high-LET and 30% cure after photons. The results for the total group fail to achieve significance but if the subgroup of 40 patients had been selected they would have demonstrated a significant margin in favour of neutrons. It would be even more confusing if the majority (160) of the patients actually did worse with high-LET therapy: suppose 45% were cured with high-LET but 55% were cured with photons. Now the whole trial (Table 19.1B) reveals nothing at all but would still conceal an important subgroup. Rational patient selection is thus an important principle in relation to any modality that may improve treatment in only a minority of cases.

In spite of the potential difficulties demonstrated by Table 19.1, some clinical indications for fast neutron therapy have emerged. These have been summarized by Wambersie *et al.* (1994) as listed in Table 19.2. Neutrons may be of some benefit in treating x-ray-resistant tumours, slowly growing tumours and some advanced cancers that perhaps contain a high proportion of hypoxic cells. Wambersie has estimated that up to 10–15% of patients currently receiving radiotherapy would benefit from neutron therapy using modern high-energy isocentric machines, *if those patients could be identified reliably*. The patients who might benefit from high-LET therapy are going to be those whose cancers are radioresistant to current megavoltage x-ray treatment.

19.7 THE PHYSICAL BASIS FOR CHARGED-PARTICLE THERAPY

With conventional x-ray therapy, absorbed dose increases very rapidly within the short distance in which electronic equilibrium ('build-up') occurs, and then decreases exponentially with increasing penetration. Figure 19.10A shows central-axis depth doses from ^{60}Co γ-rays and from x-rays generated by a 6 MV linear accelerator (Fowler, 1981). Neutrons are also uncharged and their depth–dose characteristics are similar: modern high-energy neutron therapy beams have a penetration that is comparable to 4 MV x-rays. The only rationale for neutron therapy is therefore radiobiological, as discussed earlier.

By contrast, ion beams (i.e. incident beams of *charged* particles) *increase* their rate of energy deposition as they slow down with increasing penetration, finally stopping and releasing an intense burst of ionization called the Bragg peak. As an example, curve *1* in Figure 19.10B shows the depth–dose distribution of a primary beam of 160 MeV protons. The broad peak is obtained by superimposing on curve *1* four other beams of different intensities and ranges (curves *2, 3, 4, 5*), achieved by passing the primary beam through a rotating wheel with sectors of

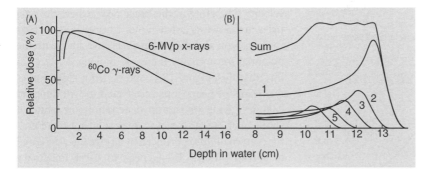

Figure 19.10 *The different depth–dose characteristics of (A) photons and (B) proton beams of different intensities and ranges, achieved by passing a primary beam (1) through plastic absorbers.*

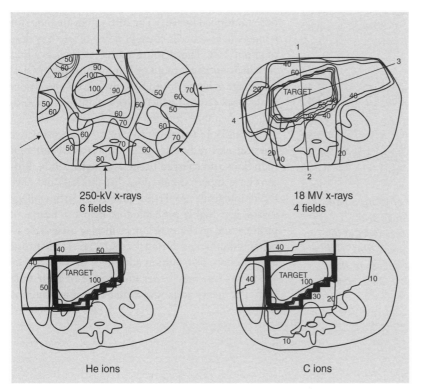

Figure 19.11 *Comparison of treatment plans for the radiotherapy of a case of pancreas carcinoma using charged particle beams or photons. From Bewley (1989), with permission.*

different thickness of plastic sheet. This spread-out peak (*Sum*) can be adjusted to cover the tumour volume and therefore increase the ratio of tumour-to-normal-tissue dose compared with conventional photon therapy (Raju, 1980).

Figure 19.11 shows some possible treatment plans with heavy-ion beams of helium and carbon nuclei, using carcinoma of the pancreas as an example. The improvement given by the He ions over 18 MV x-rays is as dramatic as the comparison between 18 MV and

250 kVp x-rays. The mean doses to the spinal cord and kidney are almost zero for He ions, 50% for 18 MV x-rays and 70% for 250 kVp x-rays. Uniformity over the tumour is 2–3%, 5% and 15%, respectively.

Carbon ions give a similar dose distribution to He ions but in addition they have a higher LET and RBE in the Bragg peak, which in suitable tumours (see above) might also confer a radiobiological advantage. The LET of a charged particle is proportional to the square of its charge divided by the square of its

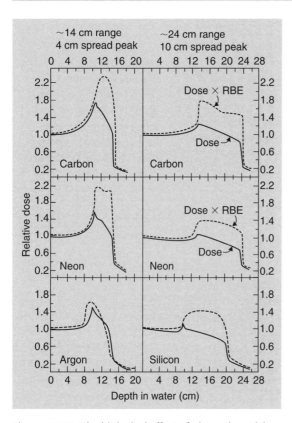

velocity. Therefore in the Bragg peak, where the particles are slowing down rapidly, heavy ions such as carbon, neon and silicon have very high LET, with the potential for a greatly increased biological effect. To illustrate this, Figure 19.12 shows depth–dose curves for beams of heavy ions accelerated to two different energies giving maximum penetrations in tissue of about 14 or 24 cm. In each case the solid line represents the pattern of dose produced by a ridge filter designed to spread out the Bragg peak to cover imaginary tumours of 4 or 10 cm, respectively. This is a similar 'peak-spreading' technique to that described in Figure 19.10B. However, the dotted line shows the distribution of *biologically effective dose*, which is physical dose multiplied by RBE. The RBE values are those for Chinese hamster cells corresponding to an x-ray dose of about 2 Gy. This demonstrates that for heavy ions (not high-energy protons or helium ions) the physical advantage of better dose distribution in the spread-out Bragg peak can be further enhanced by the radiobiological advantage from the higher LET.

Figure 19.13 conveniently summarizes the relative physical and radiobiological properties of different radiations and charged particles (Fowler, 1981). Protons have superb depth–dose distributions and have radiobiological properties similar to orthovoltage x-rays: it is highly probable that light-ion beams of protons and perhaps helium will play a key role in better radiotherapy during the next 20 years. Neutrons have no dose distribution advantage over megavoltage x-rays but may be useful because of their high LET. The heavy ions give better dose distributions

Figure 19.12 *The biological effect of charged particle beams is increased further in the Bragg peak. Depth–dose curves are shown for three types of ion beam, each with a 4 cm or 10 cm spread peak. Full lines show the dose distribution; broken lines show the biologically effective dose (i.e. dose × RBE). From Blakely (1982), with permission.*

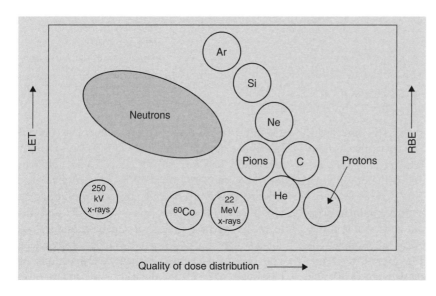

Figure 19.13 *The radiations available for radiation therapy differ in the quality of beam that they produce, also in RBE. Based on Fowler (1981).*

than x-rays and also a higher LET, depending on the particle. Argon ions have a high LET but in practice they break up so readily that only limited penetration is useful. Carbon, neon and silicon ions seem to be the most promising of the heavy ions at the present time and if heavy-ion therapy has a future it will probably be with these particles (Castro, 1995).

19.8 SUMMARY OF THERAPEUTIC CONCLUSIONS

Neutrons are the commonest type of particle beam so far used for radiotherapy but the clinical results obtained are controversial. To some extent this reflects the poor dose distributions and beam delivery systems of the early experimental neutron facilities. It is therefore essential that further work with clinical neutron radiotherapy should use facilities with isocentric beam delivery and multi-leaf or multi-rod collimation. The benefits that have been claimed for neutrons are indicated in Table 19.2. Much of the clinical work with heavy ions has taken place at the Lawrence Berkeley Laboratory in California. Some benefit in some tumours has been claimed although the very high cost of this treatment means that it would have to be restricted to a few large centres each serving a large population (Wambersie *et al.*, 1994). Proton beams are probably the most attractive radiation at the present time. They are not excessively expensive and have greatly improved dose distributions compared with photons. Over 20 000 patients have now been treated with proton beams since the early experimental tests at Berkeley and Uppsala in the 1950s. There is broad agreement that proton therapy can be particularly valuable in choroidal melanoma and in tumours very close to the spinal cord. Many centres world-wide now have proton facilities with full isocentric beam delivery, either operational or coming on line soon, and full randomized trials are expected to be undertaken in a wider range of clinical conditions with these clinic-based machines.

KEY POINTS

1. x- and γ-rays are sparsely ionizing radiations with a low linear energy transfer (LET). Some particle radiations (e.g. neutrons, α-particles or heavy ions) have a high LET.
2. High-LET radiations are *biologically* more effective per Gy than low-LET radiations. This is measured by the relative biological effectiveness (RBE). For most high-LET radiations at therapeutic dose levels, RBE is in the range of 2–10.
3. RBE increases as the LET increases up to about $100 \, \text{keV} \, \mu\text{m}^{-1}$, above which RBE decreases because of cellular overkill. The oxygen enhancement ratio (OER) also decreases rapidly over the same range of LET.
4. RBE increases as the dose is reduced *in vitro*, or the dose *per fraction* is reduced *in vivo*. In late-responding tissues, this increase occurs more rapidly than in early-responding tissues.
5. High-LET radiations may be clinically useful in carefully selected cases.
6. Heavy particles such as He, C and Ne ions, have a high LET and in addition they have improved physical depth–dose distributions.
7. Proton beams provide the best improvement in dose distribution for the lowest cost; their RBE is similar to that of low-energy photons.

BIBLIOGRAPHY

Barendsen GW (1968). Responses of cultured cells, tumours and normal tissues to radiations of different linear energy transfer. *Curr Topics Radiat Res Q* **4**: 293–356.

Bewley DK (1989). *The Physics and Radiobiology of Fast Neutron Beams*. Adam Hilger, Bristol.

Blakely EA (1982). Biology of Bevelac beams: cellular studies. In: *Pion and Heavy Ion Radiotherapy: Pre-clinical and Clinical Studies* (ed. Skarsgard LD), pp. 229–50. Elsevier, New York.

Britten RA, Warenius HM, Parkins C, and Peacock JH (1992). The inherent cellular sensitivity to 62.5 MeV neutrons of human cells differing in photon sensitivity. *Int J Radiat Biol* **61**: 805–12.

Castro JR (1995). Results of heavy ion radiotherapy. *Radiat Environ Biophys* **34**: 45–8.

Chapman JD (1980). Biophysical models of mammalian cell inactivation by radiation. In: *Radiation Biology in Cancer Research* (eds Meyn RE, Withers HR), pp. 21–32. Raven Press, New York.

Fowler JF (1981). *Nuclear Particles in Cancer Treatment.* Adam Hilger, Bristol.

Goodhead DT (1988). Spatial and temporal distribution of energy. *Health Phys* **55**: 231–40.

Goodhead DT (1989). The initial physical damage produced by ionizing radiation. *Int J Radiat Biol* **56**: 623–34.

Joiner MC (1988). A comparison of the effects of p(62)-Be and d(16)-Be neutrons in the mouse kidney. *Radiother Oncol* **13**: 211–24.

Joiner MC, Johns H (1987). Renal damage in the mouse: the effect of d(4)-Be neutrons. *Radiat Res* **109**: 456–68.

Raju MR (1980). *Heavy Particle Radiotherapy.* Academic Press, New York.

Wambersie A, Richard F, Breteau N (1994). Development of fast neutron therapy worldwide. *Acta Oncol* **34**: 261–74.

Withers HR, Thames HD, Peters LJ (1982). Biological bases for high RBE values for late effects of neutron irradiation. *Int J Radiat Oncol Biol Phys* **8**: 2071–6.

FURTHER READING

Alpen EL (1998). *Radiation Biophysics*, 2nd edn. Academic Press, San Diego.

Bewley DK (1989). *The Physics and Radiobiology of Fast Neutron Beams.* Adam Hilger, Bristol.

Engenhart-Cabillic R, Wambersie A (1998). Fast neutrons and high-LET particles in cancer therapy. *Recent Results in Cancer Research*, Vol. 150. Springer-Verlag, Berlin.

Fowler JF (1981). *Nuclear Particles in Cancer Treatment.* Adam Hilger, Bristol.

Goodhead DT (1988). Spatial and temporal distribution of energy. *Health Phys* **55**: 231–40.

Nordic Conference on Neutrons in Research and Cancer Therapy (1994). *Acta Oncol* **33**: 225–327.

Wambersie A, Auberger T, Gahbauer RA, Jones DT, Potter R (1999). A challenge for high-precision radiation therapy: the case for hadrons. *Strahlenther Onkol* **175**(Suppl 2): 122–8.

20

The combination of radiotherapy and chemotherapy

FIONA A STEWART AND HARRY BARTELINK

20.1 THE OBJECTIVES OF COMBINED MODALITY THERAPY

Virtually all classes of chemotherapeutic agents have been used in combined modality clinical trials involving one or more drugs plus a full course of radiotherapy. The main aim of such trials is an improvement in local control and/or eradication of distant metastases. To be successful, the combined modality regimen must achieve these objectives without exceeding normal-tissue tolerance. The introduction of a second modality (chemotherapy) potentially increases both the spectrum and magnitude of normal-tissue toxicities compared with radiotherapy alone. In order to evaluate the benefit of combined modality treatments, the concept of therapeutic gain is therefore essential. A therapeutic gain is achieved if the combined modality regimen results in improved tumour response, with respect to either agent alone, when the regimens are evaluated at comparable levels of overall toxicity (see Section 1.6). Any increase in toxicity from the combination arm should be taken into

account when assessing the therapeutic gain. Unfortunately, clinical trials are seldom designed in a way that allows this to be done.

The strategy outlined in Figure 20.1 is the minimum scale of study necessary to demonstrate a therapeutic gain and to exclude the possibility that the gain in tumour control seen in the combined modality arm could have been obtained merely by increasing the radiation dose. A three-arm trial is envisaged, with a radiation dose D_1 given alone or combined with chemotherapy, the third arm consisting of an increased radiation dose alone, D_2. This strategy assumes that 'toxicity' can be ascribed a single numerical value, which is an oversimplification since the addition of chemotherapy may introduce new toxicities as well as enhancing the radiation damage. In the example shown in Figure 20.1, the higher radiation dose D_2 produces a greater level of toxicity than the lower dose D_1. Adding chemotherapy to the lower radiation dose also increases toxicity, but to a lesser extent than the radiation dose D_2. The tumour response from the combined radiation plus chemotherapy is greater

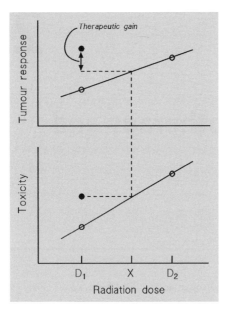

Figure 20.1 *Scheme for the identification of an improved therapeutic strategy in clinical research. Open symbols show the tumour response and toxicity associated with radiation alone (doses D_1 and D_2). Solid symbols show the results with chemotherapy added to radiation dose D_1.*

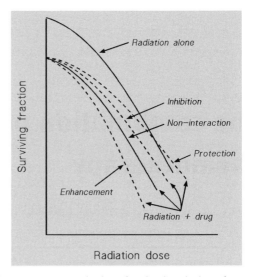

Figure 20.2 *A terminology for the description of interactive processes between a cytotoxic drug and radiation. From Steel (1979), with permission.*

than could be expected from an equitoxic dose of radiation alone. Hence, in this example there is a therapeutic gain. If a three-arm trial is not done and the combined modality arm results in both increased toxicity and increased tumour response, then the existence of a therapeutic gain must be in doubt.

20.2 EXPLOITABLE MECHANISMS IN COMBINED RADIOTHERAPY AND CHEMOTHERAPY

The first step in identifying exploitable mechanisms for combined modality therapy is to define whether the modalities are interactive (one modality modifying the response of the other) or non-interactive (each modality exerting its own independent effect). A suggested terminology of these processes is described in Figure 20.2. If chemotherapy results in a fixed amount of cell kill, shifting the dose–response curve for radiation to a lower surviving fraction without changing its shape, then the combination is *non-interactive*. If the steepness of the radiation

dose–response curve is also increased by the addition of chemotherapy, this may be called *enhancement* of response; if it is decreased, this is *inhibition*, and in the extreme case where the combination gives less effect than radiation alone, this is *protection*. Interaction between radiotherapy and chemotherapy is, however, not a prerequisite for a therapeutic gain. Some mechanisms, both interactive and non-interactive, which may be exploited to obtain a therapeutic gain, are briefly described below.

Spatial co-operation

This term describes the use of radiotherapy and chemotherapy to target disease in different anatomical sites. The commonest situation is where radiation is used to treat the primary tumour and chemotherapy is added to deal with systemic spread. There is an analogous situation in leukaemia where chemotherapy is the main treatment and radiotherapy is used to deal with disease in a 'seclusion site' such as the brain.

If spatial co-operation is effective, this should result in a reduction of distant failures after the combined therapy. The successful exploitation of spatial co-operation depends critically on the effectiveness of the chemotherapy used. In the common solid tumours, chemotherapy seldom achieves a surviving fraction better than 10^{-4}. Even small metastatic deposits of 0.1 g may contain 10^7–10^8 tumour cells and, if the majority of these are also clonogenic, standard chemotherapy may fail to control even a small amount of disseminated disease. For spatial co-operation to succeed more widely, we need more effective drugs or methods of specifically targeting existing drugs to the tumour to allow dose escalation.

Independent cell kill

This term describes the simple concept that if two effective therapeutic modalities can both be given at full dose then, even in the absence of interactive processes, the tumour response (total cell kill) should be greater than that achieved with either agent alone. For this mechanism to be exploited, the radiotherapy and chemotherapy should have non-overlapping toxicities and the chemotherapy should not enhance normal-tissue damage within the radiation field. Such a situation may be obtained by temporal separation of the two modalities but, even if this can be achieved without a negative influence on tumour control, the patient will probably have to tolerate a wider range of toxic reactions. This needs to be taken into account when assessing the overall benefit. If independent cell killing can be successfully exploited, it could potentially lead to both improved local control and reduced distant failure, without any interactions between the modalities.

Debulking

This concept involves the use of several cycles of chemotherapy to shrink the primary tumour prior to radiotherapy, often referred to as neoadjuvant chemotherapy. The rationale is that a smaller tumour will be easier to cure by radiotherapy because of a reduced cell number. Debulking may also lead to improved oxygenation and a consequent increase in radiosensitivity. Chemotherapy debulking is occasionally combined with a reduction in the radiotherapy treatment volume, to limit normal-tissue damage and permit an increase in radiation dose to the residual tumour. However, this is only possible in very chemosensitive tumours, e.g. lymphomas and childhood tumours.

The disadvantage of debulking schedules is that they involve a delay in starting radiotherapy.

Radiotherapy is usually the more effective of the two modalities and where this is the case it is unwise to delay it, particularly for rapidly proliferating tumour types like head and neck carcinomas. There is also the possibility that chemotherapy will, by debulking the tumour, stimulate tumour cell repopulation, which would be detrimental to tumour control by radiotherapy (see Section 14.4).

Enhanced tumour response

In addition to the non-interactive mechanisms discussed above, there are several mechanisms by which radiotherapy and chemotherapy may interact either directly, to give an alteration in the shape of the cell survival curve, or indirectly by killing subpopulations resistant to the other modality.

Several commonly used chemotherapy agents have been shown to inhibit the repair of radiation damage. Examples are cisplatin, bleomycin, adriamycin and hydroxyurea. These drugs, like radiation, produce DNA damage which is manifest as DNA breaks, adducts and intercalation. For cisplatin, there is also an increase in the number of radiation-induced strand breaks. This might occur by conversion of radiation-induced single-strand breaks (SSB) to double-strand breaks (DSB) during the repair of DNA-platinum adducts. Inhibition of repair, or the conversion of SSB to DSB, has the effect of steepening the radiation survival curve and leads to an enhanced response (Figure 20.2). Enhancement that occurs as a result of repair inhibition will be more pronounced in fractionated schedules than for single doses. A major problem with repair inhibition as an exploitable mechanism for obtaining a therapeutic gain, is the lack of evidence for a *selective* anti-tumour effect. For this strategy to be effective some sort of tumour drug targeting may be required.

Chemotherapy may also influence the radiation response indirectly by selective killing of a specific subpopulation of tumour cells, e.g. in radioresistant phases of the cell cycle (late S and G1), leaving a synchronized population of radiosensitive cells. Such an approach can be effective *in vitro* and in pre-clinical studies using single doses of radiotherapy for rapidly growing murine tumours, but it is unlikely to be exploitable in combination with fractionated daily radiotherapy and clinical trials have been disappointing.

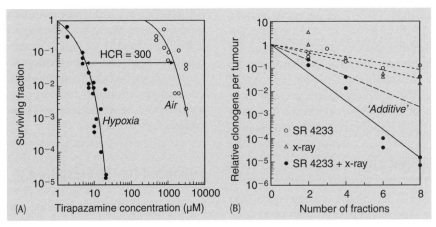

Figure 20.3 *(A) Dose–response curves for tirapazamine cell killing of murine SCVII cells exposed to drug for 90 minutes under hypoxic (closed symbols) or oxic conditions (open symbols). The hypoxic cytotoxicity ratio (HCR) is 300. (B) Response of SCVII tumours to 2–7 doses of tirapazamine alone (open symbols), 2–8 fractions of x-rays alone (open triangles) or their combination (closed symbols). Mice were treated* in vivo *and tumours excised for* in vitro *assessment of cell survival of 12 hours after the last treatment. The combination treatment caused greater cell killing than would be predicted from a simple addition of cell killing after each agent alone. Redrawn from Brown (1993), with permission.*

A more attractive approach is drug targeting of hypoxic (radioresistant) tumour cells (see Section 16.3). Several bioreductive drugs have been developed for clinical use, which are much more effective at killing hypoxic cells than well-oxygenated cells. This offers therapeutic potential in combination with radiotherapy, since hypoxia is much less prevalent in normal tissues than in tumours and hypoxic cells are radioresistant. The leading compound among such bioreductive drugs is tirapazamine (TPZ) which kills hypoxic cells at drug concentrations 50–300 times lower than oxic cells (Figure 20.3A). Under hypoxic conditions TPZ is metabolized to a highly toxic free radical, which produces DNA strand breaks. In the presence of oxygen the drug is back-oxidized to the non-toxic parent compound. Non-toxic doses of TPZ in combination with fractionated irradiation of mouse tumours results in an increased response to radiation, which appears to be greater than the sum of the two individual agents, even though there is no direct interaction between the modalities (Figure 20.3B). Theoretical calculations indicate that a hypoxic toxin that can kill 50% of hypoxic cells with each administration should be more effective in combination with fractionated radiotherapy than fully oxygenating the tumour (Brown and Koong, 1991). TPZ also causes enhanced cell killing in combination with

cisplatin under hypoxic conditions. In this case, there does appear to be a direct interaction between the DNA damage produced by TPZ and cisplatin, probably at the level of repair of DNA cross-links.

TPZ therefore shows much promise as a drug for combined modality cancer treatment. Randomized phase III trials have been started for TPZ combined with cisplatin (in non-small-cell lung cancer, NSCLC), in combination with radiotherapy (in head and neck cancer and glioblastoma) or with radiotherapy plus cisplatin (in head and neck and cervix cancers).

20.3 SEQUENCING OF CHEMOTHERAPY AND RADIOTHERAPY IN RELATION TO NORMAL-TISSUE TOXICITY

There is a large body of experimental data that demonstrates that normal-tissue damage after combined modality treatment is strongly influenced by the sequence and timing of the modalities. Many commonly used drugs cause substantial increase in normal-tissue radiation injury when the modalities are given in close sequence but not when they are separated in time. Drugs that inhibit repair of radiation injury (Section 20.2) produce maximum enhancement when they are given at the same time as

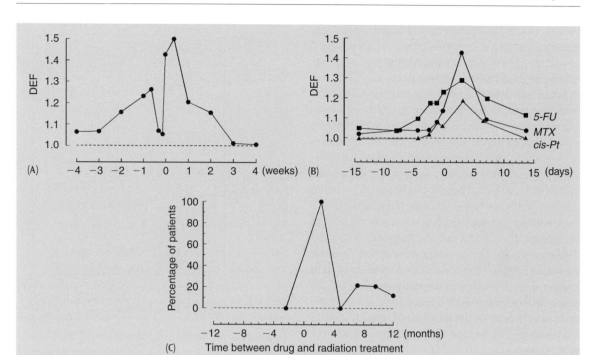

Figure 20.4 *Three examples of the results of time-line studies of the combined effects of cytotoxic drugs and radiation. (A) Cylophosphamide and pelvic irradiation in mice. (B) 5-FU, methotrexate or cisplatin and pelvic irradiation in mice (both from Pearson and Steel, 1984). (C) Normal-tissue damage in patients treated for testicular teratoma with radiation and combination chemotherapy. From Yarnold* et al. *(1983), with permission.*

radiation and these effects will be most pronounced in fractionated schedules. The risk of severe normal-tissue reactions is even greater when the drug also has a specific toxicity for tissues within the radiation field, e.g. bleomycin or adriamycin and lung toxicity, cisplatin and kidney toxicity. Drugs that inhibit proliferation will also increase toxicity in rapidly dividing tissues when delivered during a course of radiotherapy, whereas their effect is much less if given after the acute radiation reaction has healed. Dactinomycin, for example, inhibits repopulation in irradiated intestine, skin and oral mucosa. When it is given to mice in the gap between split-course irradiations it causes a marked increase in tissue damage. Similar effects would be expected to occur in clinical radiotherapy.

Investigations of the influence of temporal separation between drugs and radiation in tissue (or tumour) response are sometimes referred to as the 'time-line approach'. This methodology seeks to quantify the drug-induced increase in radiation effect as a function of the time interval between

modalities. Such an approach is illustrated in Figure 20.4, showing data from pre-clinical and clinical studies where chemotherapy was given at various times before or after various doses of pelvic irradiation. In the experimental studies (panels A and B) the normal-tissue damage after combined modality schedules was compared with that after radiation alone and dose-enhancement factors (DEF: the ratio of radiation doses without drug and with drug for a fixed level of tissue damage) were calculated for each drug-radiation interval. In the clinical study the percentage of patients with severe late morbidity after combined chemotherapy and radiotherapy was scored in relation to the interval between treatments. In each case, drugs and irradiation in close sequence were more damaging than when separated by days (pre-clinical) to weeks (clinical). The basic message from these and many other similar studies is that chemotherapy given concurrently with radiotherapy results in the highest probability of increased normal-tissue complications. Separation of the two modalities in time usually reduces this risk.

The above observation would argue against the simultaneous use of chemotherapy and radiotherapy. However, concurrent chemotherapy radiotherapy schedules are actually emerging as the most effective in terms of clinical tumour response (Section 20.6), with significantly less benefit for drugs given before (*neoadjuvant*) or after (*adjuvant*) radiotherapy in many tumour types. Apparently, the disadvantages of sequential chemotherapy/radiotherapy, e.g. prolonged overall treatment times, outweigh the advantage of reduced toxicity. It should be noted, however, that morbidity scoring is often lacking, or done in a very rudimentary way, which precludes assessment of therapeutic gain. If the use of concurrent combined modality is to be successfully pursued without exceeding normal-tissue tolerance, this may well require some reduction in the radiation dose for the combined treatment. Such a reduction must be made cautiously because of the steepness of tumour-control relationships (see Section 10.4). A proper assessment of therapeutic gain, including any increased normal-tissue toxicity, is essential when evaluating the true benefit of combined modality trials.

20.4 NOVEL MOLECULAR TARGETS FOR ENHANCED RADIATION RESPONSE

An exciting development in cancer therapy is the increased understanding of cellular growth factors and signalling pathways for control of cell proliferation, differentiation and angiogenesis. Many of these pathways are activated in tumours or in inflammatory tissue but not in healthy normal tissue, offering the potential for drug targeting. Specific molecular targets are also being identified for tumour radiosensitization via activated oncogenes. Some examples of these new approaches are described below.

The signal transduction pathway that has received the greatest attention in this regard is the ErbB receptor tyrosine kinase family. The ErbB-1 receptor EGFR (epidermal growth factor receptor) is highly expressed in many epithelial tumours and overexpression correlates with an aggressive (invasive) and radioresistant phenotype. EGFR blocking antibodies have been developed that inhibit tumour proliferation and angiogenesis, inhibit DNA repair and promote apoptosis in cells over-expressing the receptor.

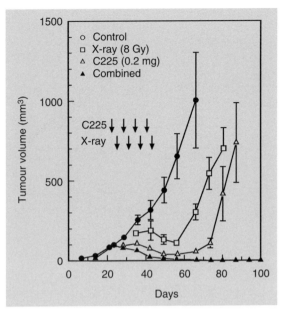

Figure 20.5 *Inhibition of tumour regrowth after treatment of SCC-1 xenografts (in nude mice) with four injections of monoclonal antibody C225 alone, or 4 × 8 Gy irradiation alone, or 4 × C225 with radiation. The combination of radiation and EGFR-blocking antibody inhibited regrowth of the tumours for at least 100 days. Redrawn from Huang and Harari (2000), with permission.*

Pre-clinical studies have demonstrated that the blocking antibody C225 in combination with fractionated irradiation of head and neck xenografts in nude mice gives long-term tumour control, whereas either agent alone is less effective (Figure 20.5). It is not possible to conclude that a greater than additive response was achieved in the example shown. Each agent alone produced some delay in tumour growth and there is no information on the response to higher doses of radiation alone.

Interpretation of the combined response to two agents in terms of supra-additivity is actually very complex and requires information on the dose effect relationships of each agent individually. If dose–response curves are non-linear, as is usually the case in cancer therapy, there is no unique description of an additive response. There is an area of uncertainty whose magnitude depends upon the non-linearity of the responses to each individual agent. The extent of the uncertainty can be evaluated by the use of an isobologram, which is an isoeffect plot of the doses of

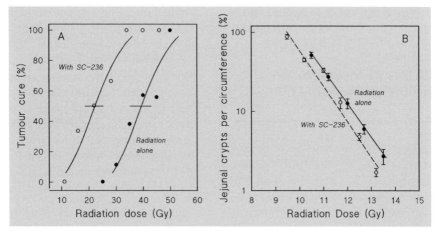

Figure 20.6 *Radiation dose–response curves for local control of FSA tumours in mice (panel A), or survival of jejunum crypt cells in mice (panel B), after treatment with single doses of radiation alone (closed symbols) or radiation and the COX-2 inhibitor SC-'236. SC-'236 caused marked sensitization of tumour response but no significant increase in intestinal cell killing. Redrawn from Kishi* et al. *(2000), with permission.*

two agents that together give a fixed biological effect. These issues are further discussed by Steel and Peckham (1979). The data shown in Figure 20.5 and other pre-clinical studies do, however, demonstrate that non-toxic doses of antibodies blocking EGFR can increase the radiation response of tumours that over-express the receptor. C225 is now being tested in combination with radiotherapy in phase III trials for head and neck cancer.

Similarly, over-expression of the ErbB-2 receptor (HER-2/neu) occurs in about 30% of all human breast cancers and antibodies blocking this receptor lead to growth arrest and radiosensitization in over-expressing cells. The antibody herceptin is now in clinical trial for women with receptor-positive breast cancer.

Another specific tumour target for drug development is the cyclo-oxygenase pathway (COX). COX enzymes are required for the synthesis of prostaglandins, which are implicated in the initiation and growth of tumours. The COX-1 enzyme is constitutively expressed in all tissues but COX-2 expression is inducible and is restricted to inflammatory and tumour tissue. As with EGFR over-expression, COX-2 is associated with an aggressive phenotype and tumour progression, especially in colon cancers that produce high levels of prostaglandins. Selective inhibitors of COX-2 have been developed that are effective in preventing the growth of colonic polyps in patients with familial adenomatous polyposis (FAP) and that inhibit tumour growth in mouse

models of human cancer. COX-2 inhibitors also cause a marked increase in radiosensitivity of murine tumours, without any modification of radiosensitivity in healthy intestine (Figure 20.6). COX-2 inhibitors are now being evaluated as radiosensitizers in randomized trials for prostate cancer.

Mutated oncogenes offer an alternative approach for molecular targeting and radiosensitization. An example of this is *ras*, which is mutated in 30% of human tumours. Over-expression of the RAS protein depends on post-translational prenylation and is associated with increased radioresistance. Inhibitors of this process, e.g. farnesyle transferase inhibitors (FTI), can reverse the transformation and cause increased radiosensitivity, which is dependent on RAS status. Some inhibition of tumour growth that is independent of RAS status also occurs (Cohen-Jonathan *et al.*, 2000). FTI in combination with radiotherapy have recently entered clinical trial for head and neck cancer.

The above are just a few of the novel molecular targets that offer possibilities for specific tumour radiosensitization. Anti-angiogenic or anti-vascular based therapies are further potential tumour-specific therapies that are well suited for combination with radiotherapy. Although these approaches are already being tested in the clinic, there is currently very little information on their effects in normal tissues. Much more pre-clinical work needs to be done, using clinically relevant, fractionated irradiation schedules in combination with these new agents, to asses the effects on both tumour control and normal-tissue damage.

20.5 PROBLEMS IN ASSESSING THE EFFICACY OF COMBINED MODALITY TRIALS

Methodological issues can sometimes make it difficult to interpret the value of combined modality treatments (Tannock, 1989, 1996). Much of the published literature concerns reports of small, non-randomized trials in which the outcome of treatment is compared with retrospective series where patients were treated with radiotherapy or surgery alone. It is virtually impossible to evaluate the therapeutic benefit of such studies, even if stringent efforts are made to match patients on the basis of various prognostic factors. The major factors identified by Tannock as introducing bias in such comparisons are as follows:

- *Patient selection* often occurs because only those patients who are fit to receive the relatively toxic combined modality schedules will be entered into the trial. If this selected patient group is compared with all patients previously treated with radiotherapy alone, this will inevitably introduce bias in favour of the new treatment.
- *Stage migration* is another problem associated with the use of historical controls, particularly when there is a long time interval between the studies. Improved diagnostic and detection methods such as CT or NMR scanning help to detect smaller amounts of metastatic disease and have the effect of shifting patients into higher-stage (i.e. more metastatic) categories. This leads to apparent improvements for each stage but no change in overall survival.
- *The duration of follow-up* may be shorter for a new study than for the historical controls. Initial tumour response is often good in combined modality studies but early differences between control and combined modality arms tend to decrease with longer follow-up. Single-arm studies that make an early evaluation of tumour response and compare actuarial survivals with historical controls after short follow-up are therefore very unreliable.
- *Small numbers of patients* included in trials is another serious problem in evaluating many

studies, including randomized trials. In order to detect an improvement in survival of 15% with 90% confidence, approximately 300–400 patients randomized to control and test arms are required. Few published series contain enough patients to be able to detect such an improvement with statistical significance. Finally, even large randomized trials cannot be properly evaluated in terms of therapeutic gain if the toxicity in the combined arm is greater than in the control arm. Comparisons of treatment outcome should be made at equivalent levels of toxicity.

Tannock (1989, 1996) concluded from his review of the literature that the methodology used in the majority of published trials did not allow conclusions to be made on the possible benefits of combined modality treatment, but only about toxicity and feasibility.

20.6 CURRENT STATUS OF COMBINED MODALITY THERAPY

Head and neck cancer

A meta-analysis of published results from 54 randomized controlled trials of combined chemotherapy and radiotherapy in head and neck cancer (Munro, 1995) demonstrated a modest (6.5%) overall improvement in survival (95%, confidence interval (CI) 3.1–9.9%) in favour of combined modality therapy. Chemotherapy concurrent with radiotherapy gave a larger increase in survival of 12.1% (CI 5–19%), whereas the survival benefit from neoadjuvant chemotherapy was less (3.7%, CI 0.9–6.5%).

A more recent patient-based analysis of 70 randomized trials (Pignon *et al.*, 2000) essentially confirmed the earlier literature-based analysis. The main meta-analysis (over 10 000 patients) demonstrated a significant 5-year overall survival benefit of 4% in favour of combined modality ($P < 0.0001$). Concurrent chemotherapy regimens gave the largest improvement (8%) and neoadjuvant or adjuvant regimens gave only small, non-significant benefits (2% and 1%, respectively). A separate analysis of six trials comparing neoadjuvant with concurrent or alternating chemotherapy (radiotherapy given during breaks in chemotherapy), demonstrated a significant benefit in favour of the concurrent regimens.

Published meta-analyses only compare survival benefits and local tumour control for combined chemotherapy trials versus radiotherapy alone or radiotherapy with surgery. No information is given on relative risks for normal-tissue damage and morbidity. Several individual trials have reported increased morbidity in combined modality trials in head and neck cancer, particularly for regimens including bleomycin and adriamycin or for concurrent chemotherapy trials in which the same radiotherapy dose is given in both arms. A recent German multicentre trial (Budach *et al.*, 2001) compared accelerated radiotherapy alone with a reduced dose of accelerated radiotherapy and concurrent mitomycin C (MMC) and fluorouracil (5-FU). This trial demonstrated a 10% increase in survival ($P = 0.05$) in favour of the combined modality arm without any increase in early or late toxicity. The combination of concurrent chemotherapy and radiotherapy was more effective than a 10% increase in radiation dose at equitoxic levels of normal-tissue damage.

Lung cancer

A patient based meta-analysis of 52 randomized trials (almost 10 000 patients) comparing chemotherapy with no chemotherapy for non-small-cell lung cancer has been published (Non-small-cell Lung Cancer Collaboration Group, 1995). Older trials using alkylating agent chemotherapy combined with surgery for early-stage disease actually gave higher mortality rates than surgery alone. However, there were small but significant benefits for more modern combined modality regimens containing cisplatin compared with radiotherapy alone or surgery alone, both for early and locally advanced disease (4% and 5% increase in survival at 2 years).

Some trials using concomitant cisplatin-based regimens have demonstrated much larger improvement in local control and survival (Figure 20.7) (Schaake-Koning *et al.*, 1992). In one randomized trial where hyperfractionated radiotherapy was given with or without concurrent carboplatin and etoposide (Jeremic *et al.*, 1996) there was a large improvement in 4-year recurrence-free survival (42% versus 19%), with no increase in acute or late toxicity.

For limited-stage small-cell lung cancer, irradiation of the chest has led to improved local control in many studies (relative to chemotherapy alone).

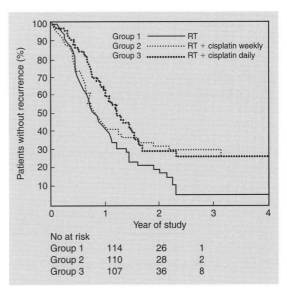

Figure 20.7 *Disease-free survival in patients with non-small-cell lung cancer treated with cisplatin and radiotherapy (RT) was significantly longer than in patients treated with radiotherapy alone (P = 0.015 overall). RT + weekly cisplatin was not significantly different from RT alone (P = 0.15), but RT + daily cisplatin gave significantly improved disease-free survival (P = 0.003) and overall survival (P = 0.009). From Schaake-Koning* et al. *(1992), with permission.*

Alternating chemotherapy–radiotherapy schedules have produced some of the best results ever reported for this disease, with 3-year survival of 26% (Tubiana, 1989), although a high incidence of severe toxicity is reported in some more recent trials.

Gastrointestinal cancer

The most promising results for combined modality studies in cancers of the gastrointestinal tract have been obtained with concomitant irradiation and chemotherapy regimens including 5-FU and either MMC or cisplatin. The RTOG has recently published results from a randomized study of locally advanced oesophageal cancer, which demonstrated a large benefit for treatment with concurrent 5-FU, cisplatin and radiotherapy (50 Gy) versus a higher dose (67 Gy) of radiotherapy alone (27% versus 0% 5-year survival; $P < 0.001$; Al-Sarraf *et al.*, 1997). The study was continued using the combination schedule only and 3-year survival rates of 30% confirmed the original result.

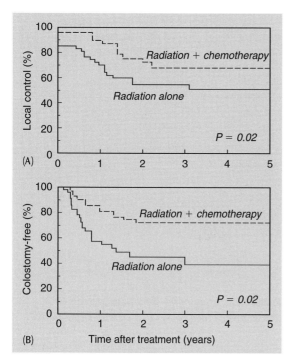

Figure 20.8 *Loco-regional control (panel A) and colostomy-free interval (panel B) in patients with locally advanced anal cancer, randomized to receive radiotherapy alone (solid lines) or radiotherapy with concomitant 5-FU and MMC. The combined treatment led to a significant improvement in both local control (P = 0.02) and colostomy-free interval (P = 0.002). Redrawn from Bartelink* et al. *(1997a), with permission.*

Regimens containing 5-FU have sometimes also demonstrated improved local control and survival in rectal cancer when used postoperatively with radiotherapy. Other trials have, however, not always confirmed this survival advantage, despite increased toxicity. The clearest indication for the use of combined modality in rectal cancer is for patients with Dukes' stage C tumours, where the chemotherapy appeared to delay metastatic spread.

Two randomized trials for anal cancer (UKCCCR, 1996; Bartelink *et al.*, 1997a) demonstrated significant improvement in local control and colostomy-free survival for concurrent chemotherapy and radiotherapy (5-FU infusion with MMC) versus radiotherapy alone (Figure 20.8). A randomized RTOG trial confirmed that the inclusion of MMC in the chemotherapy schedule gave significantly better results than 5-FU and radiotherapy (Flam *et al.*, 1996). This

approach has now been widely adopted as a method of improving local control and avoid mutilating surgery, although overall survival remains unchanged.

Breast cancer

Post-mastectomy radiotherapy reduces the risk of local recurrence from about 30% to 10% in patients with invasive breast cancer. In high risk, pre-menopausal women with positive axillary nodes, adjuvant chemotherapy after mastectomy significantly reduces the risk of distant metastases. Radiotherapy combined with postoperative chemotherapy further reduces loco-regional recurrence and analysis of Danish trials (over 1700 patients) also indicates an improved 10-year survival of 54% versus 45% (Overgaard *et al.*, 1997).

Combined chemotherapy and radiotherapy also reduces the risk of local recurrence and disease-free survival for early breast cancer after breast-conserving surgery. Even a single course of chemotherapy given immediately after surgery has been shown to be effective and such a schedule does not require any delay in starting the radiotherapy (Elkhuizen *et al.*, 2000). However, the benefit of adjuvant chemotherapy is less apparent in women with early-stage disease without any known risk factors (such as young age, elevated p53 status, multifocal disease), since they have a very high survival rate even without chemotherapy. Adjuvant tamoxifen is useful in women with oestrogen-receptor-positive tumours. Concurrent chemotherapy is rarely used for early breast cancer because of increased toxicity and poor cosmetic results.

Combination chemotherapy and radiotherapy has been tested in numerous trials for advanced, inoperable breast cancer. The claims for positive results based on uncontrolled trials have, however, generally not been confirmed in randomized trials, although delayed recurrence without improved survival is seen in some studies. The largest of these randomized trials (Bartelink *et al.*, 1997b) demonstrated a significant improvement in short-term survival for adjuvant chemotherapy but with longer follow-up this difference was no longer significant. Adjuvant hormone therapy did give a significant increase in long-term survival, with a 25% reduction in the death hazard ratio. The best results were in women who received both adjuvant chemotherapy and hormone therapy, with a 35% reduction in the death hazard ratio (Figure 20.9).

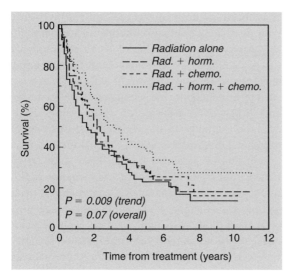

Figure 20.9 *Survival curves for patients with locally advanced breast cancer treated with radiotherapy alone (solid curve) or with adjuvant chemotherapy (short dashes), adjuvant hormone therapy (long dashes) or chemotherapy and hormone therapy (dotted line). Chemotherapy was combination cyclophosphamide, methotrexate and 5-FU. Hormone therapy was tamoxifen for post-menopausal women and ovarian irradiation plus prednisolone for pre-menopausal women. Multivariate analysis of results at 8 years after trial closure demonstrated a significant improvement in survival for patients treated with hormone therapy (P = 0.04) or hormone therapy and chemotherapy (P = 0.02) but not for chemotherapy alone (P = 0.21). Redrawn from Bartelink et al. (1997b), with permission.*

Cancer of the cervix

Until recently the usefulness of combined chemotherapy and radiotherapy for advanced cervical cancer was dubious. The majority of published trials with chemotherapy given before or after radiotherapy demonstrated no significant benefit, and at least one of the larger trials showed a significantly worse survival in the combined modality arm (Tattersall *et al.*, 1995). However, a series of large randomized trials has recently demonstrated a significant survival advantage for concurrent chemotherapy and radiotherapy, with a consistent 30–50% reduction in the relative risk of death compared with radiotherapy alone (Thomas, 1999). The cisplatin-based schedules were superior to

hydroxyurea and weekly, single-agent cisplatin was generally less toxic than multi-drug schedules.

Concomitant chemotherapy and radiotherapy is now standard treatment for bulky cervical cancer in North America, although some questions remain on which chemotherapy schedules should be used and whether the combination schedules offer benefits for all stages of disease. Some of the positive published trials have used relatively low radiation doses or prolonged overall treatment times. Some doubt therefore remains on the magnitude of benefit for concomitant chemotherapy with 'optimal' radiotherapy regimens.

Bladder cancer

Survival rates for locally advanced bladder cancer are poor due to both local recurrence and metastatic spread. Standard treatment is cystectomy with or without radiotherapy. Combined radiation and chemotherapy has been tested with the aim of bladder conservation and reduced metastatic spread. Early pilot studies generally suggested benefits for the combined modality approach but results from the first large randomized trials were disappointing. Neither response rates nor survival were improved by the addition of doxorubicin and 5-FU to radiotherapy. Some of the more recent trials using cisplatin-based regimens do indicate a modest improvement in local control and increased survival for T3/T4 cancers. Results from the large EORTC/MRC trial (BA06/30894 trial, 1999) show a 5% improvement in loco-regional disease-free interval at 3 years, in favour of neoadjuvant chemotherapy (cisplatin, methotrexate and vinblastine). Median survival was prolonged by 6 months, which represents a 5%, non-significant, increase in overall survival. This limited gain was offset by a 1% additional mortality due to chemotherapy. Confirmation of these results in other randomized trials, possibly using alternative chemotherapy schedules, must be awaited before neoadjuvant chemotherapy can be considered as standard treatment for invasive bladder cancer.

Summary of clinical results

Modest gains in tumour response (10–20%) can be achieved with combined modality treatments for several cancer sites. The improvement usually comes from increased local tumour control, which may also lead to improved survival, rather than a decrease in distant metastases. Results for tumour response are generally better for concurrent chemotherapy rather than sequential treatments. However, few of the published trials have scored normal-tissue morbidity and evaluated tumour response at equitoxic dose levels. Some of the published clinical trials demonstrating a gain in favour of combined modality have used suboptimal regimens (e.g. protracted overall treatment times or low total doses) in the radiotherapy-alone arm. Care should therefore be taken in interpretation of the clinical information on combined modality treatments, since not all of the reported improvement in tumour response will translate into a therapeutic gain when compared with optimal radiotherapy alone.

20.7 FUTURE PERSPECTIVES

Advances have been made in recent years with combined modality treatment but the gains are still modest for the majority of solid adult tumours. New drugs with increased activity against the major tumour types are needed, as well as methods for targeting these drugs to tumours. Current approaches include intraperitoneal or intrathecal or intra-arterial drug administration. One example of such targeting is the RADPLAT protocol for advanced head and neck cancer (Kumar and Robbins, 2001). This protocol involves intra-arterial high-dose cisplatin, with systemic thiosulphate rescue, combined with concurrent radiotherapy. Good loco-regional control rates were achieved with organ preservation. Survival is also good when compared retrospectively with conventional treatments, although randomized trials have not yet been done.

Conjugation of cytotoxic drugs to tumour-seeking carriers, and pH- or hypoxia-dependent cyto-toxins also offer possibilities for tumour targeting. Alternatively, cytokines can sometimes be used to stimulate normal-tissue proliferation and recovery, for instance with high-dose chemotherapy and bone marrow transplant regimens for leukaemia. This approach allows drug escalation to levels that would otherwise produce life-threatening toxicity.

Prediction of those patients most likely to benefit from combined modality therapy is also a worthwhile goal (see Chapter 22). If patients who are resistant to chemotherapy could be identified before treatment, this would prevent unnecessary toxicity in this group and the benefits of combined modality therapy could be better evaluated in the remaining chemosensitive group. Current efforts to develop such tests include the measurement of DNA damage and drug–DNA adducts, or chromosome damage. An example of this is antibody staining of cisplatin–DNA adducts, which can be done on buccal cell smears of patients. A small pilot study in 27 patients undergoing concurrent cisplatin and radiotherapy for NSCLC indicated that patients with intense adduct staining had significantly longer survival than those with light staining (Van de Vaart *et al.*, 2000). If confirmed in larger studies, this may be a useful approach for identifying those patients most likely to benefit from combined cisplatin and radiotherapy schedules. Expression profiling, using new micro-array technology, may soon also be able to be used to identify those patients with poor risk factors who would be most likely to benefit from combined modality treatments in general.

As mentioned above (Section 20.4), there are now a number of molecular targets that are being exploited to specifically radiosensitize tumours that over-express the target, e.g. COX-2 or activated oncogenes such as *ras*. Antibodies are also being developed which can block signalling pathways involved in tumour cell proliferation, differentiation and angiogenesis, e.g. EGFR. Many of these novel approaches are already being tested in clinical trials and they offer the potential for much more specific tumour targeting than conventional chemotherapy. Since these agents are cytostatic rather than cytotoxic when used alone, they are likely to be most effective when combined with a cytotoxic agent such as radiotherapy. Further pre-clinical evaluation of these agents is required, using clinically relevant tumour and normal-tissue models and fractionated irradiation schedules. This should provide the basis for a rational translation of these new approaches to the clinic.

KEY POINTS

1. A therapeutic gain is achieved if tumour response after combined modality treatment is increased relative to either agent alone, when

the regimens are evaluated at comparable levels of toxicity.

2. Interaction between drugs and radiation is not a prerequisite for therapeutic gain. Spatial co-operation, independent additive cell kill, or independent killing of subpopulations resistant to the other modality may also lead to a therapeutic gain.

3. Interactions between drugs and radiotherapy are time-dependent. Concurrent chemotherapy gives the best chance of improved response in several cancers (e.g. head and neck, cervix) but may lead to an increase in acute normal-tissue damage. Any increased toxicity must be taken into account when evaluating the therapeutic gain.

4. Modest gains in loco-regional control and/or survival (usually <15%) have been achieved with concomitant chemotherapy and radiotherapy in cancers of head and neck, cervix, anus, oesophagus and in NSCLC.

5. Novel molecular targets are now being exploited to obtain more specific tumour targeting of combined modality treatments.

BIBLIOGRAPHY

Al-Sarraf M, Martz K, Herskovic A *et al.* (1997). Progress report of combined chemoradiotherapy versus radiotherapy alone in patients with esophageal cancer: an intergroup study. *J Clin Oncol* **15**: 277–84.

Bartelink H, Roelofsen F, Eschwege F *et al.* (1997a). Concomitant radiotherapy and chemotherapy is superior to radiotherapy alone in the treatment of locally advanced anal cancer: results of a phase III randomized trial of the European organization for research and treatment of cancer radiotherapy and gastrointestinal cooperative groups. *J Clin Oncol* **15**: 2040–9.

Bartelink H, Rubens RD, Van der Schueren E, Sylvester R (1997b). Hormonal therapy prolongs survival in irradiated locally advanced breast cancer: a European organization for research and treatment of cancer randomized phase III trial. *J Clin Oncol* **15**: 207–15.

BA06/30894 Trial (1999). Neoadjuvant cisplatin, methotrexate, and vinblastin chemotherapy for muscle invasive bladder cancer: a randomised controlled trial. *Lancet* **354**: 533–40.

Brown JM (1993). SR 4233 (tirapazamine): a new anticancer drug exploiting hypoxia in solid tumours. *Br J Cancer* **67**: 1163–70.

Brown JM, Koong A (1991). Therapeutic advantage of hypoxic cells in tumors: a theoretical study. *J Natl Cancer Inst* **83**: 178–85.

Budach VG, Haake K, Stueben G *et al.* (2001). Accelerated chemoradiation to 70.6 Gy is more effective than accelerated radiation to 77.6 Gy alone. Two-year results of a German multicenter randomized trial (Aro 95-6). *Proc ASCO* **20**: 224.

Cohen-Jonathan E, Muschel RJ, McKenna WG *et al.* (2000). Farnesyltransferase inhibitors potentiate the antitumor effect of radiation on a human tumor xenograft expressing activated HRAS. *Radiat Res* **154**: 125–32.

Elkhuizen PH, van Slooten HJ, Clahsen PC *et al.* (2000). High local recurrence risk after breast-conserving therapy in node-negative premenopausal breast cancer patients is greatly reduced by one course of perioperative chemotherapy: a European Organization for Research and Treatment of Cancer Breast Cancer Cooperative Group Study. *J Clin Oncol* **18**: 1075–83.

Flam M, John M, Pajak TF *et al.* (1996). Role of mitomycin in combination with fluorouracil and radiotherapy, and of salvage chemoradiation in the definitive nonsurgical treatment of epidermoid carcinoma of the anal canal: results of a phase III randomized intergroup study. *J Clin Oncol* **14**: 2527–39.

Huang SM, Harari PM (2000). Modulation of radiation response after epidermal growth factor receptor blockade in squamous cell carcinomas: inhibition of damage repair, cell cycle kinetics, and tumor angiogenesis. *Clin Cancer Res* **6**: 2166–74.

Jeremic B, Shibamoto Y, Acimovic L, Milisavljevic S (1996). Hyperfractionated radiation therapy with or without concurrent low-dose daily carboplatin/etoposide for stage III non-small-cell lung cancer: a randomized study. *J Clin Oncol* **14**: 1065–70.

Kishi K, Peterson S, Petersen C *et al.* (2000). Preferential enhancement of tumor radioresponse by a cyclooxygenase-2 inhibitor. *Cancer Res* **60**: 1326–31.

Kumar P, Robbins KT (2001). Treatment of advanced head and neck cancer with intra-arterial cisplatin and concurrent radiation therapy: the RADPLAT protocol. *Curr Oncol Rep* **3**: 50–65.

Munro AJ (1995). An overview of randomized controlled trials of adjuvant chemotherapy in head and neck cancer. *Br J Cancer* **71**: 83–91.

Non-small-cell Lung Cancer Collaborative Group (1995). Chemotherapy in non-small cell lung cancer: a meta-analysis using updated data on individual patients from 52 randomized clinical trials. *Br Med J* **311**: 899–909.

Overgaard M, Hansen PS, Overgaard J et al., for the Danish Breast Cancer Cooperative Group 82b Trial (1997). Postoperative radiotherapy in high-risk premenopausal women with breast cancer who receive adjuvant chemotherapy. *N Engl J Med* **337**: 949–55.

Pearson AE, Steel GG (1984). Chemotherapy in combination with pelvic irradiation: a time-dependence study in mice. *Radiother Oncol* **2**: 49–55.

Pignon JP, Bourhis J, Domenge C, Designé L on behalf of the MCH-NC Collaborative Group (2000). Chemotherapy added to locoregional treatment for head and neck squamous-cell carcinoma: three meta-analyses of updated individual data. *Lancet* **355**: 949–55.

Schaake-Koning C, Van den Bogaert W, Dalesio O et al. (1992). Effects of concomitant cisplatin and radiotherapy on inoperable non-small-cell lung cancer. *N Eng J Med* **326**: 524–30.

Steel GG (1979). Terminology in the description of drug-radiation interactions. *Int J Radiat Oncol Biol Phys* **5**: 1145–50.

Steel GG, Peckham MJ (1979). Exploitable mechanisms in combined radiotherapy-chemotherapy: the concept of additivity. *Int J Radiat Oncol Biol Phys* **5**: 85–91.

Tannock IF (1989). Combined modality treatment with radiotherapy and chemotherapy. *Radiother Oncol* **16**: 83–101.

Tannock IF (1996). Treatment of cancer with radiation and drugs. *J Clin Oncol* **14**: 3156–74.

Tattersall MHN, Lorvidhaya V, Vootiprux V et al. (1995). Randomized trial of epirubicin and cisplatin chemotherapy followed by pelvic radiation in locally advanced cervical cancer. *J Clin Oncol* **13**: 444–51.

Thomas GM (1999). Improved treatment for cervical cancer: concurrent chemotherapy and radiotherapy. *N Engl J Med* **340**: 1198–2000.

Tubiana M (1989). The combination of radiotherapy and chemotherapy: a review. *Int J Radiat Biol* **55**: 497–511.

UKCCCR (1996). Epidermoid anal cancer: results from the UKCCCR randomised trial of radiotherapy alone versus radiotherapy, 5-fluorouracil, and mitomycin. UKCCCR Anal Cancer Trial Working Party. UK Coordinating Committee on Cancer Research. *Lancet* **348**: 1049–54.

Van de Vaart P, Belderbos J, de Jong D et al. (2000). DNA-adduct levels as a predictor of outcome for NSCLC patients receiving daily cisplatin and radiotherapy. *Int J Cancer* **89**: 160–6.

Yarnold JR, Horwich A, Duchesne G et al. (1983). Chemotherapy and radiotherapy for advanced testicular non-seminoma. *Radiother Oncol* **1**: 91–9.

21

Retreatment tolerance of normal tissues

FIONA A STEWART

21.1 INTRODUCTION

Curative radiotherapy usually involves treating a small volume of normal tissue, immediately surrounding the tumour, to the limit of tolerance. In addition there will be a much larger volume of normal tissue, perhaps involving other organs, that receives a lower radiation dose, as a result of shielding techniques or non-overlapping fields. The composite effect of these differing radiation exposures to normal tissues will be to produce a level of morbidity that is the maximum that the therapist judges to be tolerable by the patient. This is what we mean by normal-tissue tolerance (see Section 5.1). The actual value of tolerance dose will depend on the organ, fractionation, field size and concomitant treatments, as well as the performance status of the patient (see Section 11.5).

It is sometimes necessary to consider retreatment of areas that have already received radiation therapy, because of either tumour recurrence or the appearance of a new primary or metastases within the previously irradiated field. Second tumours are particularly common in head and neck cancer, where it has been estimated that up to 30% of patients

will develop new primary tumours within 10 years. Decisions regarding the safe retreatment dose are very complex and depend on the degree of overlap of treatment fields and the timing and extent of tissue regeneration (in relation to the interval between treatments), as well as the extent of residual normal-tissue damage present after the regenerative process is complete. Other important factors are the presence of distant metastases and whether the patient is to be retreated with curative or palliative intent. The risk of normal-tissue damage developing after re-irradiation is much greater than after the initial treatment. These risks have to be weighed against the morbidity that could result from no re-irradiation, or from any alternative means of retreatment. Surgery of heavily irradiated tissues is, for example, often difficult.

This chapter summarizes the main findings from experimental studies on the retreatment tolerance of normal tissues. In order to compare data on different normal tissues using various fractionation regimens, the results have been recalculated in terms of the biologically effective dose (BED) using linear-quadratic (LQ) fractionation concepts (see Section 12.10). For each study we have recalculated the BED for a defined level of tolerance and this is referred to as the BED$_t$. The intensity of both the initial treatment and the retreatment is specified as a percentage of the BED$_t$. A summary of clinical data for re-irradiation is also given (Sections 21.9 and 21.10).

21.2   SKIN

Published data for re-irradiation tolerance of acute skin reactions in rodents are consistent in demonstrating very good recovery from the initial damage with restoration of almost full radiation tolerance within 8 weeks (Figure 21.1). Recovery is faster after initial treatments that are below tolerance. The extent and time-course of this recovery fits well with the known time-scale for the proliferative response of epithelial cells after irradiation (see Section 4.4). Accelerated proliferation in irradiated rodent skin occurs from about 8 days after treatment, depending on dose. A certain level of cell depletion is required to trigger this accelerated proliferation, which is then maintained until the original cell number is restored and tissue regeneration is complete. This occurs more rapidly after low radiation doses (i.e. after less cell killing) than after high doses. Some results demonstrate that repeated re-irradiation with large doses progressively reduces retreatment tolerance, consistent with some reduction in stem-cell density of the epidermis.

Fewer data are available for an analysis of late radiation effects after re-irradiation of the skin but some results suggest a poorer retreatment tolerance (50–70% BED$_t$) than for acute reactions (Figure 21.2).

This is not a universal finding, however, and other studies have demonstrated very good retreatment tolerance of both rat and pig skin for late deformity end-points. Re-irradiation tolerance for late skin reactions is probably only markedly compromised when these reactions are consequential to a severe acute reaction (see Section 4.2), rather than representing a true independent late response.

Re-irradiation tolerance for acute damage in other rapidly dividing mucosal tissues, such as intestine,

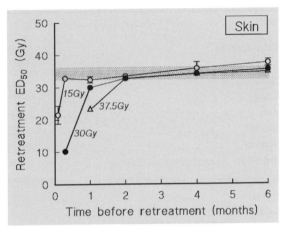

Figure 21.1 *Retreatment tolerance of mouse skin. The vertical scale gives the retreatment dose required for a specified level of skin damage (ED$_{50}$ for desquamation) at different times after priming treatments with 15–37.5 Gy. The shaded area shows the range of ED$_{50}$ doses for the same level of skin damage for previously untreated mice. Adapted from Terry* et al. *(1989), with permission.*

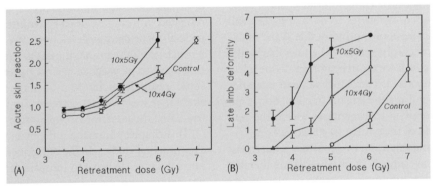

Figure 21.2 *Differences in retreatment tolerance for acute skin reactions (A) or late limb deformity (B) after irradiation of mouse hind limbs. Re-irradiation was at 6 months after 10 × 4 Gy, 10 × 5 Gy or no previous irradiation. Retreatment tolerance for late deformity was much less than for acute skin reactions. Redrawn from Brown and Probert (1975), with permission.*

are in general agreement with results for skin. There are currently no pre-clinical data available to determine the retreatment tolerance for late bowel complications after previous irradiation.

21.3 BONE MARROW

Depletion of the various cellular compartments of the bone marrow after irradiation is rapidly followed by a regenerative phase. After whole-body irradiation with single doses of up to 4 Gy, recovery of the stem cells (colony-forming units, CFU-S) to near normal levels occurs in about 2–4 weeks. After higher doses, a sustained depletion of CFU-S may occur, although this is masked by their ability to maintain a normal content of peripheral blood cells through increased proliferation of committed precursor cells. However, repeated injury such as re-irradiation can reduce the stem-cell pool to below a critical level. The CFU-S which survive repeated irradiations also have a reduced capacity for self-renewal. In such circumstances any additional insult could tip the balance towards severe bone marrow insufficiency. It can be concluded that some recovery of retreatment tolerance does occur in bone marrow if sufficient time is allowed for stem-cell regeneration, but estimates of the level of recovery based on mature peripheral blood cells can be very misleading.

21.4 LUNG

Experimental studies in mice demonstrate good recovery of re-irradiation tolerance in the lung for the endpoint of lethal pneumonitis. Recovery is similar to that seen in rapidly dividing tissues such as the skin and intestine, despite the slow turnover times of most lung cell types. Mice given initial doses of 6–8 Gy to both lungs (approximately 30–50% of the BED_t for pneumonitis) could be re-irradiated with doses equivalent to 100% BED_t at 4–8 weeks (Terry et al., 1988). Recovery was slower after higher initial doses, and after initial doses in excess of 70% of the BED_t the full re-irradiation tolerance was never achieved (Figure 21.3).

Two separate waves of lethality occur in mice after thoracic irradiation (see Figure 4.5). The first, at 12–16 weeks, is characterized by histologically

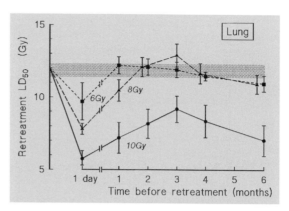

Figure 21.3 *Retreatment tolerance of the mouse lung. The vertical scale gives the LD_{50} for retreatment at the indicated times after priming treatment with 6, 8, or 10 Gy. The shaded area shows the range of LD_{50} values for previously untreated animals. Adapted from Terry et al. (1988), with permission.*

identifiable pneumonitis, whereas later deaths are associated with increased collagen deposition and fibrosis in the lungs of some strains of mice (Travis et al., 1980). The remarkably good re-irradiation tolerance of lung that has been demonstrated in experimental studies only applies for the pneumonitis phase. It is likely that retreatment tolerance for late lung damage may be poorer, although few quantitative data are available.

The time-course for recovery and retreatment tolerance of radiation-induced pneumonitis is consistent with the early increase in proliferation of type II pneumocytes seen at 2–8 weeks after irradiation (see Section 4.4). The proliferation of these cells is apparently able to fully compensate for cell loss after low radiation doses. Re-irradiation after high doses leads to an earlier onset of pneumonitis, particularly for retreatment after a short interval. This is consistent with the target-cell population being nearer to a critical level of cell depletion and requiring longer for repopulation.

21.5 SPINAL CORD

Therapists are understandably cautious of re-irradiating the spinal cord because of the disastrous consequences (myelopathy and paralysis) of exceeding tolerance. It has also been assumed that long-term regeneration will not be effective in such a

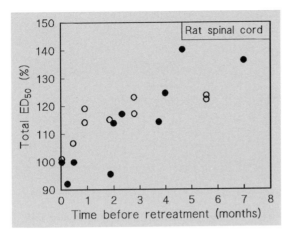

Figure 21.4 *Long-term recovery after irradiation of rat cervical cord. The total cumulative isoeffective dose (for 50% paresis) is expressed as a percentage of BED$_t$ and as a function of the interval between initial and re-irradiation dose. Data are for 3-week-old (○) and adult (●) rats; adapted from Ruifrok* et al. *(1992), White and Hornsey (1980), van der Kogel* et al. *(1982), with permission.*

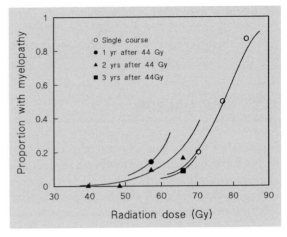

Figure 21.5 *Retreatment tolerance of the monkey spinal cord. At 2–3 years after an initial dose of 44 Gy (i.e 60% of BED$_t$), a further 66 Gy (85% of BED$_t$) could be delivered with less than 20% incidence of myelopathy for the same level of damage. All treatments were given with 2.2 Gy per fraction. From Ang* et al. *(2001), with permission.*

slowly proliferating tissue. However, there is now substantial experimental evidence that indicates that some long-term recovery does occur in the irradiated cord and that retreatment, albeit with a reduced dose, is feasible.

Analysis of data obtained on spinal cord damage in rats, mice and guinea-pigs allows three main conclusions to be made. First, re-irradiation tolerance is inversely related to the size of the initial dose. Second, retreatment tolerance increases from 2 to 26 weeks after the initial treatment and third, substantial residual injury remains, particularly after high-dose initial treatment. The maximum total dose (i.e. initial plus retreatment doses) that could be given in the rat was about 140% of the BED$_t$ for 50% paralysis after the initial treatment (Figure 21.4).

The findings from rodent studies are supported by a study of re-irradiation tolerance of monkey spinal cord (Figure 21.5). In these experiments an 8 cm length of the cervical cord was initially irradiated with 20 fractions of 2.2 Gy, which is equivalent to about 60% of the BED$_t$ for a 50% incidence of paralysis (76 Gy in 2.2 Gy fractions). After 1, 2 or 3 years, the monkeys were re-irradiated with a further 18–30 fractions of 2.2 Gy. Re-irradiation doses of 66 Gy (equivalent to about 85% BED$_t$) resulted in less

than 20% paralysis. This represents a considerable recovery of the damage induced from the initial treatment.

The increase in tolerance observed for the spinal cord with longer retreatment intervals may be related to proliferation in the putative target cells (oligo-dendrocytes and endothelial cells). Mature glial cells normally have a slow turnover with a lifespan of approximately 140 days, but a marked increase in proliferation occurs at about 21 weeks after irradiation. This is followed by a rapid decline in the glial cell numbers, which precedes the onset of white-matter necrosis. An early, transient increase in glial cell proliferation also occurs at 3 weeks after irradiation. This could be related to the early regenerative phase that has been identified in glial progenitor cells after irradiation of the rat optic nerve (van der Maazen *et al.*, 1992). The main wave of increased proliferation actually occurs rather later than the period over which dose-sparing effects are observed for retreatment in rodent models (4–14 weeks, see Figure 21.4). This late proliferative burst in glial cells may actually precipitate further damage as lethally damaged cells attempt to divide. The precise influence of stimulated proliferation of glial cells for regeneration of the spinal cord after irradiation remains unclear.

21.6 BLADDER

Studies on re-irradiation tolerance of mouse bladder have not demonstrated any recovery from late, functional damage (as measured by increased frequency of urination or reduced bladder compliance) for retreatment intervals of 12 or 40 weeks compared with short (1-day) intervals (Figure 21.6). The latent period before expression of permanent functional damage was also much shorter in animals that were re-irradiated, even after low, sub-tolerance initial doses.

The normal, untreated bladder epithelium has a very slow cell turnover time, in excess of 200 days, but it is capable of rapid proliferation in response to injury (see Section 4.4). The increase in proliferation is maximal at about 40 weeks after irradiation. Bladders re-irradiated at this time therefore have a urothelium that is in a state of rapid turnover, and damage from the second treatment is expressed without the usual delay. Despite the evidence for extensive epithelial proliferation after bladder irradiation, retreatment studies have failed to demonstrate any dose-sparing effect. Compensatory proliferation precipitates an early expression of damage without preventing or reducing the extent of late damage. This implies that epithelial damage, although involved in the initial urination

frequency response, is not the only factor that determines persistent bladder damage.

21.7 KIDNEY

The kidneys are among the most radiosensitive of organs, although the latent period before expression of functional damage may be very long, particularly after low doses. Progressive, dose-dependent development of functional damage, without apparent recovery, has been clearly demonstrated in rodents. This is consistent with clinical observations of slowly progressive renal damage, which can be expressed over periods of at least 7 years after irradiation. Based on the known profiles for development of renal radiation injury, it is perhaps obvious that re-irradiation after large initial doses is unlikely to be feasible. However, it is less obvious what the situation would be after low, sub-tolerance doses to the kidneys.

In view of the slowly progressive nature of renal radiation injury, the absence of any measurable renal dysfunction at the time of retreatment certainly

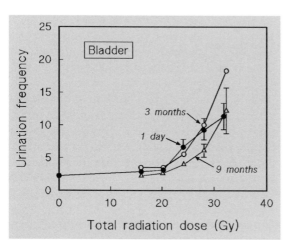

Figure 21.6 *Dose–response curves for late bladder damage after irradiation with two doses separated by 1 day (●), 3 months (○) or 9 months (△). The total dose for a given amount of damage did not increase with increasing time from first treatment. From Stewart et al. (1990), with permission.*

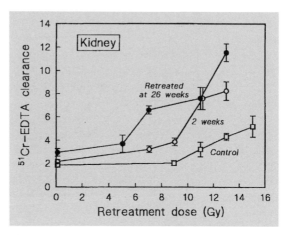

Figure 21.7 *Dose–response curves for renal damage at 35 weeks after re-irradiation. The initial treatment was 6 Gy, given at either 2 weeks (○) or 26 weeks (●) before retreatment. The response of age-matched control animals (no initial dose) is also shown. Renal damage was worse for retreatment with the longer 26-week interval than for a shorter interval, indicating progression of sub-threshold damage rather than recovery. From Stewart et al. (1989), with permission.*

cannot be interpreted as a sign that there is no latent or residual injury. Experimental studies demonstrate that doses of radiation too low to produce overt renal damage do significantly reduce the tolerance to retreatment; none of these studies has demonstrated any long-term functional recovery of the kidney. After an initial dose of only 6 Gy (25% of the BED_t), the tolerance of retreatment actually *decreases* with time (Figure 21.7). This is consistent with there being continuous progression of occult damage in the interval between treatments and implies that re-irradiation of the kidneys after any previous irradiation should be approached with extreme caution.

21.8 SUMMARY OF EXPERIMENTAL DATA

Figure 21.8 summarizes results from experimental studies for re-irradiation tolerance in four tissues where recovery following a range of initial treatments has been evaluated. Both the initial and the retreatment radiation exposures are shown as a percentage of the tolerance dose for a defined level of damage, calculated in terms of BED_t using the appropriate α/β ratio for each tissue. The dashed lines indicate the relationship that would be expected if there is full repair of sublethal injury but no proliferative

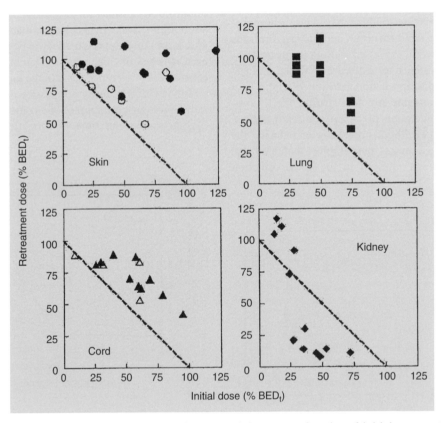

Figure 21.8 *Summary of retreatment tolerance in four normal tissues, as a function of initial treatment dose. Both the initial and retreatment doses have been calculated as a percentage of BED_t. The dashed line indicates the retreatment doses that would be expected if there is full recovery of sublethal damage but no long-term proliferative recovery. Sources: skin desquamation (●) or late deformity (○), Brown and Probert (1975), Denekamp (1975), Wondergem and Haveman (1987), Simmonds et al. (1989), Terry et al. (1989); lung pneumonitis (■), Terry et al. (1988); cervical (▲) or lumbar (△) spinal cord, Hornsey et al. (1982), van der Kogel et al. (1982), White and Hornsey (1980), Ruifrok et al. (1992), Ang et al. (1993), Mason et al. (1993), Wong et al. (1993), Lavey et al. (1994); kidney (◆), Stewart et al. (1989, 1994).*

recovery and no cell depletion between the treatments. Where data points for retreatment fall above the dashed line (in skin, lung and cord) this indicates some long-term recovery in the tissue. Where the data points fall below the dashed line (kidney), this indicates damage progression and cell depletion rather than recovery. The general conclusion is that, on the basis of studies in experimental animals, several normal tissues are able to tolerate considerable retreatment with radiation. The phenomenon is not, however, universal and care must be applied in translating this into the clinic.

21.9   CLINICAL EXPERIENCE WITH RETREATMENT OF THE HEAD AND NECK REGION

It is difficult to analyse clinical reports of retreatment tolerance in the same way as the animal data since they are based on retrospective analyses of heterogeneous groups of patients treated with a wide range of doses and irradiation techniques, sometimes in combination with chemotherapy or hyperthermia. There are, however, several reported series each with at least 50 patients retreated with radiotherapy only for recurrent head and neck cancer (Table 21.1). General conclusions from these and other smaller studies are that local control rates of over 30% can be achieved with total retreatment doses of at least 50–60 Gy but that lower doses are ineffective (local control <15%). Serious complications (mainly subcutaneous fibrosis, trismus and impaired hearing) occur in up to 60% of long-term survivors and are generally associated with higher total cumulative doses and short retreatment intervals.

The largest series (Lee *et al.*, 1997) included a total of 654 patients with recurrent undifferentiated or poorly differentiated nasopharyngeal carcinoma. Due to the number of patients included and the relative homogeneity of the group, it is possible to make more detailed analyses of the results from this series. Extent of local recurrence was the most important prognostic factor, with 35% local control for stage T1 compared with 11% for T3 recurrences. Initial and retreatment doses were calculated in terms of biologically effective dose (BED) using α/β ratios of 10 Gy for tumour control and 2 or 3 Gy for late normal-tissue damage. Using this approach, the initial treatment

dose had no influence on tumour control but the retreatment BED was significantly correlated with local control probability. The 5-year local control for T1/T2 recurrences treated with >70 Gy BED_{10} was 40% compared with only 14% for BED_{10} of <60 Gy. The risk of late complications, by contrast, was strongly associated with initial dose but was only weakly associated with retreatment dose.

Comparison of these results with well-matched groups of over 3000 patients treated with a single course of radiotherapy allow three important conclusions to be made (Lee *et al.*, 2000). First, patients re-irradiated for recurrent nasopharyngeal cancer had a significantly lower complication-free survival rate than patients who received a single course of therapy (48% versus 81% 5-year actuarial rates). Second, some recovery of normal-tissue damage did occur between the initial and re-irradiation (higher total cumulative doses were tolerated in retreatment schedules than expected from single-course data). Third, the most important determinant of late normal-tissue damage was severity of damage after the initial treatment.

21.10   CLINICAL EXPERIENCE WITH RETREATMENT OF OTHER SITES

Early experience of retreatment of recurrent cervical cancer was not encouraging. Local control and survival rates were generally poor (10–20% long-term survival) and complication rates were high (30–50%). More recent studies, in which patients had been carefully selected on the basis of volume and location of the cancer, demonstrated much better results, particularly for retreatment using brachytherapy. In these studies, long-term survivals of 60% with a severe complication rate below 15% could be achieved after full-dose retreatment (Puthawala *et al.*, 1982; Russell *et al.*, 1987). Favourable conditions were small tumour volume, second primary malignancies and retreatment with brachytherapy. Unfavourable conditions were recurrent cancer, large tumour volume and retreatment with external-beam therapy.

Retreatment of recurrent lung cancer with palliative intent (30 Gy/3 weeks) leads to improvement of symptoms (cough, dyspnoea, pain and haemoptysis) in the majority of patients and good tumour response if patients are selected on the basis of having achieved

Table 21.1 Re-irradiation of recurrent head and neck cancer

Reference	Site	Number of patients	Retreatment dose (Gy)	Local control[a] (%)	Survival[a] (%)	Complications (%)
External-beam with or without brachytherapy						
Yan et al. (1983)	NP	219	<50–>50	11	18	>29[b]
Wang (1987)	NP	51	<50–>60 ± IC boost	NS	0 < 60 Gy 45 > 60 Gy	6
Emami et al. (1987)	All except NP	52 36	<50 >50	11 25	17	28
Levendag et al. (1992)	All	55 18	18–84 EB 35–95 (incl. IC)	29 50	**20** 20	7 **17**
Pryzant et al. (1992)	NP	53	28–99 (incl. IC)	**35**	**21**[c]	**17**
Stevens et al. (1994)	All	100	19–77 ± IC	32	17[c] 37[d]	9
Lee et al. (1997)	NP	654	7.5–70 ± IC	23/32	**16**	**48**
De Crevoisier et al. (1998)	ALL	169	60–65		9[e]	>41
Teo et al. (1998)	NP	103	60–82 (incl. IC)	**15**	**8**	61
192I brachytherapy alone						
Syed et al. (1978)	All	64	45–60	48	44/2 years	30
Mazeron et al. (1987)	OP	70	50–71	**69**	14	27
Langlois et al. (1988)	T, OP	123	31–84	**59**	**24**	23

IC, intracavitary irradiation; NP, nasopharynx; NS, not stated; OP, oropharynx; P, pharyngeal wall; T, tongue.
Data in bold show actuarial estimates.

[a] Local control and survival rates are at 5 years unless otherwise specified.

[b] Complication rate for patients surviving ⩾5 years.

[c] Survival in patients with recurrent tumour.

[d] Survival in patients with new primary tumour.

[e] Most patients also received chemotherapy.

a good response to initial therapy (Montebello *et al.*, 1993). Palliative retreatment is associated with lower levels of oesophagitis than the initial treatment and no increase in pneumonitis. The retreatment doses are of course much lower than the initial doses and most patients will succumb to their disease before late damage (i.e. lung fibrosis) has time to be expressed.

Palliative re-irradiation of recurrent metastatic brain lesions, recurrent rectal cancer and breast cancer also has given significant improvement of symptoms in the majority of patients, with some long-term survivors. Modern three-dimensional treatment planning and conformal, stereotactic (brain) or intra-operative (rectum) radiotherapy reduces the risk of serious normal-tissue damage.

The limited clinical data available suggest that retreatment can be carried out in some sites and provides either effective palliation without a high incidence of morbidity or, when a full dose is given, reasonably good local control and survival with an increased risk of morbidity. In some situations this risk is probably acceptable when weighed against the alternative option of no treatment.

KEY POINTS

1. Rapidly dividing tissues are capable of proliferative recovery to completely restore the original cell numbers and full re-irradiation tolerance within a few months of irradiation. After several repeated irradiations there may be a reduced density of stem cells leading to decreased retreatment tolerance.
2. In terms of pneumonitis, the lung is capable of extensive long-term recovery after radiation doses below tolerance. Retreatment tolerance for late lung damage is less than for pneumonitis.
3. The spinal cord is capable of moderate long-term recovery, and cumulative (initial plus retreatment) doses of up to 140% of the full BED can be given if the interval before retreatment is at least 6 months.
4. Re-irradiation tolerance for late bladder damage does not increase with increasing time between treatments. The onset of late bladder

damage occurs much earlier after retreatment than after previous partial-tolerance irradiation.
5. Re-irradiation tolerance of the kidney decreases with increasing interval between treatments, indicative of continuous progression of sub-threshold damage.
6. Clinical experience confirms that re-irradiation can usefully be given in selected cases although the risk of normal-tissue complications is greater than for a single treatment.

BIBLIOGRAPHY

Ang KK, Price RE, Stephens LC *et al.* (1993). The tolerance of primate spinal cord to re-irradiation. *Int J Radiat Oncol Biol Phys* **25**: 459–64.

Ang KK, Jian G-L, Feng Y, Stephens LC, Tucker SL, Price RE (2001). Extent and kinetics of recovery of occult spinal cord injury. *Int J Radiat Oncol Biol Phys* **50**: 1013–20.

Brown JM, Probert JC (1975). Early and late radiation changes following a second course of irradiation. *Radiology* **115**: 711–16.

De Crevoisier R, Bourhis J, Domenge C *et al.* (1998). Full-dose reirradiation for unresectable head and neck carcinoma: experience at the Gustave-Roussy Institute in a series of 169 patients. *J Clin Oncol* **16**: 3556–62.

Denekamp J (1975). Residual radiation damage in mouse skin 5 to 8 months after irradiation. *Radiology* **115**: 191–5.

Emami B, Bignardi M, Spector GJ, Devineni VR, Hederman MA (1987). Reirradiation of recurrent head and neck cancers. *Laryngoscope* **97**: 85–8.

Hornsey S, Myers R, Warren P (1982). Residual injury in the spinal cord after treatment with X-rays or neutrons. *Br J Radiol* **55**: 516–19.

Langlois D, Hoffstetter S, Malissard L, Pernot M, Taghian A (1988). Salvage irradiation of oropharynx and mobile tongue about 192 iridium brachytherapy in centre Alexis Vautrin. *Int J Radiat Oncol Biol Phys* **14**: 849–53.

Lavey RS, Taylor JMG, Tward JD *et al.* (1994). The extent, time course, and fraction size dependence of mouse spinal cord recovery from radiation injury. *Int J Radiat Oncol Biol Phys* **30**: 609–17.

Lee AW, Foo W, Law SC *et al.* (1997). Reirradiation for recurrent nasopharyngeal carcinoma: factors affecting the therapeutic ratio and ways for improvement. *Int J Radiat Oncol Biol Phys* **38**: 43–52.

Lee AWM, Foo W, Law SCK et al. (2000). Total biological effect on late reactive tissues following reirradiation for recurrent nasopharyngeal carcinoma. *Int J Radiat Oncol Biol Phys* **46**: 865–72.

Levendag PC, Meeuwis CA, Visser AG (1992). Reirradiation of recurrent head and neck cancers: external and/or interstitial radiation therapy. *Radiother Oncol* **23**: 6–15.

Mason KA, Withers HR, Chiang C-S (1993). Late effects of radiation on the lumbar spinal cord of guinea pigs: retreatment tolerance. *Int J Radiat Oncol Biol Phys* **26**(4): 643–8.

Mazeron JJ, Langlois D, Glaubiger D et al. (1987). Salvage irradiation of oropharyngeal cancers using iridium 192 wire implants: 5-year results of 70 cases. *Int J Radiat Oncol Biol Phys* **13**: 957–62.

Montebello JF, Aron BS, Manatunga AK, Horvath JL, Peyton FW (1993). The re-irradiation of recurrent bronchogenic carcinoma with external beam irradiation. *Am J Clin Oncol* **16**: 482–8.

Pryzant RM, Wendt CD, Delclos L, Peters LJ (1992). Retreatment of nasopharyngeal carcinoma in 53 patients. *Int J Rad Oncol Biol Phys* **22**: 941–7.

Puthawala AA, Syed AM, Fleming PA, DiSaia PJ (1982). Re-irradiation with interstitial implant for recurrent pelvic malignancies. *Cancer* **50**: 2810–14.

Ruifrok ACC, Kleiboer BJ, van der Kogel AJ (1992). Reirradiation tolerance of the immature rat spinal cord. *Radiother Oncol* **23**: 249–56.

Russell AH, Koh W-J, Markette K et al. (1987). Radical re-irradiation for recurrent or second primary carcinoma of the female reproductive tract. *Gynecol Oncol* **27**: 226–32.

Simmonds RH, Hopewell JW, Robbins MEC (1989). Residual radiation-induced injury in dermal tissue: implications for retreatment. *Br J Radiol* **62**: 915–20.

Stevens KR, Jr, Britsch A, Moss WT (1994). High-dose reirradiation of head and neck cancer with curative intent. *Int J Radiat Oncol Biol Phys* **29**: 687–98.

Stewart FA, Luts A, Lebesque JV (1989). The lack of long term recovery and reirradiation tolerance in the mouse kidney. *Int J Radiat Biol* **56**: 449–62.

Stewart FA, Oussoren Y, Luts A (1990). Long-term recovery and reirradiation tolerance of mouse bladder. *Int J Radiat Oncol Biol Phys* **18**: 1399–406.

Stewart FA, Oussoren Y, Van Tinteren H, Bentzen SM (1994). Loss of reirradiation tolerance in the mouse kidneys with increasing time after single or fractionated partial tolerance doses. *Int J Radiat Biol* **66**: 169–79.

Syed AMN, Feder BH, George FW, III, Neblett D (1978). Iridium-192 afterloaded implant in the retreatment of head and neck cancers. *Br J Radiol* **51**: 814–20.

Teo PML, Kwan WH, Chan ATC et al. (1998). How successful is high-dose (>60 Gy) reirradiation using mainly external beams in salvaging local failures of nasopharyngeal carcinoma? *Int J Radiat Oncol Biol Phys* **40**: 897–913.

Terry NHA, Tucker SL, Travis EL (1988). Residual radiation damage in murine lung assessed by pneumonitis. *Int J Radiat Oncol Biol Phys* **14**: 929–38.

Terry NHA, Tucker SL, Travis EL (1989). Time course of loss of residual radiation damage in murine skin assessed by retreatment. *Int J Radiat Biol* **55**: 271–83.

Travis EL, Down JD, Holmes SJ, Hobson B (1980). Radiation pneumonitis and fibrosis in mouse lung assayed by respiratory frequency and histology. *Radiat Res* **84**: 133–43.

van der Kogel AJ, Sissingh HA, Zoetelief J (1982). Effect of X rays and neutrons on repair and regeneration in the rat spinal cord. *Int J Radiat Oncol Biol Phys* **8**: 2095–7.

van der Maazen RWM, Verhagen I, Kleiboer BJ, van der Kogel AJ (1992). Repopulation of O-2A progenitor cells after irradiation of the adult rat optic nerve analyzed by an in vitro clonogenic assay. *Radiat Res* **132**: 82–6.

Wang CC (1987). Reirradiation of recurrent nasopharyngeal carcinoma – treatment techniques and results. *Int J Radiat Oncol Biol Phys* **13**: 953–6.

White A, Hornsey S (1980). Time dependent repair of radiation damage in the rat spinal cord after X rays and neutrons. *Eur J Cancer* **16**: 957–62.

Wondergem J, Haveman J (1987). The effect of previous treatment on the response of mouse feet to irradiation and hyperthermia. *Radiother Oncol* **10**: 253–61.

Wong CS, Poon JK, Hill RP (1993). Reirradiation tolerance in the rat spinal cord: influence of level of initial damage. *Radiother Oncol* **26**: 132–8.

Yan JH, Hu YM, Gu Z (1983). Radiation therapy of recurrent nasopharyngeal carcinoma. *Acta Radiol Oncol* **22**: 23–8.

FURTHER READING

Morris DE (2000). Clinical experience with retreatment for palliation. *Semin Radiat Oncol* **10**: 210–21.

Nieder C, Milas L, Ang KK (2000). Tissue tolerance to reirradiation. *Semin Radiat Oncol* **10**: 200–9.

Stewart FA (1999). Re-treatment after full-course radiotherapy: is it a viable option? *Acta Oncol* **38**: 855–62.

Stewart FA, van der Kogel AJ (1994). Retreatment tolerance of normal tissue. *Semin Radiat Oncol* **4**: 103–11.

22

Individualization of therapy

ADRIAN C BEGG AND CATHARINE ML WEST

22.1 INTRODUCTION

The goal of a predictive assay is to obtain information that can be used to choose a treatment protocol, so that each individual patient will receive optimal treatment. At present, treatment choice is usually based on parameters such as tumour site, histological type, tumour stage and performance status. Within these broad categories, some tumours show a greater response to radiotherapy than others. If these tumours could be identified before treatment, alternative therapies might be selected that may give a better chance of cure than the standard therapy. A practical distinction between a prognostic and a predictive assay is that a prognostic assay gives information on the likely outcome after standard treatment, whereas a predictive assay will additionally indicate how the patient could best be treated. For example, the presence of a p53 mutation may indicate that a patient has a worse prognosis without suggesting an obvious treatment, whereas patients with high proliferative tumours could be assigned to a treatment designed to minimize this disadvantage, such as accelerated fractionation.

Individual patients also differ in their tolerance of radiation therapy. Among a group of patients given the same treatment protocol, some suffer more severe normal-tissue reactions than others. It is these severe reactors that limit the dose of radiation that can be prescribed to a group of patients. If severe reactors could be identified prior to therapy, it might be possible to improve their management (e.g. by reducing the treatment dose) as well as that of the rest of the patient group (e.g. by increasing their dose).

This chapter deals with these two aspects of the individualization of radiation therapy: predicting tumour response and predicting normal-tissue response.

What determines tumour response after radiotherapy?

Radiobiological determinants of tumour response to radiotherapy can be put into three broad categories: intrinsic radiosensitivity, proliferation rate and the extent of hypoxia. In addition to these radiobiological parameters, other factors that can determine success or failure are tumour size at the time of treatment and the metastatic potential of the tumour. Large tumours are harder to control than small tumours simply because there are more cells to kill and this will require higher doses. This will be true even if intrinsic radiosensitivity, hypoxia and repopulation rates are equal at small and large sizes. Tumour size should therefore be taken into account when assessing the performance of a predictive assay. Metastatic potential is clearly important for survival and should be considered separately from factors affecting local tumour control.

For each of the three radiobiological parameters mentioned above, there are several measurement options. Intrinsic radiosensitivity, for example, depends upon damage induced at a given dose and the extent of repair (see Section 8.5). Damage induction and repair can be measured at the DNA or chromosome level, or the genes and microenvironmental factors involved in the processes can also be studied. Alternatively, cell survival can be measured, which represents the final outcome of all these processes. Examples of end-points for measuring tumour proliferation are the thymidine-labelling index, Ki67 index, S-phase fraction and T_{pot} (see Section 2.7). The level of tumour hypoxia has been assessed using many different methods that include oxygen electrodes, hypoxia-specific probes and non-invasive imaging (see Section 15.4). As it is not known which end-point/method will provide the best response predictor, this chapter concentrates on those that have been most widely tested in human tumours.

22.2   INTRINSIC RADIOSENSITIVITY

Evidence for the importance of tumour cell radiosensitivity comes from studies of the low-dose region of the radiation survival curve obtained for cells of different histological origins. Parameters describing the initial part of the survival curves (SF_2 or the initial slope) could discriminate between cell lines derived from tumours of different histological type, grouped according to clinical radioresponsiveness. For instance, cell lines derived from lymphomas were significantly more radiosensitive than those derived from melanomas (Deacon et al., 1984; Fertil and Malaise, 1985). In experimental tumours, SF_2 measured in vitro was shown to correlate with tumour response in vivo to fractionated radiotherapy in some studies (Bristow and Hill, 1990; Rofstad, 1994) although not in all (Taghian et al., 1993). A number of groups also showed significant differences in the radiosensitivity of tumour lines derived from a single histological type.

The above data led to studies measuring the SF_2 of human tumours and relating the findings to

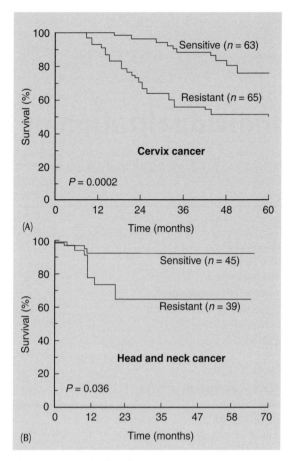

Figure 22.1 *Intrinsic radiosensitivity (SF_2), measured* in vitro *on tumour biopsy material, can predict local control in (A) cervix cancer (West et al., 1997) and (B) head and neck cancer (Bjork-Eriksson et al., 2000).*

radiotherapy response. Although only a limited number of studies have been reported, this is probably due to poor success rates in growing human tumour cells *in vitro*, and insufficient accrual of patients. Some studies used non-clonogenic assays that were easier to perform than the 'gold standard' clonogenic assay. Results of these have generally been disappointing, partly due to the inadequacy of the assays and perhaps also due to the inclusion of surgery in the treatment (Brock et al., 1990). A few studies have used a clonogenic assay in which cell suspensions from biopsies were irradiated *in vitro* and assayed by colony growth in soft agar. Studies on carcinoma of the cervix have shown that tumour cell radiosensitivity is a highly significant and independent prognostic factor for radiotherapy outcome (West et al., 1997). In the Swedish

Table 22.1 *Summary of clinical studies in which tumour-cell radiosensitivity has been measured* in vitro *using either a clonogenic or a growth assay and the results correlated with radiotherapy outcome*

Study type	Tumour type	Assay	n	P-value	Reference
Prospective	H&N	Clonogenic	84	0.036	Bjork-Eriksson *et al.* (2000)
Prospective	H&N	Clonogenic	38	NS	Stausbol-Gron & Overgaard (1999)
Prospective	Cervix	Clonogenic	128	0.0002	West *et al.* (1997)
Prospective	H&N	CAM	56	0.001	Girinsky *et al.* (1994)
Prospective	H&N	CAM	40	NS	Brock *et al.* (1992)
Retrospective*	Gliomas[†]	Clonogenic	85	NS	Taghian *et al.* (1993)
Prospective	Gliomas[†]	MTT	24	0.01	Ramsay *et al.* (1992)
Retrospective	H&N[†]	Clonogenic	34	NS	Schwartz *et al.* (1992)
Prospective	Cervix[†]	Clonogenic	33	NS	Allalunis-Turner *et al.* (1992)

H&N, head and neck; NS, $P > 0.05$.
*Combined analysis of data from three centres.
[†]Studies involved early or long-term passage cell lines rather than primary tumours.

study shown in Figure 22.1, SF_2 was measured in patients with head and neck cancer. In both cases the patients with sensitive tumour cells showed a better response, confirming the importance of tumour radiosensitivity as a prognostic factor for radiotherapy outcome (Bjork-Eriksson *et al.*, 2000). Other studies have also shown that SF_2 measurements are predictive for outcome but there are some that did not, in particular studies that established cell lines prior to assay (Table 22.1). In general, one can conclude that intrinsic tumour cell radiosensitivity is an important factor determining radiotherapy response but that we do not yet have a reliable method for its measurement in primary human tumours.

The main disadvantages of the colony assay are its poor success rate for growing human tumours in the laboratory (at best only 70% of tumours will form colonies) and the time needed to produce data (often up to 4 weeks). In recent years there have been many studies evaluating alternative assays that generate results in less than 1 week. Examples are those that measure chromosome damage (Brown *et al.*, 1992; Coco Martin *et al.*, 1999), DNA damage (Marples *et al.*, 1998), glutathione (Silvestrini *et al.*, 1997) and apoptosis. Studies comparing results of these assays with clonogenic cell death in cell lines have shown variable results, some detecting significant correlations, others not. Similarly, some assays have been used in clinical studies and yielded results that correlated with radiotherapy outcome whilst others have shown no correlation. More recent studies have looked at gene expression, mutations, or functional assays

for some of the many genes involved in the recognition and repair of radiation-induced damage to DNA, mostly in *in vitro* cell lines. Genes that have been investigated include *Ku80*, *DNA-PKcs*, *ATM*, *XRCC1*, *Rad51*, among others. The correlations with intrinsic radiosensitivity were found in most cases to be poor and few of these have been sufficiently evaluated as predictive assays for radiotherapy. However, this avenue of research is supported by the observation that the expression of a single DNA repair gene (*Ku70*) in human tumours correlates with radiotherapy outcome (Wilson *et al.*, 2000).

The conclusion based on the studies of tumour-cell radiosensitivity that have been performed so far is that cell-based assays probably have very limited clinical utility as predictive assays but have been useful in confirming at least one mechanism underlying differences in response of tumours to radiotherapy. The future may lie in obtaining a greater understanding of tumour response to radiation, and differences in gene expression profiles among tumours.

22.3 TUMOUR HYPOXIA

Tumour hypoxia is a key factor involved not only in determining resistance to treatment but also in malignant progression. Evidence for an association between measurements of hypoxia in individual human tumours and response to radiation therapy has been summarized in Section 15.4 and Table 15.2.

An important finding was the demonstration that hypoxic tumours respond poorly not only to radio-therapy but also when treated with surgery alone. This is consistent with data showing that hypoxia plays a key role in tumour progression by promoting both angiogenesis and metastasis.

There are limitations on the use of Eppendorf electrodes to measure hypoxia in human tumours, in particular that they are only suitable for studies on accessible tumours. Alternative methods with poten-tial for more widespread clinical use are therefore being sought. The efficacy of hypoxia-specific probes such as pimonidazole (Raleigh *et al.*, 2000) and EF5 (Evans *et al.*, 2000) are now being investigated clinically. Bioreduction of these drugs occurs only under hypoxic conditions, followed by binding of the reduced products to macromolecules. Bound adducts can be detected with specific antibodies, allowing measurement by immunohistochemistry (Figure 22.2) or flow cytometry. The use of fluorin-ated derivatives of such bioreductive drugs allows their detection by non-invasive PET (Rischin *et al.*, 2001), MRS and MRI methods (Aboagye *et al.*, 1998). These have the additional advantage of sam-pling the whole tumour and not just a small part of it. These drugs depend upon hypoxia for their reduc-tion, although there are factors that can influence their quantification that make them a less direct measure of hypoxia than is the case with electrodes. However, despite their potential pitfalls, it is clear that such agents hold considerable promise for quan-tifying hypoxia in human tumours. Results correlat-ing such measurements with outcome after therapy are awaited with interest.

Other methods that are being used to measure tumour hypoxia in the clinic include cross-sectional imaging methods (CT, MRI) (Cooper *et al.*, 2000) and the comet assay (Aquino-Parsons *et al.*, 1999). Gene expression studies provide surrogate intrinsic markers of hypoxia. Hypoxia is known to affect the expression of a variety of genes, many of which are suppressed but some of which are up-regulated. The main advantage of using endogenous markers for hypoxia is that it eliminates the need to inject a marker drug. Examples of such markers are HIF1α (hypoxia-inducible factor), HIF1-dependent genes such as *VEGF* (vascular endothelial growth factor), *glut-1* and *glut-3* (regulating glucose transport), and *CAIX* (regulating pH). There is much activity at the time of writing comparing intrinsic markers of hypoxia with

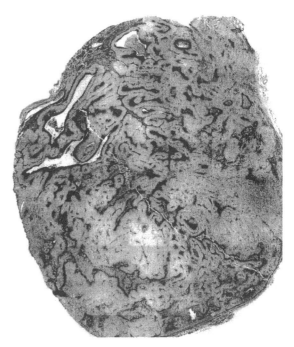

Figure 22.2 *Detection of hypoxia using the bioreductive marker pimonidazole, given 12 hours before operation to remove a squamous carcinoma of the head and neck. Immunohistochemistry with anti-pimonidazole antibody shows black regions that indicate areas of hypoxia scattered throughout the tumour (Janssen H, Begg AC, Haustermans K, unpublished).*

both other methods for measuring hypoxia and radiotherapy outcome (Figure 22.3). Although no relationship has been seen between *VEGF* expression and measurements of hypoxia in human tumours (Raleigh *et al.*, 1998; West *et al.*, 2001b), promising data have been obtained using *CAIX* (Wykoff *et al.*, 2000; Loncaster *et al.*, 2001) and *glut-1* (Airley *et al.*, 2001). In addition, measuring lactate levels in tumours (an end-point of anaerobic glycolysis known to increase under hypoxia) has been shown to predict treatment outcome (Walenta *et al.*, 2000).

Another possible surrogate marker of hypoxia is to measure tumour vascularity. This is of interest because of the known association between hypoxia and angiogenesis, and the fact that oxygen is delivered via a tumour blood supply that varies from ordered to chaotic. A variety of methods have been used to score vascularity, including intercapillary distance, vascular density, hotspots, and the proportion of tumour areas greater than a fixed distance from a

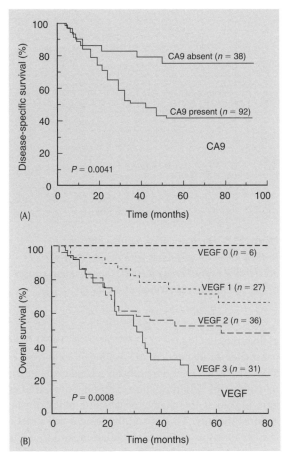

Figure 22.3 *Expression of hypoxia-related endogenous markers can predict outcome after radiotherapy for cervix cancer. (A) Carbonic anhydrase-IX (CA9; Loncaster et al., 2001); (B) vascular endothelial growth factor (VEGF; Loncaster et al., 2000).*

vessel. Some of these methods have shown a positive correlation with outcome, others negative, and this is a difficult area at the present time (West *et al.*, 2001b).

22.4   TUMOUR CELL REPOPULATION

The importance of tumour proliferation is most clearly shown by the higher doses required to control a tumour when overall treatment time is increased (see Figure 14.3). Further evidence comes from studies showing loss of local control as a result of gaps in treatment, whether planned or unplanned. There is also increasing evidence from randomized trials

that accelerated regimens can improve outcome (see Section 14.4).

Methods available for measuring tumour proliferation have been described in Section 2.9. These include measurement of mitotic index, labelling index with thymidine analogues, the proportion of cells in the S phase of the cell cycle by DNA flow cytometry, tumour potential doubling time and using antibodies to detect proliferation-associated proteins. The majority of clinical radiotherapy studies to date have sought to measure T_{pot}. Use of this parameter was encouraged by the fact that estimates of effective doubling times for repopulation, derived from clinical studies with different overall times, were similar in magnitude to pre-treatment T_{pot} values, despite the fact that results in experimental tumours were not encouraging. T_{pot} is relatively easy to measure clinically, whereas measurement of other kinetic parameters such as the cell cycle time or volume double time may be difficult or impractical. A considerable number of studies on T_{pot} have been carried out, some of which showed a relationship with outcome while most did not. A multicentre analysis of over 470 head and neck cancer patients treated with radiotherapy alone showed a lack of significance of T_{pot} as a predictor (Begg *et al.*, 1999). Labelling index was a significant prognostic factor in the univariate analysis of this multicentre study (Figure 22.4) and a number of other studies have shown a significant although usually weak correlation between labelling index and radiotherapy outcome.

The conclusion from these studies is that pre-treatment T_{pot} estimates are not sufficiently robust for determining tumour cell proliferation during radiotherapy. Labelling index also appears unlikely to provide a strong predictor. The lack of correlation with radiotherapy outcome, however, should not be interpreted as showing that proliferation is unimportant but rather that T_{pot} is not the best way of measuring it.

Most flow-cytometry studies have failed to discriminate satisfactorily between normal and malignant cells, clearly a serious weakness. Some investigators have combined an immunohistochemical measurement of labelling index, where malignant cells can be distinguished morphologically, with DNA synthesis time measured by flow cytometry. This is probably more accurate than using flow cytometry for both parameters, especially for diploid tumours where normal/malignant distinctions cannot be made on the basis of DNA content. Use of this approach could lead to improved evaluation of clinical correlations.

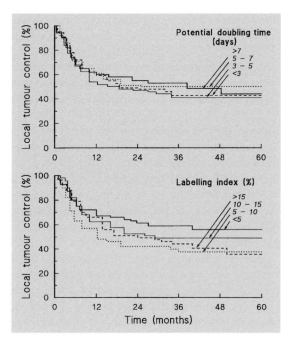

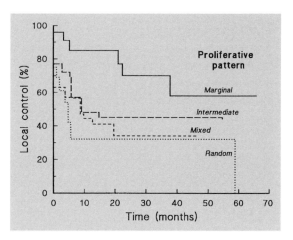

Figure 22.5 *The tissue proliferative pattern after BrdUrd labelling correlates with outcome after accelerated radiotherapy (CHART) for squamous cancer of the head and neck (Wilson et al., 1995).*

Figure 22.4 *Correlation between pre-treatment cell kinetic parameters and local tumour control after radiotherapy for advanced head and neck cancer in a multicentre study (Begg et al., 1999). In univariate analyses, labelling index (LI) was significant (P = 0.02) although T$_{pot}$ was not. In a multivariate analysis, neither parameter reached significance.*

More recently, as the complex mechanisms involved in cell cycle regulation are unravelled, an increasing number of gene products have been identified that may serve as possible markers of cell proliferation. Examples are cell-cycle regulatory proteins, including cyclins (D1, E, A), cyclin-dependent kinases (ckd1, cdk2) and cyclin-dependent kinase inhibitors (p16, p27). In addition, knowledge of growth stimulatory and inhibitory pathways mediated by growth factors and cytokines via membrane receptors (e.g. the epidermal growth factor receptor, EGFR) is increasing and could be used in the future to help predict not only proliferation rates but also changes in proliferation rate in response to damage.

Finally, there are two examples where kinetic parameters have been used in a setting not strictly designed to measure proliferation rates. Some investigators have shown that the pattern of IdUrd or BrdUrd labelling, whether marginal, random or mixed, correlates with outcome in certain situations,

as illustrated in Figure 22.5 (Wilson *et al.*, 1995). This parameter is independent of labelling index and other kinetic parameters, and is probably related to the extent or pattern of differentiation. Second, some studies have looked at the change of labelling index during or after therapy. This is simply using a cell kinetic marker to assess response to radiation, and thus the aim is to predict radiosensitivity rather than proliferation rate.

22.5 PREDICTION OF NORMAL-TISSUE TOLERANCE

The existence of individuals with extreme sensitivity to ionizing radiation was first realized with the publication of a study showing the hypersensitivity of fibroblasts cultured from a patient with ataxia telangiectasia (Taylor *et al.*, 1975). This was followed by several reports showing that severely over-reacting patients had hypersensitive fibroblasts. These individuals are rare (Burnet *et al.*, 1998) and the small numbers have no impact on doses routinely given to radiotherapy patients. However, in the 1980s there was increasing evidence for a range of radiosensitivities within the 'normal' population without known genetic syndromes. Significant differences between individuals were found in radiosensitivity of fibroblasts taken from normal donors (Little *et al.*, 1988).

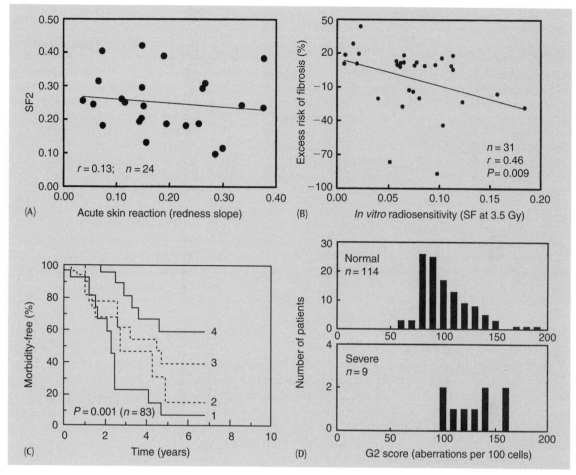

Figure 22.6 *The results of four studies aiming to predict radiotherapy damage to normal tissues, using fibroblasts or lymphocytes. (A) Intrinsic radiosensitivity of fibroblasts* in vitro *failed to predict early reactions (Begg et al., 1993) but (B) showed a significant correlation with late tissue damage (Johansen et al., 1994). (C) Intrinsic radiosensitivity of lymphocytes was significantly correlated with late morbidity in cervix cancer patients (West et al., 2001a) (patients were stratified according to SF$_2$ quartiles with 1 < 0.25, 2 < 0.30, 3 < 0.40 and 4 > 0.40; in the analysis shown all morbidity was used, i.e. mild, moderate and severe); also (D) with severe reactions in breast cancer patients (Barber et al., 2000). These results indicate the contribution of target-cell radiosensitivity to normal-tissue reactions but the assays are impractical for routine clinical use.*

Further evidence for differences in cellular radiosensitivity as a determinant of normal-tissue response to radiotherapy came from studies showing that inherent differences between individuals dominated normal-tissue reactions over and beyond other contributing factors (Turesson *et al.*, 1996). It is probably the 5% most sensitive individuals within a patient population that limit the dose that can safely be applied in radiotherapy, assuming that these patients suffer bad reactions because of high intrinsic radiosensitivity

and not because of dosimetric errors. As it is not known beforehand who these patients are, radiation doses to many patients may be too low, jeopardizing their chance of cure.

In the 1990s, studies were carried out to test whether the severity of normal-tissue damage could be predicted from the *in vitro* radiosensitivity of normal cells. In general, no correlations were seen with acute radiation effects (Figure 22.6A), but several small studies showed correlations between fibroblast radiosensitivity

Table 22.2 *Radiosensitivity as a predictor of normal-tissue damage: correlation with late effects in larger studies using radiosensitivity measured with cell-based assays*

Study type	Tumour type	Cell type	Assay	n^a	P-value	Reference
Retrospective	Breast	Fibroblast	Clonogenic	104	0.19	Peacock *et al.* (2000)
Retrospective	Breast	Fibroblast	Clonogenic	79	0.13	Russell *et al.* (1998)
Retrospective	Breast	LCL[b]	MTT[c]	56	<0.02	Ramsay and Birrell (1995)
Retrospective	Breast	Fibroblast	Clonogenic	31	0.009	Johansen *et al.* (1994)
Retrospective	Breast/H&N	Fibroblast	Clonogenic	46	0.005	Oppitz *et al.* (2001)
Prospective	H&N	Fibroblast	Clonogenic	17	0.0013	Geara *et al.* (1993)
Prospective	H&N	Lymphocyte	LDA[d]	21	NS	Geara *et al.* (1993)
Prospective	H&N	Fibroblast	Clonogenic	25	0.50	Rudat *et al.* (1997)
Prospective	Cervix	Lymphocyte	LDA[d]	83	0.002	West *et al.* (2001a)

NS, Non-significant.

[a] Number of patients included in study.

[b] Lymphoblastoid cell lines.

[c] MTT, a tetrazolium-based colorimetric cell growth assay.

[d] LDA, limiting dilution assay; a type of clonogenic assay.

and the severity of late effects (Burnet *et al.*, 1992; Geara *et al.*, 1992; Johansen *et al.*, 1994). The results of the latter study are summarized in Figure 22.6B. Disappointingly, many subsequent larger studies have failed to confirm these findings (Table 22.2). There have been two large studies using peripheral blood lymphocytes (Ramsay and Birrell, 1995; West *et al.*, 2001a; see Table 22.2) and both showed that their radiosensitivity correlated with the severity of late effects (Figure 22.6C).

As with tumour radiosensitivity, there is continuing interest in evaluating rapid assays, including the measurement of chromosome damage (Russell *et al.*, 1995; Slonina *et al.*, 2000) or DNA damage (Kiltie *et al.*, 1999). The results of Barber *et al.* (2000) based on studies of G2 chromosomal radiosensitivity are shown in Figure 22.6D. Although some significant correlations with late effects have been reported, other studies have shown no relationship. A general problem with assays studied to date is that experimental variability has been relatively large compared with inter-individual differences in radiosensitivity. As for radiosensitivity studies on tumours, there is interest in looking at the many possible genes that determine the radiosensitivity of an individual at both the gene and protein levels (Appleby *et al.*, 1997; Carlomango *et al.*, 2000). Such studies are likely to expand with the increasing use of microarray technology.

Although clonogenic survival is a crucial concept for tumour control, it may be less significant for late

normal-tissue damage. The radiosensitivity of fibroblasts from a fibrosis-prone mouse strain was found by Dileto and Travis (1996) to be identical to that from a fibrosis-resistant strain. There is therefore increasing interest in seeking other factors that can influence the response of normal tissues to radiation. Cytokines are known to play an important role in the development of radiation injury in normal tissues (Rodemann and Bamberg, 1995). TGF-β is a key cytokine in fibrosis development (see Section 4.3), influencing fibroblast proliferation and differentiation, and plasma levels of this cytokine have been shown to correlate with radiation-induced lung damage in patients (Anscher *et al.*, 1998). This is a growing and important area of research and increased understanding of the molecular pathogenesis of radiation injury may lead to better predictions of the radiation response of normal tissues.

22.6 HOW ACCURATE MUST AN ASSAY BE?

When deciding whether to base treatment decisions on the results of a predictive assay, its accuracy in terms of false positives and false negatives must be considered. Consider, for example, using an assay for tumour cell proliferation to select patients for conventional radiotherapy or accelerated radiotherapy with dose reduction. If a high proliferation rate is predicted, then accelerated fractionation would be the choice. However, a false-positive result (the tumour actually having a slow proliferation rate) would lead to an unnecessary dose reduction that would compromise the probability of cure for that patient. Statistical procedures therefore need to be applied when assessing an assay, such as defining ROC (receiver-operating characteristics; sensitivity versus specificity) curves. Such calculations indicate the effect on morbidity and tumour control for the whole population but are unfortunately rarely done. The P-value for a correlation with outcome is not sufficient for assessing the clinical usefulness of an assay.

22.7 HOW SHOULD CLINICIANS RESPOND TO PREDICTION RESULTS?

If and when reliable predictive assays are developed, their use will depend on available alternative treatments. The following are some examples of possible courses of action. Patients with very hypoxic tumours could be assigned to treatments that include hypoxia-modifying or hypoxia-exploiting agents, such as ARCON or tirapazamine (see Section 16.8). Tumours with fast proliferation rates will be candidates for accelerated fractionation, or radiotherapy given together with drugs designed to combat proliferation, such as EGFR inhibitors. Patients with radioresistant tumours may benefit from switching to an alternative therapeutic modality such as surgery or chemotherapy, combined chemoradiotherapy or the radiation dose to the tumour could be increased using some form of conformal radiotherapy. If reliable predictive information is available on normal-tissue sensitivity, possible strategies would be to reduce the radiation dose for radiosensitive individuals, to offer a radio-protective agent (only if the agent does not also protect tumours), or to use a post-radiotherapy approach such as anti-TGF-β antibodies or antisense oligonucleotides.

22.8 THE FUTURE

More successful prediction will undoubtedly come through better understanding of tumour and normal-tissue biology and radiobiology. Knowledge of the genetic basis of radiosensitivity has increased enormously in the Past few years (see Section 9.4), and continued rapid progress can be expected. This knowledge has yet to be applied to the prediction of therapeutic responses. The field of 'array technology' can be expected to play a significant role: mRNA microarrays in which the expression of many thousands of genes can be measured simultaneously seems to be a promising development. It is a technology that has already provided some success in improving prognosis in a number of disease areas. Protein and tissue array technologies are also developing fast and could usefully complement cDNA or oligomer array data. One of the problems of the predictive assay studies to date has been that they have mostly been limited to one parameter. In view of the complex nature of tumour and normal-tissue responses to radiation therapy, these technologies clearly have great potential, allowing the simultaneous study of genes that are associated with such characteristics as hypoxia, proliferation, radiosensitivity or differentiation.

KEY POINTS

1. For tumours, there is evidence that intrinsic radiosensitivity, proliferation and hypoxia are important determinants of radiotherapy outcome.
2. For normal tissues, the radiosensitivity of target cells is a key aspect, but other important factors such as cytokine production may have a useful role in individualizing treatment choices.
3. Reliable and clinically applicable predictive assays are not yet available for the known primary determinants of tumour or normal-tissue responses.
4. Future progress depends on better understanding of the molecular and cell biology of the radiation response and is likely to be aided by modern molecular techniques such as array technology.

BIBLIOGRAPHY

Aboagye EO, Kelson AB, Tracy M, Workman P (1998). Preclinical development and current status of the fluorinated 2-nitroimidazole hypoxia probe N-(2-hydroxy-3,3,3-trifluoropropyl)-2-(2-nitro-1-imidazolyl) acetamide (SR 4554, CRC 94/17): a non-invasive diagnostic probe for the measurement of tumor hypoxia by magnetic resonance spectroscopy and imaging, and by positron emission tomography. *Anticancer Drug Des* **13**: 703–30.

Airley RA, Loncaster J, Davidson SE *et al.* (2001). Glucose transporter Glut-1 expression correlates with tumor hypoxia and predicts metastasis-free survival in advanced carcinoma of the cervix. *Clin Cancer Res* **7**: 928–34.

Allalunis-Turner MJ, Day RS, Pearcey RG, Urtasun RC (1992). Radiosensitivity testing in gynecological tumors and malignant gliomas. In: *Radiation Research: a Twentieth Century Perspective* (eds Dewey WC, Edington M, Fry RJM, Hall EJ, Whitmore GF), Vol. 2, pp. 712–15. Academic Press, San Diego.

Anscher MS, Kong FM, Andrews K *et al.* (1998). Plasma transforming growth factor β1 as a predictor of radiation pneumonitis. *Int J Radiat Oncol Biol Phys* **41**: 1029–35.

Appleby JM, Barber JB, Levine E *et al.* (1997). Absence of mutations in the ATM gene in breast cancer patients with severe responses to radiotherapy. *Br J Cancer* **76**: 1546–9.

Aquino-Parsons C, Luo C, Vikse CM, Olive PL (1999). Comparison between the comet assay and the oxygen microelectrode for measurement of tumor hypoxia. *Radiother Oncol* **51**: 179–85.

Barber JB, Burrill W, Spreadborough AR *et al.* (2000). Relationship between in vitro chromosomal radiosensitivity of peripheral blood lymphocytes and the expression of normal-tissue damage following radiotherapy for breast cancer. *Radiother Oncol* **55**: 179–86.

Begg AC, Russell NS, Knaken H, Lebesque JV (1993). Lack of correlation of human fibroblast radiosensitivity *in vitro* with early skin reactions in patients undergoing radiotherapy. *Int J Radiat Biol* **64**: 393–405.

Begg AC, Haustermans K, Hart AA *et al.* (1999). The value of pretreatment cell kinetic parameters as predictors for radiotherapy outcome in head and neck cancer: a multicenter analysis. *Radiother Oncol* **50**: 13–23.

Bjork-Eriksson T, West C, Karlsson E, Mercke C (2000). Tumor radiosensitivity (SF2) is a prognostic factor for local control in head and neck cancers. *Int J Radiat Oncol Biol Phys* **46**: 13–19.

Bristow RG, Hill RP (1990). Comparison between *in vitro* radiosensitivity and *in vivo* radioresponse in murine tumor cell lines. II: *In vivo* radioresponse following fractionated treatment and *in vitro/in vivo* correlations. *Int J Radiat Oncol Biol Phys* **18**: 331–45.

Brock WA, Baker FL, Wike JL, Sivon SL, Peters LJ (1990). Cellular radiosensitivity of primary head and neck squamous cell carcinomas and local tumor control. *Int J Radiat Oncol Biol Phys* **18**: 1283–6.

Brock WA, Brown BW, Goepfer J, Peters LJ (1992). In vitro radiosensitivity of tumor cells and local tumor control by radiotherapy. In: *Radiation Research: a Twentieth Century Perspective* (eds Dewey WC, Edington M, Fry RJM, Whitmore GF), pp. 969–99. Academic Press, San Diego.

Brown JM, Evans J, Kovacs MS (1992). The prediction of human tumour radiosensitivity *in situ*: an approach using chromosome aberrations detected by fluorescence *in situ* hybridization. *Int J Radiat Oncol Biol Phys* **24**: 279–86.

Burnet NG, Nyman J, Turesson I *et al.* (1992). Potential for improving radiotherapy cure rates by predicting normal-tissue tolerance from *in vitro* cellular radiation sensitivity. *Lancet* **339**: 1570–1.

Burnet NG, Johansen, J, Turesson I, Nyman J, Peacock JH (1998). Describing patients' normal tissue reactions: concerning the possibility of individualising radiotherapy dose prescriptions based on potential predictive assays of normal tissue radiosensitivity. *Int J Cancer* **79**: 606–13.

Carlomagno F, Burnet NG, Turesson I *et al.* (2000). Comparison of DNA repair protein expression and activities between human fibroblast cell lines with different radiosensitivities. *Int J Cancer* **85**: 845–9.

Coco Martin JM, Mooren E, Ottenheim C *et al.* (1999). Potential of radiation-induced chromosome aberrations to predict radiosensitivity in human tumour cells. *Int J Radiat Biol* **75**: 1161–8.

Cooper RA, Carrington B, Loncaster JM *et al.* (2000). Tumour oxygenation levels correlate with dynamic contrast-enhanced MRI parameters in carcinoma of the cervix. *Radiother Oncol* **57**: 53–9.

Deacon J, Peckham MJ, Steel GG (1984). The radioresponsiveness of human tumours and the initial slope of the cell survival curve. *Radiother Oncol* **2**: 317–23.

Dileto CL, Travis EL (1996). Fibroblast radiosensitivity *in vitro* and lung fibrosis *in vivo*: comparison between a fibrosis-prone and fibrosis-resistant mouse strain. *Radiat Res* **146**: 61–7.

Evans SM, Hahn S, Pook DR *et al.* (2000). Detection of hypoxia in human squamous cell carcinoma by EF5 binding. *Cancer Res* **60**: 2018–24.

Fertil B, Malaise EP (1985). Intrinsic radiosensitivity of human cell lines is correlated with radioresponsiveness of human tumors: analysis of 101 published survival curves. *Int J Radiat Oncol Biol Phys* **11**: 1699–707.

Geara FB, Peters LJ, Ang KK *et al.* (1992). Intrinsic radiosensitivity of normal human fibroplasts and lymphocytes after high- and low-dose-rate irradiation. *Cancer Res* **52**: 6348–52.

Geara FB, Peters LJ, Ang KK, Wike JL, Brock WA (1993). Prospective comparison of *in vitro* normal cell radiosensitivity and normal-tissue reactions in radiotherapy patients. *Int J Radiat Oncol Biol Phys* **27**: 1173–9.

Girinsky T, Bernheim A, Lubin R *et al.* (1994). *In vitro* parameters and treatment outcome in head and neck cancers treated with surgery and/or radiation: cell characterization and correlations with local control and overall survival. *Int J Radiat Oncol Biol Phys* **30**: 789–94.

Johansen J, Bentzen SM, Overgaard J, Overgaard M (1994). Evidence for a positive correlation between *in vitro* radiosensitivity of normal human skin fibroblasts and the occurence of subcutaneous fibrosis after radiotherapy. *Int J Radiat Biol* **66**: 407–12.

Kiltie AE, Ryan AJ, Swindell R *et al.* (1999). A correlation between residual radiation-induced DNA double-strand breaks in cultured fibroblasts and late radiotherapy reactions in breast cancer patients. *Radiother Oncol* **51**: 55–65.

Little JB, Nove J, Strong LC, Nichols WW (1988). Survival of human diploid skin fibroblasts from normal individuals after X-irradiation. *Int J Radiat Biol* **54**: 899–910.

Loncaster J, Cooper RA, Logue JP, Davidson SE, West CML (2000). Vascular endothelial growth factor (VEGF) expression is a prognostic factor for radiotherapy outcome in advanced carcinoma of the cervix. *Br J Cancer* **83**: 620–5.

Loncaster J, Harris A, West CML (2001). CA IX expression, a potential new intrinsic marker of hypoxia: correlations with tumour oxygen measurements and prognosis in locally advanced carcinoma of the cervix. *Cancer Res* **61**: 6394–9.

Marples B, Longhurst D, Eastham AM, West CM (1998). The ratio of initial/residual DNA damage predicts intrinsic radiosensitivity in seven cervix carcinoma cell lines. *Br J Cancer* **77**: 1108–14.

Oppitz U, Baier K, Wulf J, Schakowski R, Flentje M (2001). The *in vitro* colony assay: a predictor of clinical outcome. *Int J Radiat Biol* **77**: 105–10.

Peacock J, Ashton A, Bliss J *et al.* (2000). Cellular radiosensitivity and complication risk after curative radiotherapy. *Radiother Oncol* **55**: 173–8.

Raleigh JA, Calkins-Adams DP, Rinker LH *et al.* (1998). Hypoxia and vascular endothelial growth factor expression in human squamous cell carcinomas using pimonidazole as a hypoxia marker. *Cancer Res* **58**: 3765–8.

Raleigh JA, Chou SC, Calkins-Adams DP, Ballenger CA, Novotny DB, Varia MA (2000). A clinical study of hypoxia and metallothionein protein expression in squamous cell carcinomas. *Clin Cancer Res* **6**: 855–62.

Ramsay J, Birrell G (1995). Normal-tissue radiosensitivity in breast cancer patients. *Int J Radiat Oncol Biol Phys* **31**: 339–44.

Ramsay J, Ward R, Bleehen NM (1992). Radiosensitivity testing of human malignant gliomas. *Int J Radiat Oncol Biol Phys* **24**: 675–80.

Rischin D, Peters L, Hicks R, Hughes P, Fisher R, Hart R, Sexton M, D'Costa I, von Roemeling R (2001). Phase-I trial of concurrent tirapazamine, cisplatin, and radiotherapy in patients with advanced head and neck cancer. *J Clin Oncol* **19**: 535–42.

Rodemann HP, Bamberg M (1995). Cellular basis of radiation-induced fibrosis. *Radiother Oncol* **35**: 83–90.

Rofstad EK (1994). Fractionation sensitivity (alpha/beta ratio) of human melanoma xenografts. *Radiother Oncol* **33**: 133–8.

Rudat V, Dietz A, Conradt C, Weber KJ, Flentje M (1997). *In vitro* radiosensitivity of primary human fibroblasts. Lack of correlation with acute radiation toxicity in patients with head and neck cancer. *Radiother Oncol* **43**: 181–8.

Russell NS, Artlett CF, Bartelink H, Begg AC (1995). Use of fluorescence *in situ* hybridization to determine the relationship between chromosome aberrations and cell survival in eight human fibroblast strains. *Int J Radiat Biol* **68**(2): 185–96.

Russell NS, Grummels A, Hart AA *et al.* (1998). Low predictive value of intrinsic fibroblast radiosensitivity for fibrosis development following radiotherapy for breast cancer. *Int J Radiat Biol* **73**: 661–70.

Schwartz JL, Beckett MA, Mustafi R, Vaughan ATM, Weichselbaum RR (1992). Evaluation of different in vitro assays of inherent sensitivity as predictors of radiotherapy response. In *Radiation Research: a Twentieth Century Perspective* (eds Dewey WC, Edington M, Fry RJM, Hall EJ, Whitmore GF), Vol. 2, pp. 716–21. Academic Press, San Diego.

Silvestrini R, Veneroni S, Benini E *et al.* (1997). Expression of p53, glutathione S-transferase-pi, and Bcl-2 proteins and benefit from adjuvant radiotherapy in breast cancer. *J Natl Cancer Inst* **89**: 639–45.

Slonina D, Klimek M, Szpytma T, Gasinska A (2000). Comparison of the radiosensitivity of normal-tissue cells with normal-tissue reactions after radiotherapy. *Int J Radiat Biol* **76**: 1255–64.

Stausbol-Gron B, Overgaard J (1999). Relationship between tumour cell *in vitro* radiosensitivity and clinical outcome after curative radiotherapy for squamous cell carcinoma of the head and neck. *Radiother Oncol* **50**: 47–55.

Taghian A, Ramsay J, Allalunis-Turner J *et al.* (1993). Intrinsic radiation sensitivity may not be the major determinant of the poor clinical outcome of glioblastoma multiforme. *Int J Radiat Oncol Biol Phys* **25**: 243–9.

Taylor AM, Harnden DG, Arlett CF *et al.* (1975). Ataxia telangiectasia: a human mutation with abnormal radiation sensitivity. *Nature* **258**: 427–9.

Turesson I, Nyman J, Holmberg E, Oden A (1996). Prognostic factors for acute and late skin reactions in radiotherapy patients. *Int J Radiat Oncol Biol Phys* **36**: 1065–75.

Walenta S, Wetterling M, Lehrke M *et al.* (2000). High lactate levels predict likelihood of metastases, tumor recurrence, and restricted patient survival in human cervical cancers. *Cancer Res* **60**: 916–21.

West CM, Davidson SE, Roberts SA, Hunter RD (1997). The independence of intrinsic radiosensitivity as a prognostic factor for patient response to radiotherapy of carcinoma of the cervix. *Br J Cancer* **76**: 1184–90.

West CML, Davidson SE, Elyan SAG *et al.* (2001a). Lymphocyte radiosensitivity is a significant prognostic factor for morbidity in carcinoma of the cervix. *Int J Radiat Oncol Biol Phys* **51**: 10–15.

West CML, Loncaster JA, Cooper RA, Wilks DP, Bromley M (2001b). Tumor vascularity: a histological measure of angiogenesis and hypoxia. *Cancer Res* **61**: 2907–10.

Wilson CR, Davidson SE, Margison GP, Jackson SP, Hendry JH, West CML (2000). Expression of Ku70 correlates with survival in carcinoma of the cervix. *Br J Cancer* **83**: 1702–6.

Wilson GD, Dische S, Saunders MI (1995). Studies with bromodeoxyuridine in head and neck cancer and accelerated radiotherapy. *Radiother Oncol* **36**: 189–97.

Wykoff CC, Beasley NJ, Watson PH *et al.* (2000). Hypoxia-inducible expression of tumor-associated carbonic anhydrases. *Cancer Res* **60**: 7075–83.

Glossary of terms in radiation biology

α/β ratio: The ratio of the parameters α and β in the linear-quadratic model; used to quantify the fractionation sensitivity of tissues (*q.v.*).

Accelerated fractionation: Reduction in overall treatment time; a schedule in which the average rate of dose delivery exceeds the equivalent of 10 Gy per week in 2 Gy fractions.

Acute hypoxia: Low oxygen concentrations associated with the transient closing and opening of blood vessels. Sometimes called *transient* hypoxia.

Additive: A situation in which the effect of a combination is the sum of the effects of the separate treatments (= 'independent cell kill').

Analogue: A chemical compound structurally similar to another but differing by a single functional group.

Angiogenesis: The process of formation of new blood vessels.

Apoptosis: A mode of rapid cell death after irradiation in which the cell nucleus displays characteristic densely staining globules and some at least of the DNA is subsequently broken down into internucleosomal units. Sometimes postulated to be a 'programmed' and therefore potentially controllable process.

Autoradiography: Use of a photographic emulsion to detect the distribution of a radioactive label in a tissue specimen.

Biologically effective dose (BED): In fractionated radiotherapy, the total dose that would be required in very small dose fractions to produce a particular effect, as indicated by the linear-quadratic equation. Otherwise known as extrapolated total dose (ETD). BED values calculated for different α/β ratios are not strictly comparable. For time-dose calculations, EQD_2 (equivalent dose in 2 Gy fractions) is preferred (see Section 13.1).

BNCT: Boron neutron capture therapy.

Brachytherapy: Radiotherapy using radioactive sources inserted into a body cavity or through needles into tissues.

Cell-cycle time: The time between one mitosis and the next.

Cell loss factor (ϕ): The rate of cell loss from a tumour, as a proportion of the rate at which cells are being added to the tumour by mitosis. Usually calculated by the relation: $\phi = 1 - T_{pot}/T_d$, where T_{pot} is potential doubling time and T_d is the cell population doubling time.

CHART: Continuous hyperfractionated accelerated radiotherapy.

Chromosomal instability: An effect of irradiation in which chromosomal aberrations continue to appear through many cell generations.

Chronic hypoxia: Persistent low oxygen concentrations such as exist in viable tumour cells close to regions of necrosis.

Clonogenic cells: Cells that have the capacity to produce an expanding family of descendents (usually at least 50). Also called 'colony-forming cells' or 'clonogens'.

Colony: The family of cells derived from a single clonogenic cell.

Complementation: Identification of whether a (radiosensitive) phenotype in different mutants is due to the same gene. Studied by means of cell fusion.

Direct action: Ionization or excitation of atoms within DNA leading to free radicals, as distinct from the reaction with DNA of free radicals formed in nearby water molecules.

D_0: A parameter in the multi-target equation: the radiation dose that reduces survival to e^{-1} (i.e. 0.37) of its previous value on the exponential portion of the survival curve.

Dose-modifying factor (DMF): When a chemical or other agent acts as if to change the dose of radiation, DMF indicates the ratio: (dose without/dose with) the agent for the same level of effect. Similarly:

Dose-reduction factor (DRF) or **sensitizer enhancement ratio (SER)**.

Dose rate effect: Decreasing radiation response with decreasing radiation dose rate.

Double trouble: A hotspot within a treatment field receives not only a higher dose but also a higher dose per fraction, which means that the biological effectiveness of the dose is also greater.

Doubling time: Time for a cell population or tumour volume to double its size.

Early normal-tissue responses: Radiation-induced normal-tissue damage that is expressed in weeks to a few months after exposure. Generally due to damage to parenchymal cells. α/β ratio tends to be large.

ED_{50}: Radiation dose that produces a specified effect in the normal tissues of 50% of animals ('effect-dose-50%').

Elkind repair: Recovery of the shoulder on a survival curve when irradiation follows several hours after a priming dose.

EQD_2: Equivalent total dose in 2 Gy fractions.

Exponential growth: Growth according to an exponential equation: $V = V_0 \exp(kt)$. The volume doubling time is constant $[= (\log_e 2)/k]$.

Extrapolated total dose (ETD): Calculated isoeffect dose when the dose rate is very low, or when fraction size is very small (*see* Biologically effective dose).

Extrapolation number: A parameter in the multi-target equation: the point on the survival scale to which the straight part of the curve back-extrapolates.

Field-size effect: The dependence of normal-tissue damage on the size of the irradiated area; also known as 'volume effect'.

FISH: Fluorescence *in situ* hybridization. Fluorescent dyes are attached to specific regions of the genome, thus aiding the identification of chromosomal damage.

Flexible tissues: Non-hierarchical cell populations in which function and proliferation take place in the same cells.

Flow cytometry: Analysis of cell suspensions in which a dilute stream of cells is passed through a laser beam. DNA content and other properties are measured by light scattering and fluorescence following staining with dyes or labelled antibodies.

Free radical: A fragment of a molecule containing an unpaired electron, therefore very reactive.

Genomic or genetic instability: Tendency for genetic changes to increase with time, in tumours or in any cells after irradiation.

gray (Gy): The special name for the SI unit of absorbed dose, i.e. kerma. $1\,Gy = 1\,joule\,kg^{-1}$. The gray has replaced the previous unit, the rad ($1\,Gy = 100\,rad$).

Growth delay: Extra time required for an irradiated tumour to reach a given size, compared with an unirradiated tumour.

Growth fraction: The proportion of cells in a population that are cycling.

Hierarchical tissues: Cell populations comprising a lineage of stem cells, proliferating cells, and mature cells. The mature cells do not divide.

Hyperbaric oxygen (HBO): The use of high oxygen pressures (2–3 atmospheres) to enhance oxygen availability in radiotherapy.

Hyperfractionation: Increase in number of fractions and reduction in dose per fraction below a conventional level of 1.8–2.0 Gy.

Hyperthermia: The use of heat treatments above normal physiological temperatures to treat cancer.

Hypofractionation: The use of dose fractions substantially larger than the conventional level of $\sim 2\,Gy$.

Hypoxia: Low oxygen tension; usually the very low levels that are required to make cells maximally radioresistant. Sometimes used to mean **anoxia** ($=$ literally, the complete absence of oxygen).

Incomplete repair: Increased damage from fractionated radiotherapy when the time interval between doses is too short to allow complete recovery.

Indirect action: Damage to DNA by free radicals formed through the ionization of nearby water molecules.

Inducible response: A response to irradiation that is modified by a small dose of radiation given shortly before.

Initial slope: The steepness of the initial part of the oxic cell survival curve, sometimes indicated by the surviving fraction at 2 Gy.

Interphase death: The death of irradiated cells before they reach mitosis.

Ionization: The process of removing electrons from (or adding electrons to) atoms or molecules, thereby creating ions.

Isoeffect plots: Graphs of the total dose for a given effect (e.g. ED_{50}) plotted, for instance, against dose per fraction or dose rate.

Labelling index: Proportion or percentage of cells within the S phase, and therefore labelled by [^{3}H]thymidine or other precursors such as bromodeoxyuridine.

Late normal-tissue responses: Radiation-induced normal-tissue damage that in humans is expressed months to years after exposure. Generally due to damage to connective-tissue cells. α/β ratio tends to be small (<5 Gy).

Latent period or latency interval: Time between irradiation and expression of injury.

$LD_{50/30}$: Radiation dose to produce lethality in 50% of animals by 30 days; similarly $LD_{50/7}$ etc.

Linear energy transfer (LET): The rate of energy loss along the track of an ionizing particle. Usually expressed in keV μm^{-1}.

Linear-quadratic (LQ) model: Model in which the effect (E) is a linear-quadratic function of dose (d): $E = \alpha d + \beta d^2$. For cell survival: $S = \exp(-\alpha d - \beta d^2)$.

Log-phase culture: A cell culture growing exponentially.

Mean inactivation dose ($\bar{D}$): An estimate of the average radiation dose to inactivate a cell. It is calculated as the area under the survival curve, plotted on linear coordinates.

Mitotic death: Cell death associated with a post-irradiation mitosis.

Mitotic delay: Delay of entry into mitosis, or accumulation in G2, as a result of treatment.

Mitotic index: Proportion or percentage of cells in mitosis at any given time.

Multi-target equation: Model that assumes the presence of a number of critical targets in a cell, all of which require inactivation to kill the cell. Survival is given by: $S = 1 - [1 - \exp(D/D_0)]^n$.

Non-stochastic effect: An effect where the severity increases with increasing dose, perhaps after a threshold region.

NTCP: Normal-tissue complication probability.

NSD: Nominal standard dose in the Ellis formula.

Oxygen enhancement ratio (OER): The ratio of dose given under anoxic conditions to the dose resulting in the same effect when given under oxic conditions.

Photodynamic therapy: Cancer treatment using light to activate a photosensitizing agent, thereby releasing cytotoxic free radicals.

Plateau-phase cultures: Cell cultures grown to confluence so that proliferation is markedly reduced (= 'stationary phase').

Plating efficiency: The proportion or percentage of *in vitro* plated cells that form colonies.

Potential doubling time (T_{pot}): The predicted cell population doubling time in the assumed absence of cell loss.

Potentially lethal damage (PLD): Cellular damage that is recovered during the interval between treatment and assay, especially under suboptimal growth conditions.

Prodromal phase: Signs and symptoms in the first 48 hours following irradiation of the central nervous system.

Quasi-threshold dose (D_q): Point of extrapolation of the exponential portion of a multi-target survival curve to the level of zero survival: $D_q = D_0 \ln(n)$.

Radio-responsiveness: A general term, indicating the overall level of clinical response to radiotherapy.

Radiosensitivity: The radiation dose required to produce a defined level of cell inactivation. Usually indicated by the surviving fraction at 2 Gy (i.e. SF_2) or by the parameters of the linear-quadratic or multi-target equations.

Radiosensitizer: In general, any agent that increases the sensitivity of cells to radiation. Most commonly applied to electron-affinic chemicals that mimic oxygen in fixing free-radical damage.

Reassortment or Redistribution: Return towards a more even cell-age distribution, following the selective killing of cells in certain phases of the cell cycle.

Recovery: An increase in cell survival as a function of time during or after irradiation (*see* Repair).

Regression rate: The rate at which a tumour shrinks during or after treatment.

Relative biological effectiveness (RBE): Ratio of dose of a reference radiation quality (usually 250 keV x-rays) and dose of a test radiation that produces equal effect.

Reoxygenation: The process by which surviving hypoxic clonogenic cells become better oxygenated during the period after irradiation of a tumour.

Repair: Restoration of the integrity of damaged macromolecules (*see* Recovery).

Repair saturation: Explanation of the shoulder on cell survival curves on the basis of the reduced effectiveness of repair after high radiation doses.

Reproductive integrity: Ability of cells to divide many times and thus be 'clonogenic'.

SF_2: Surviving fraction at 2 Gy.

Sievert (Sv): Dose equivalent in radiation protection. Dose in Gy is multiplied by a radiation quality factor.

Slow repair: Long-term recovery that takes place on a time-scale of weeks to months.

Spatial co-operation: The use of radiotherapy and chemotherapy to hit disease in different anatomical sites.

Spheroid: Clump of cells grown together in tissue-culture suspension. Not usually a colony.

Split-dose recovery (SLD recovery): Decrease in radiation effect when a single radiation dose is split into two fractions separated by times of up to a few hours (= Elkind recovery, or recovery from sublethal damage).

Stem cells: Cells capable of self-renewal and of differentiation to produce all the various types of cells in a lineage.

Stochastic effect: An effect where the incidence, but not the severity, increases with increasing dose (e.g. carcinogenesis).

Sublethal damage: Non-lethal cellular injury that can be repaired, or accumulated with further dose to become lethal.

Supra-additivity or synergism: A biological effect due to a combination that is greater than would be expected from the addition of the effects of the component agents.

Target cell: A stem cell whose death contributes to a reduction in growth or tissue function.

Target theory: The idea that the shoulder on cell survival curves is due to the number of unrepaired lesions per cell.

Targeted radiotherapy: Treatment of disseminated cancer by means of drugs that localize in tumours and carry therapeutic amounts of radioactivity.

TBI: Total-body irradiation.

TCD_{50}: The radiation dose that gives a 50% tumour control probability.

TCP: Tumour control probability.

TER: Thermal enhancement ratio; the ratio of radiation doses that produces the same biological effect (without heat)/(with heat).

TGF: Therpeutic gain factor; the ratio of TER values in tumour/normal tissue.

Therapeutic index: Tumour response for a fixed level of normal-tissue damage.

Thermal dose: A function of temperature and heating time that is thought to relate well to biological effect.

Thermotolerance: The observation that an initial heat treatment reduces the effect of a second heat treatment given shortly afterwards.

Time–dose relationships: The dependence of isoeffective radiation dose on the duration (and number of fractions) in radiotherapy.

Time factor: In calculations of the response of tumours to fractionated radiotherapy, the time factor describes the change in isoeffective total dose that follows an increase or decrease in the overall treatment duration.

Tolerance: The maximum radiation dose or intensity of fractionated radiotherapy that the therapist judges to be acceptable. Usually expressed in dose units. Actual values will depend on fractionation, field-size, concomitant treatments, etc.

Transient hypoxia: Low oxygen concentrations associated with the transient closing and opening of blood vessels. Sometimes called *acute* hypoxia.

Tumour bed effect (TBE): Slower rate of tumour growth after irradiation due to stromal injury in the irradiated 'vascular bed'.

Tumour cord: Sleeve of viable tumour growing around a blood capillary.

Volume doubling time: Time for a tumour to double in size.

Volume effect: Dependence of radiation damage to normal tissues on the volume of tissue irradiated.

Xenografts: Transplants between species; usually applied to the transplantation of human tumours into immune-deficient mice and rats.

Index

Page numbers in **bold** refer to the Glossary